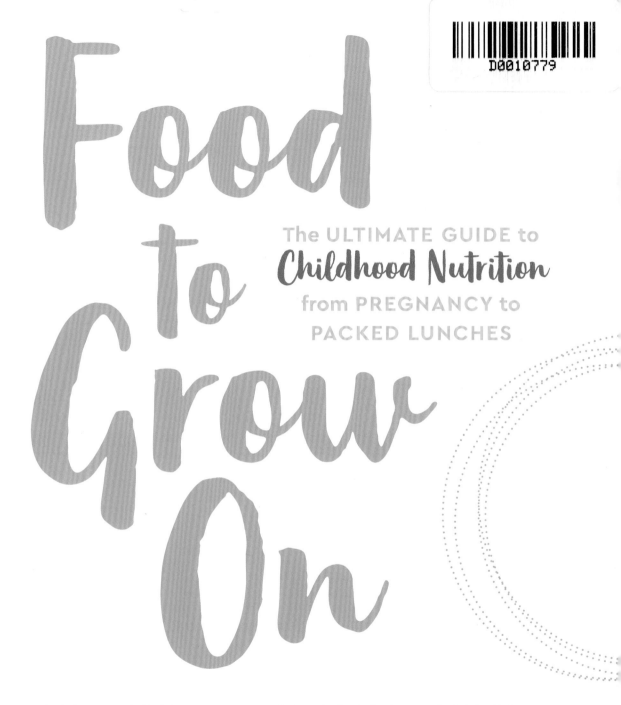

Food to Grow On

The ULTIMATE GUIDE to
Childhood Nutrition
from PREGNANCY to PACKED LUNCHES

By SARAH REMMER, RD and CARA ROSENBLOOM, RD

appetite
by RANDOM HOUSE

Appetite by Random House® and colophon are registered trademarks of Penguin Random House LLC.

Library and Archives Canada Cataloguing in Publication is available upon request.
The Helderleigh Foundation Edition ISBN: 978-0-525-61189-9
Original ISBN: 978-0-525-60999-5
eBook ISBN: 978-0-525-61003-8

Photography by Shannon Hutchison Photography and food styling by Sylvia Kong
Cover photography c/o Getty Images: (top right); yacobchuk;
(middle) miodrag ijnjatovic; (bottom right) Natalia Klenova/EyeEm
Photographs c/o Getty Images: page ii, Walter B. McKenzie; page vi, Cavan Images;
page 31, Igor Emmerich; page 48, sturti; page 60, Anna Bizon; page 101, Jose Pelaez Inc;
page 109, JGI/Jamie Grill; page 133, Toshiro Shimada; page 219, D-Keine; page 325, Tetra Images;
page 348, Carlos. G Lopez; page 335, SolStock; page 362, PeopleImages
Photographs c/o Shutterstock: page 17, Halfpoint; page 66, Monkey Business Images;
page 125, Trendsetter Images; page 284, nadianb; page 356, bbarnard
Illustrations by Talia Abramson and Leah Springate, and c/o Vecteezy: biggorilla298
Book design by Leah Springate
Printed and bound in China

Published in Canada by Appetite by Random House®,
a division of Penguin Random House Canada Limited.

www.penguinrandomhouse.ca

10 9 8 7 6 5 4 3 2 1

appetite
by RANDOM HOUSE

Penguin
Random House
Canada

Sarah: To my children, Ben, Lylah, and James, for always inspiring me, challenging me, and cheering me on. I love you!

Cara: To my daughter, Kasey, and son, Aubrey, you bring me endless amounts of joy. Thank you for making me laugh every day. I love you.

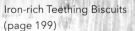

Iron-rich Teething Biscuits (page 199)

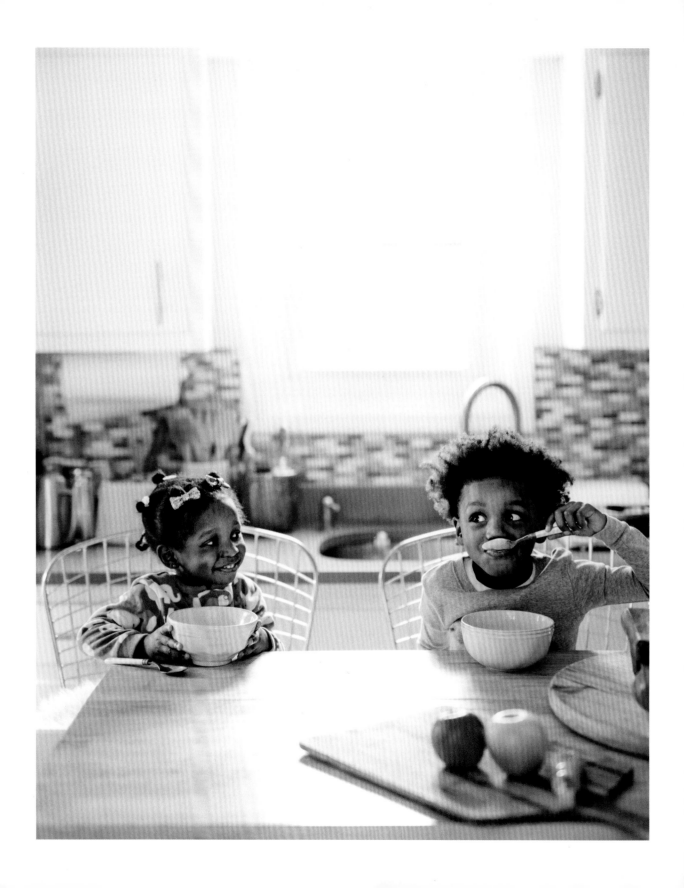

Contents

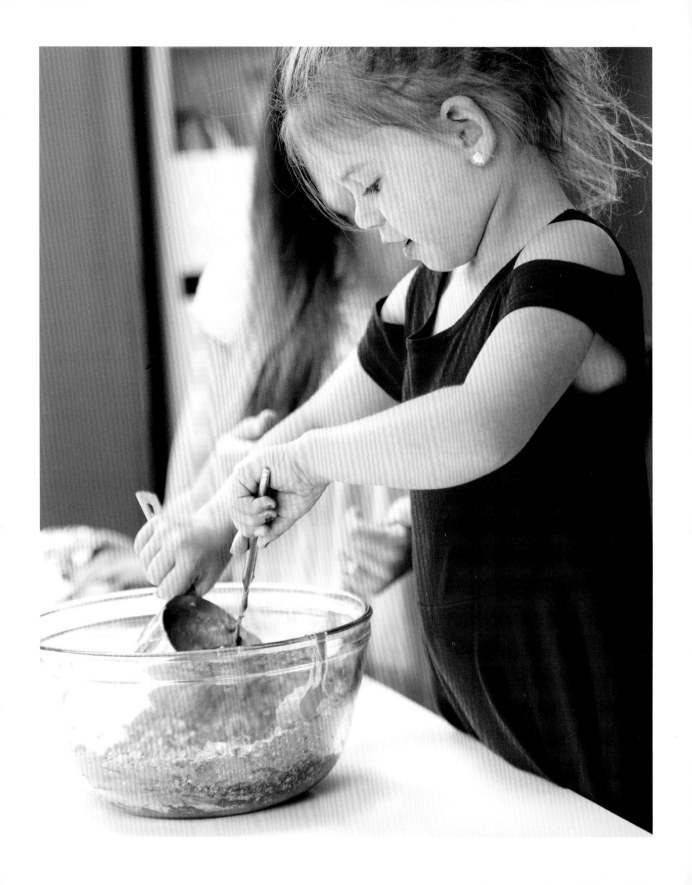

Introduction

We are so honored to have written this book, and are thrilled to share it with you. Our goal is to help you survive and thrive in the early days and years of feeding your child (because they sure can be confusing and overwhelming!). We figured there should be an expert guide to this important time as parents play such a huge role in shaping their children's eating habits for life. So we looked for one, but couldn't find it; there wasn't a credible, extensive, easy-to-navigate, question-and-answer guide to feeding kids written by registered dietitians—until now! In a perfect world, you'd be granted your very own personal dietitian when you become pregnant, and have access to them until your child is school-age (and beyond!). But because that's not reality, you have us! Dietitians in your hands. Inside this book, you'll find all the information you need to feed and nourish your child—and yourself—from the moment you find out a baby is on the way until you're sending them off to school with lunchbox in tow.

Parents have so many questions about nutrition, and as moms and trusted experts in childhood nutrition, we have valuable knowledge to share. In this book, we will help you figure out what you should and shouldn't eat while pregnant. We'll support you postpartum (sneak preview: it can be &%#&^% hard!), whether you decide to breastfeed or bottle-feed or both. We'll help you through weaning your baby and the transition to solid foods. We'll give you information on what your little one's nutritional needs are from birth to the age of 6. We'll help you decide what foods you should serve to your baby, toddler, and child on a daily and weekly basis. And we won't stop there because healthy eating extends way beyond *what* kids eat into *how* they eat as well. Mealtimes can be a challenge when it comes to young kids (we get this as moms ourselves!). That's why we will also focus on *when, where,* and *how* to feed your child, in addition to *what* to feed your child. We'll explain how to set mealtime boundaries and meal and snack schedules. We'll talk about why family dinners matter (and how to facilitate them without losing your mind). And we'll look at how to help your child feel empowered to make nutritious food choices on their own, and learn to love a variety of foods long-term.

> **Healthy eating extends way beyond *what* kids eat into *how* they eat as well.**

Have you ever seen one of those kids who happily munches away on raw vegetables? Or one who chooses water over juice? Or one who eats a piece of cake and leaves a little behind because their tummy is full? We'll help you raise those kids (hint: it starts when they are babies, and YOU play a big role). We'll also give you peace of mind that your child is okay if they go through a phase of refusing vegetables, even for months (because it happens, and it's normal!), and help create a positive, healthy feeding relationship between you and your child for life.

Who we are

We are dietitians, yes. We see clients, read research articles, go to nutrition conferences, and talk with colleagues and other health professionals regularly. We pride ourselves on staying on top of the latest research, news, and trends when it comes to nutrition and health. But we are parents too. We've experienced the joys of feeding as well as the challenges. We've cried trying to breastfeed a newborn, we've stressed about whether our toddlers were getting enough nutrients for growth and development, and we've almost lost our sh*t trying to get our picky eaters to eat. We get it. We're not perfect, nor do we claim to know *all* of the answers to every feeding challenge you'll encounter. But we know a lot, not only from our education and professional experience, but from raising 5 little eaters between us.

WE ADMIT IT: WE LOVE NUTRITION!

When it comes to what to eat during pregnancy and feeding your child as they grow, we are huge proponents of good nutrition, for obvious reasons! As dietitians, we believe in *whole* foods because they are nutrient-rich and come with many health benefits. We believe in maximizing nutrition at every meal and snack and working toward optimal nutrition for each family member every day. But . . . we get that eating this way 100% of the time isn't realistic (or fun!). We realize that there are going to be store-bought, packaged foods, takeout dinners, birthday parties, holidays, and plenty more opportunities for treats. This is real life. And we take that into account with all of the advice we give. In other words, we're realists too.

CARA SAYS: *I'm a mom of 2 kids—my daughter, Kasey, is 14 and my son, Aubrey, is 10. I've been a dietitian since 2000, and spent the first 3 years of my career working at the world-renowned Hospital for Sick Children (SickKids) in Toronto. After having children, I started my own nutrition communications business, and I've been happily working from home, packing school lunches, doing laundry, and juggling this business since 2007. I write about nutrition for newspapers, magazines, blogs, and* *apps. I have a unique blend of book learning (a Bachelor of Science in Food and Nutrition), hands-on teaching experience, and real-world experience, so it makes sense that I can relate to what you're going through!*

SARAH SAYS: I'm a mom to 3 kids—Ben, 10, Lylah, 7, and James, 5—and I've been a dietitian since 2006. I've spent most of my time in private practice, counseling individuals and families on nutrition, feeding, and wellness. I'm the founder of The Centre for Family Nutrition based in Calgary, Alberta, and create nutrition and health content for families on my blog and social media platforms as well as for various websites, magazines, and news outlets. I also work with companies that align with my philosophy on eating and feeding, and am passionate about empowering parents to raise happy and healthy kids. My expertise stems not only from my years of education and experience, but also from being in the "trenches" myself. I really, truly, for real get it!

How to use this book

Like any great page-turner, you won't be able to put this down. Brew some coffee or tea, get cozy, and dive in. Wait, what? You're not going to read a book on pregnancy and feeding children from cover to cover?! Fair enough! How about this: start with the introduction and read about our overall approach to feeding and nutrition. Then flip to the chapter that corresponds to the stage you're currently in or the challenge you're currently facing. There you will get age-appropriate information that will leave you think-ing, "How the heck did they know?" You'll find each chapter is structured the same way:

INTRODUCTION: At the beginning of each chapter, you'll get an overview of the stage you and/or your child are currently in. Here we'll cover developmental milestones, nutritional breakdowns, and which foods should be eaten, why and how.

QUESTIONS: We know you're busy. There's a good chance you won't be lazing in the bubble bath with ample time to read a whole chapter, so we've divided the chapters into the specific questions you may have—like: "Which nutrients (and foods) should I be getting more of now that I'm pregnant?" "What should I avoid eating or drinking while breastfeeding?" "My child eats a total of about 6 foods. How can I expand her palate?" Just flip to the question, get the answer, and keep the book handy until your next quandary arises. Done and done!

BREAKOUTS: Within the questions we break the information down even further:

 We Got You: Non-judgmental words of support, parent to parent.

 Reality Check: The not-so-obvious but very real truths about food, nutrition, and feeding that will help you understand them a little better (and hopefully help you breathe a sigh of relief!).

 Problem Solved: Real stories from parents and clients we have worked with over the years, which show how specific nutrition problems were solved.

 Deep Dive: Some people want the tip of the iceberg—"what to do"—while others want the "why to do it" too. Here we answer the "why" for those who are curious, diving deeper into more detailed scientific explanations.

 Shades of Gray: In some circumstances, nutrition information is not fully developed. In these cases, we'll tell you both sides of the story and let you decide what's best for you and your family.

 Sarah Says and Cara Says: Anecdotes about our own pregnancies and experiences raising and feeding children.

? **We Asked!** We used social media to ask questions to folks just like you. Pregnant women, new parents, and seasoned moms and dads weighed in and answered our questions about their own unique food habits and ideas, and we've shared their responses throughout.

10 **Top 10 Tips:** The last page of every chapter recaps our top 10 takeaways for that particular age or stage.

RECIPES: You'll also find some simple and delicious recipes scattered throughout the book, developed with the whole family in mind. Please note, unless otherwise specified:

- **Milk:** Use anything you have in your fridge (e.g., non-fat or whole cow's milk, soy milk, any other plant-based milk).

- **Yogurt:** Use Greek (any fat content you want) as it has more protein and less sugar than plain yogurt, and a creamy and thick consistency (Icelandic or skyr yogurts are good options too).

- **Salt:** Babies, toddlers, and children require less salt than adults and the recipes were developed with this in mind; feel free to add more salt to adult portions to suit your taste buds.

- **Sugar:** It is not recommended that children consume sugar (e.g. brown sugar, maple syrup etc.) before the age of 2. If a recipe calls for it, assume it is geared towards those older than 2.

AND THEN: After all that, if you still can't find what you're looking for, we're online to help! Join our amazing social communities, filled with other parents like you.

Sarah
www.sarahremmer.com
Sarah Remmer Nutrition Consulting
@sarahremmer

Cara
www.wordstoeatby.ca
Words to Eat By
@cararosenbloom

What We Believe

In a nutshell, we believe that babies, toddlers, and even young kids intuitively know how to eat and how much to eat. As parents, it's our job to nurture this intuition and ensure that we're providing nutritious food choices at appropriate intervals throughout the day. It's also our job to encourage our kids to continue to be intuitive eaters, even when outside influences come into play (think friends, or shiny, colorful, sugary cereal boxes in the grocery store, or holidays like Halloween). As our children's role models we should also be facilitating a positive eating environment, setting boundaries, and modeling healthy eating practices ourselves. Sounds like a lot, doesn't it? Fear not—this is where we come in—we've got your back!

Pregnancy and postpartum

Nutrition is key both before and after delivering your baby. During pregnancy, you're

Fed is best. A happy and relaxed mom = a happy and well-fed baby.

growing a human inside of you, and you have to keep yourself well-nourished too. That's a big job! And after baby's arrival, your nutritional needs don't slow down. Not only are you healing and recovering from delivery, but now you're also potentially producing breastmilk (assuming you *can* and *want* to breastfeed), which requires additional nutrients and calories. No need to stress, though—it's fairly easy to meet your nutrient requirements if you do a bit of planning and mindful eating. We've got you! We've been there when it comes to things like pregnancy-related nausea, constipation, and heartburn, so we've got lots of tips on how to manage those pesky side effects of pregnancy, as well as lots of advice on healthy weight gain during pregnancy *and* weight loss after baby. But no diets or deprivation—that's just not our style!

Baby 0 to 6 months

Fed is best! We are certainly not strangers to the dilemma and pressure of whether to breastfeed or formula-feed. We've been through it all—breastfeeding, expressing, pumping, formula-feeding, blocked ducts, mastitis, and crying uncontrollably while experiencing any combination of the above . . . you name it, we've done it. So, although we both strongly encourage breastfeeding and work with moms to go that route if they can, we also know that it can be tough stuff. When it comes down to it, we believe that fed is best—whether it's via boob or bottle, breastmilk or formula—and we know this for sure: a happy and relaxed mom = a happy and well-fed baby. We give you lots of tips and advice for each and every which way you choose to feed your baby. And, whether breast or bottle, we always encourage "responsive feeding" (read more on page 44).

Baby 6 to 12 months

There is no single "right way" to introduce solids to your baby, whether you want to start with traditional spoon-feeding or try baby-led weaning (letting baby self-feed with finger foods right from the start). We support either way (or a combo) wholeheartedly. We just believe that it's important that baby be introduced to a wide variety of tastes and textures within the first couple of months of starting solid foods, and that *all* feeding be led by baby's cues (aka responsive feeding). Babies should be encouraged to trust their bodies when it comes to eating and to self-regulate their appetite. The best way to help them do this is to establish a healthy feeding routine, let them lead, and not pressure or coax them to eat. Don't worry—we walk you through everything when we get there.

> **There is no single "right way" to introduce solids to your baby.**

Toddlers and kids 1 to 6 years

We're big fans of Ellyn Satter's Division of Responsibility (sDOR) in feeding, which is a brilliant concept about the roles of parents and children when it comes to feeding (read more on page 41). The sDOR takes the pressure off of both parents and kids and encourages kids to eat intuitively, listen to their bodies, love a variety of foods, and establish a long-term healthy relationship with food.

We're also strong believers in the power of family meals for kids of all ages. Heck, we encourage you to include babies at the table even before they're ready for solids! This is where children learn how to eat, develop a love for food, have a chance to bond with parents, and learn what's "normal" when it comes to eating. It is also wonderful for children to feel as though they have some say in (or a hand in) what's being served or made. We'll chat about how to do that (without losing your mind!) later on.

A variety of nutritious food choices, from whole grain crackers to berries.

Foods to Choose

There are so many different ways to eat. We all have different preferences, budgets, customs, religious beliefs, allergies or intolerances, and ethical philosophies, and this affects the foods we choose to eat and to feed our kids. As parents it's your job to choose and prepare the food your child will eat, and that's a big, important job because your child's health—both in the short and long term—is highly influenced by the foods they eat. A healthy diet paired with an active lifestyle reduces your child's future risk of developing heart disease, type 2 diabetes, dementia, osteoporosis, high blood pressure, high cholesterol, and certain types of cancer. That doesn't mean there's no room for treats—trust us, no one expects perfection—but nutritious foods (i.e., foods that will deliver the nutrients that you and your child need) are so important for kids. Read much more about nutrition needs for all ages on pages 23 to 39.

> ♥ **WE GOT YOU!**
>
> There isn't one single way of eating, and what works for one person might not work for the next. We're not critical of any kind of eating plan as long as it serves you well and is *nutritious* and *sustainable*.

Whole food

The best food choice you can make for you and your family is to focus on serving nutrient-rich whole foods. Preparing a variety of whole foods every day will help you and your child thrive. In this book, we talk a lot about whole foods, nutritious processed foods, and ultra-processed foods, so it's important to explain the difference:

Whole foods: Foods like vegetables, fruit, fish, poultry, eggs, meat, whole grains, beans, nuts, and seeds. They should form the bulk of your diet and fill your plate at most meals.

Nutritious processed foods: Foods like canned tuna, jarred tomato sauce, or cheese are not to be feared. These foods are made relatively simply by adding oil, salt, or sugar, and contain just a few ingredients. They are convenient, healthy, and a great part of your menu.

Ultra-processed foods: Foods like chips, cookies, cereal, hotdogs, chicken nuggets, candy, ice cream, soft drinks, fries, noodle soups, and boxed mac and cheese. These foods are the result of industrial formulations of a long list of cheap ingredients that you may not recognize or understand. The purpose of this type of intense processing is to create foods that are uber-convenient, shelf-stable, great tasting, and profitable. But these foods are low in nutrients so should not make up a large part of your menu.

Foods to Choose

Below you'll see a list of whole foods to focus on most of the time, nutritious processed foods you can serve regularly, and ultra-processed foods to limit.

Whole foods (serve most often)	Nutritious processed foods (serve regularly)	Ultra-processed foods (limit)
• Vegetables and fruits: fresh, frozen, or dried • Fruit: fresh, frozen, or dried • Fish, poultry, meat, seafood, eggs • Legumes: chickpeas, kidney beans, black beans, lentils, tofu, edamame, peanuts • Dairy: milk, kefir, plain yogurt • Nuts: almonds, cashews, pecans, nut butter • Seeds: hemp, pumpkin, sesame, sunflower, chia • Whole grains: barley, brown rice, oats, quinoa, wholegrain wheat, polenta, rice, wheat • Herbs and spices	• Canned vegetables and fruits • Jarred tomato sauce • Canned fish like light flaked tuna, salmon, sardines • Canned beans or lentils • Nuts or seeds with added salt • Cheese • Fresh breads, bagels, pita, naan, roti, flatbread • Chicken or turkey deli meat • Fruit cups	• Frozen chicken and fish nuggets, fingers, and sticks • Hotdogs and sausages • Instant noodle soups • Powdered pasta dishes • Ice cream • Store-bought baked goods • Mass-produced breads • Sweetened breakfast cereals • Sweetened yogurts or yogurt drinks and tubes • Salty snacks like chips, pretzels, cheesies, tortillas • Sweet drinks such as soda, lemonade, iced tea • Sweet treats like cookies, cakes, candy, chocolate

LIMIT ULTRA-PROCESSED FOODS

Your family's diet should not be dominated by ultra-processed foods. Once in a while? For sure. Three meals a day, every day? No. Studies show that diets filled with ultra-processed foods are linked to an increased risk of developing heart disease, metabolic syndrome, and some types of cancer. Try to limit serving ultra-processed foods wherever you can. Unfortunately, children's diets are currently FILLED with ultra-processed foods.

- The average American child over the age of one gets almost 60% of calories from ultra-processed foods.[1] That means more than half of their diet is filled with cookies, candy, hotdogs, soft drinks, pizza, fries, and chips. Not good.
- Canadians are the second-largest consumers of ultra-processed foods. Kids between the ages of 2 and 9 get 51.9% of their daily calories from ultra-processed foods.[2]

If an overreliance on ultra-processed foods sounds like your child's current diet, don't feel bad or guilty about it! You probably didn't know there was such a big difference between nutritious processed and ultra-processed foods. Just start to make small changes and add and replace processed foods with more whole foods. For example, prepackaged chicken nuggets can be replaced with our recipe for Crispy Baked Chicken Fingers (page 292).

Mealtimes

When it comes to meals, it's important to include balance and variety. What we mean by "balance" is a balance of nutrients coming from different foods, which will help you to meet your and/or your child's nutrient needs by the end of the day or week. Ideally, an adult's plate should look like the diagram opposite to maximize nutrition. Kids should be served and offered a good variety of these foods too. Ratios aren't as important for kids—it's more about offering variety and letting them

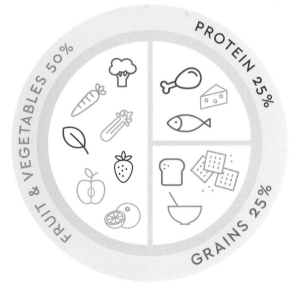

explore and eat what they'd like in the amounts that feel right to them. A simple way to structure kids' meals is to include at least one food from these 3 groups at each meal:

Fruits and vegetables: Aim for a variety of these with lots of different colors and textures. Vegetables and fruits are jam-packed full of essential vitamins and minerals, as well as fiber. Choose fresh or frozen (frozen are just as nutritious!). Does your child refuse to eat veggies? Flip to page 279.

Protein-rich foods: Choose nutrient-dense proteins such as lean meats, poultry, low-mercury fish (see the Reality Check opposite), beans, lentils, eggs, milk, yogurt, cheese, cottage cheese, eggs, tofu, tempeh, peanuts and other nuts, and seeds. These not only help to build and repair muscles and other body tissues, but also help to fill you up quicker, keep you fuller longer, and sustain your energy levels.

Grains: Choose *whole grains* most of the time, as these are minimally processed and offer more nutrition than their white, processed counterparts (think whole grain versus white bread, brown versus white rice, and whole grain versus white pasta). Grains like these provide carbohydrates for energy, as well as vitamins, minerals, and fiber.

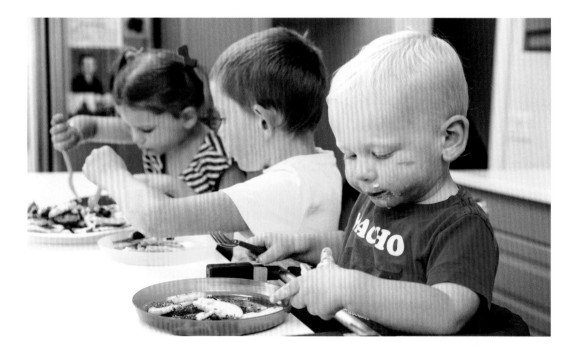

Mealtime Combinations

As busy parents, we like it when something is simplified or made into a list. Who doesn't like a good list?! Use this chart for ideas on combining fruits and vegetables, proteins, grains, and starches. Choose at least one from each column!

Vegetables and fruits	Protein-rich	Grains
• Apples and pears • Berries • Broccoli and cauliflower • Citrus: oranges, etc. • Leafy greens • Raw veggie sticks: carrot, cucumber, peppers, etc. • Roasted root vegetables: beets, parsnip, sweet potato, etc. • Sandwich toppers: tomato, lettuce, etc. • Stir-fried veggies: peppers, mushrooms, snow peas, etc. • Stone fruit: peaches, etc. • Tropical fruit: banana, mango, pineapple, etc.	• Beans: edamame, black, kidney, etc. • Cheese • Eggs • Fish and seafood: halibut, salmon, shrimp, etc. • Lentils: red, black, or green • Peas: chickpeas, black-eyed peas, split peas, etc. • Meat: beef, lamb, pork, etc. • Nuts and nut butters • Poultry: chicken, turkey, etc. • Seeds: pumpkin, sesame, sunflower, etc. • Tofu • Yogurt: Greek or skyr	• Basmati or brown rice • Oats or oatmeal • Pot barley • Quinoa • Sweet potato or yam • Wheat berries • Whole grain bread • Whole grain corn tortillas • Whole grain crackers • Whole grain waffles or pancakes • Whole grain pasta • Wild rice

REALITY CHECK: MERCURY IN FISH

Pregnant and breastfeeding women need to watch their mercury intake (see pages 75, 84 and 135), and low-mercury fish is always the best choice to serve children. Here is a note on the mercury content in different fish (read more about tuna on page 84):

- **Higher mercury fish:** albacore tuna, big eye tuna, king mackerel, marlin, orange roughy, shark, swordfish, tilefish.
- **Lower mercury fish:** anchovies, catfish, haddock, herring, salmon, skipjack tuna, tilapia, trout, sardines, sole.

Plant-based eating

Plant-based diets are becoming increasingly popular because they are good for your health and good for the planet. What do we mean by plant-based? Simply, a diet filled with foods that come from plants, like vegetables, fruit, beans, lentils, grains, nuts, and seeds. Plant-based diets don't necessarily have to be strictly vegan or vegetarian, although some are. You can follow a mainly plant-based diet and enjoy animal foods moderately too! Nutritious, plant-based diets can decrease the risk of heart disease, high blood pressure, type 2 diabetes, and certain cancers. You can start gradually by including more plant-based foods and increasing these if it feels right for you and your family. Or even just try a meatless meal once or twice a week!

> **WE GOT YOU!**
>
> The decision to raise a vegan, vegetarian, or plant-based child is a personal one—if you follow this type of diet, you may want your child to as well. A plant-based diet can definitely meet the nutritional needs for you and your child, as long as it is properly planned. Read all about it on pages 207 to 209 and 349 to 350.

ULTRA-PROCESSED PLANT-BASED FOODS

There are now plenty of ultra-processed foods made from plants. Eating more chickpeas, lentils, almonds, and peanuts is great—that's plant-based eating at its best. But simply choosing ultra-processed plant-based versions of fast food is not! Ultra-processed veggie burgers, veggie dogs, and snacks have been crowned with an undeserved health halo because they are "made from plants"—don't believe the hype. Once plant food is ultra-processed, it's no longer as nutritious. It's better to choose whole foods rather than ultra-processed foods, even if both come from plants.

Gluten-free diets

Some diets are followed for medical reasons, such as a gluten-free diet. It's meant for people with celiac disease or gluten sensitivity. Gluten is a protein naturally found in wheat, barley, and rye. That includes foods like spelt, triticale, couscous, pasta, bread, rolls, buns, pita, cookies, cakes, crackers, and pies made with gluten-containing flours. There are also many products that *may* contain gluten, such as (but not limited to) processed meats, French fries, hydrolyzed vegetable protein, modified food starch, natural flavoring, soy sauce, vegetable gum, cooking spray, canned soups and soup mixes, and some salad dressings.

If you don't have celiac disease or gluten sensitivity, there's no clinically established reason to follow a gluten-free diet. And there's no good evidence to suggest that a gluten-free diet will help with overall health.

Snacks

Snacks make their way into your child's diet around 9 to 12 months of age, when meals alone are no longer enough to sustain them throughout the day. Snacks are meant to fill nutritional gaps between meals. They're NOT meant to replace meals or sustain your child all day, every day (which could easily happen—kids love snacks a lot). Think of snacks as mini meals that consist of 2 to 3 different foods, served in smaller quantities than you would at mealtime. We encourage you to include a bit of protein plus a fruit or vegetable and/or a whole grain (e.g., cheese and whole grain crackers, or a whole grain mini pita, hummus, and grapes). Serve fruits or vegetables often to help make sure your child eats lots of them each day. For adults, snacks should serve the same purpose as they do for kids: to fill nutritional gaps. When choosing your own snacks, choose a protein-rich food and add a fruit or vegetable to balance it out.

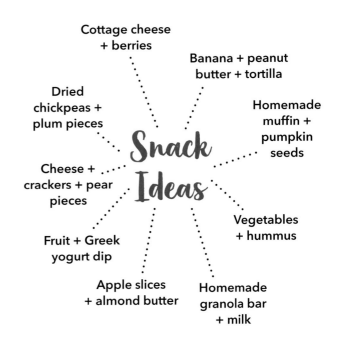

Snack Ideas

Cottage cheese + berries

Banana + peanut butter + tortilla

Dried chickpeas + plum pieces

Homemade muffin + pumpkin seeds

Cheese + crackers + pear pieces

Vegetables + hummus

Fruit + Greek yogurt dip

Apple slices + almond butter

Homemade granola bar + milk

WE GOT YOU!

Make sure you recognize the difference between a snack and a treat. A snack is a mini meal made of whole foods like vegetables, fruits, nuts, seeds, yogurt, etc. A treat is something more indulgent that you're not relying on for nutrition, like chocolate, chips, cake, ice cream, etc.

Sweets and treats

We're dietitians, but we're also both chocoholics. We believe that the occasional indulgence in something that you absolutely love—whether that's a little chocolate, potato chips, or candy—is not a bad thing. In fact, we encourage indulging in your most loved foods, and discourage making any food "forbidden" or strictly limited. Just make sure that it's something that you can really enjoy and savor. Treats shouldn't displace any of the nutrient-dense foods in your diet, and you should eat them mindfully. This is especially true when you're pregnant or breastfeeding, because of your increased nutritional needs.

When it comes to children, treats and sweets shouldn't be served until after the age of 2 (okay, so maybe on their first birthday—c'mon . . . who can resist the cute birthday cake photo op?). After the age of 2, our very best advice is that treats should be served *randomly for fun*. They shouldn't be forbidden or villainized, but they also shouldn't be served all of the time (which means they eventually become expected). We talk specifically about treats and babies on page 37, toddlers on pages 253 and 294, and kids on pages 340 and 353.

Drinks

We're big fans of water, and we're not alone. In 2019, a joint statement from the Academy of Nutrition and Dietetics, the American Academy of Pediatric Dentistry, the American Academy of Pediatrics, and the American Heart Association advised that kids should drink mostly water, with some milk, and limit their intake of sugary beverages such as soda and juice. That statement was for kids, but can equally apply to adults too. Since coffee and tea are 99% water, those are good choices for adults too, as long as you don't exceed certain caffeine levels, especially while pregnant (see page 87).

REALITY CHECK

Juice contains excess calories and sugar that children don't need—it fills them up with little nutritional value. Did you know that an 8-ounce juice box contains 6 teaspoons of sugar? It has as much sugar as soda, iced tea, or other sweetened drinks. It's liquid candy! The bit of vitamin C it contains does not make it a health food!

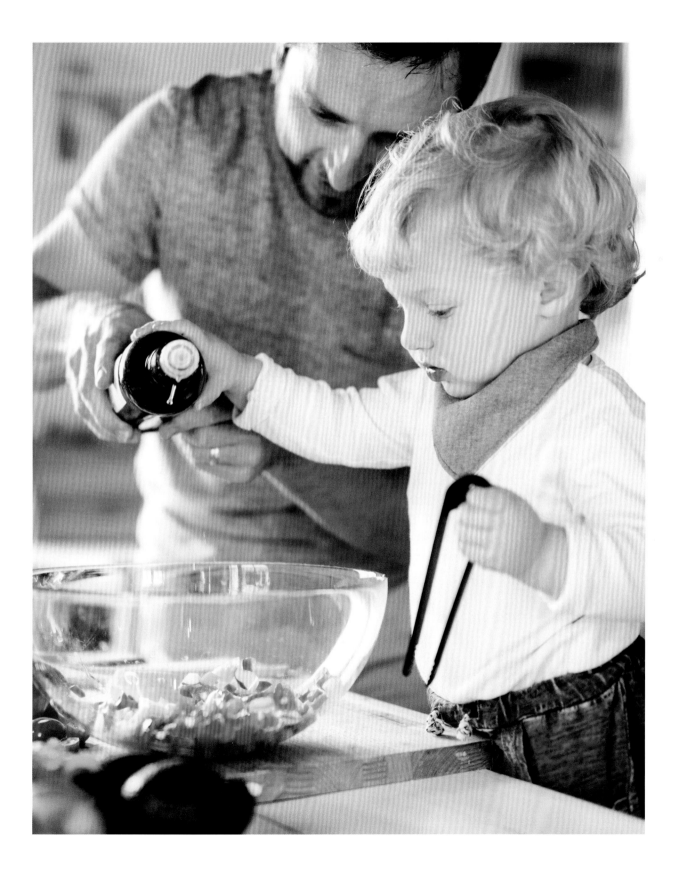

Eating Organic

From meat to milk to vegetables to processed snacks, many foods are now available as both conventionally grown and organically grown. In the US and Canada, organic farming is regulated, and specific approved methods must be used for a product to bear the USDA Organic or Canada Organic logo. The demand for organic foods is huge, largely because consumers are worried about the potential effects of chemicals such as pesticides and GMOs in conventional farming (more on those in the pages that follow). This is a valid concern, especially when you're growing a little human inside of you or are feeding a growing family. Here is what we think you should do when making the decision about eating organic.

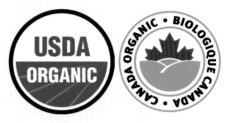

REALITY CHECK

Remember, organic is a method of farming, not a health claim; organic does not necessarily mean "healthier." Many people see the organic logo on food packages and assume it means the food is good for them. That's not necessarily the case! Think about it: if you take organic flour, organic butter, and organic sugar to make cookies, they are still cookies! The cookies are not magically healthier because they are organic. They are still cookies that are high in fat and sugar but low in fiber, vitamins, and minerals.

What does "organic" mean?

All farmers have the same end-goal: to grow or raise the best quality food. Both conventional and organic farmers must follow government regulations and standards. Farmers that grow or raise organic food have these rules to follow:

- Use natural processes to protect soil
- Use organic seeds
- Practice crop rotation to prevent soil erosion

- Provide animals with living areas that encourage natural behavior, such as grazing
- Do not use GMOs (this means an organic farmer can't plant GMO seeds, an organic cow can't eat GMO corn as feed, and an organic food producer can't use any GMO ingredients in their products)
- Do not use most synthetic pesticides, fertilizers, or growth hormones

WHAT ARE GMOs?

The World Health Organization categorizes GMOs as plants or animals that have had their genetic material (DNA) altered in a way that does not occur naturally by mating or natural recombination. It's high-level science here! So why the heck are researchers modifying food? Some good reasons: to make them more tolerant to different types of weather; to increase crop yield to feed more people; and to make them more resistant to insects and pests, thus reducing the need for pesticides.

According to the USDA, genetically modified soybeans and corn account for 90% of GMO crops.[3] Other GMO crops include:

- Cotton (to make cottonseed oil)
- Canola seeds (used for making canola oil)
- Sugar beets (used to make sugar, but different than sugar cane)
- Papayas
- Alfalfa
- Arctic apples (they don't turn brown when you cut into them)
- Bruise-free potatoes

Scientists are working on GMO wheat, but it is not currently available for sale.

WHAT ABOUT PESTICIDES?

Pesticides are used to reduce damage to plants from weeds, rodents, and insects. Pesticides can either be synthetic (factory-made) or natural (used in organic farming). Wait, what? Yup, organic farming still uses pesticides! They are different than the

SHADES OF GRAY: GMOs

Some people are anti-GMO, right? Why is that? Well, it's a relatively new science. The first GMO crop came to market in 1994, so that's not a long time to establish a safety record. Some people are concerned that without long-term studies, we don't know how GMOs will affect human health. To date, the USDA and Health Canada have deemed GMOs to be safe based on short-term studies. Some people don't feel this is enough, so they choose non-GMO products only. It's really up to you.

pesticides used in conventional farming, but organic farmers still need to ward off insects, etc.. To do this, they use things like copper sulfate and rotenone.

The best-ever-gold-star pesticide would destroy pests without harming humans, other plants, animals, or the environment. Scientists are always working on improving pesticides, but unfortunately that perfect pesticide does not exist yet.

DEEP DIVE: PESTICIDES

The word "pesticide" strikes fear in people and is synonymous with "toxin" or "poison." Of course, pesticides can be toxic when consumed at ultra-high doses, but the USDA, Health Canada, and the US Environmental Protection Agency say you should not be concerned about the low dose found on food.

Government agencies test pesticide levels in foods to ensure that the amount of pesticide residue is tiny, then add a 10-fold to 100-fold safety net for food that is actually released for public consumption. So pesticide levels are very, very, very low. However, some studies link exposure to organophosphate pesticides to increased risks of ADHD, lower IQ in children, low birthweight, and early gestation among newborns. These studies do not show cause and effect (i.e., they do NOT show clearly that pesticides CAUSE low IQ), but they do show a correlation (which means kids with lower IQ also had more pesticide residue in their blood/urine samples, but could have 10 other things as well).[4]

Of course, skeptics say that governments may not be testing the right things to truly predict the potential dangers from long-term, low-level exposure from a mix of many pesticides. That's why the choice to eat conventionally grown or organic foods is up to you. There's no perfect answer to suit everyone.

SO SHOULD I EAT ORGANIC?

This is 100% your personal choice. There are valid arguments in favor of each side, but there's no clear answer. If you decide to go organic, that's great! However, if you choose to select only a few foods to buy organic—or none at all—that's awesome too! Above all, try to eat nutritious, whole foods most of the time. And know that you can have a very healthy and nutritious diet—organic or not!

Eating Organic Pros and Cons		
Pros:	Neutral:	Cons:
• Organic meat and dairy tend to have higher levels of omega-3 fat • Organic fruits and vegetables tend to have more antioxidants • Organic farming may be more beneficial for the planet	• Vitamin and mineral content is largely the same • Some say organic food tastes better, but taste is subjective! • The levels of synthetic pesticides are higher in conventionally grown foods but whether small doses of pesticides over time are detrimental is unclear	• Organic food costs more than conventionally grown food • Some natural and organic pesticides may be just as harmful as synthetic pesticides—this is unknown • Organic farming alone cannot feed the whole planet because it's often small-scale production

Examples of nutrient-rich foods, like egg, kale, almonds, and our Yummy Salmon Bites on page 317

Important Nutrients

The food that your family eats should be—for the most part—whole foods, because these are the most nutrient-rich (read more about this on pages 9 and 10). But what does "nutrient-rich" actually mean? Well, nutrient-rich foods are those that contain the essential nutrients for our growth and development. Each nutrient (e.g. protein, calcium, dietary fat, etc.) plays a different and important role in being, and growing, a healthy human. Although *all* nutrients are important during the stages of pregnancy, postnatal, infancy, and childhood, we've highlighted a few particularly important ones here to give you an understanding of why they are important and what they provide the body. We don't want to scare you with a whole bunch of numbers here, but we've included them in the Nutritional Breakdowns charts on pages 364 to 372 for those of you who want to dive deeper.

Protein

WHY IS IT IMPORTANT?
Protein is important for everyone, regardless of age or stage. It provides building blocks for the growth and repair of the cells in your muscles, organs, skin, and nails. Your body also uses protein to make enzymes and hormones.

SOURCES OF PROTEIN
Fish, meat, poultry, tofu, beans, lentils, peas, nuts, seeds, eggs, and dairy foods (yogurt, milk, and cheese). See the chart on page 364.

Dietary fat

WHY IS IT IMPORTANT?
Dietary fat is part of the body's cells. It helps support brain and nerve function and is essential for ensuring the body absorbs fat-soluble vitamins such as vitamins A, D, E, and K. Some dietary fats are considered essential, which means you need to get them

via food (omega-3 fat is an example; see below). Dietary fat makes you feel fuller longer because it takes a while to digest, unlike sugar and other refined carbs, which are digested quickly, leaving you hungry again soon (read more on page 32).

SOURCES OF FAT

Good fats: Monounsaturated and polyunsaturated fats found in healthful plant and seafood sources, such as oily fish, nuts, seeds, oils, olives, and avocados.

Controversial fats: Saturated fats found in butter, cheese, cream, fatty meat, coconut oil, and palm oil. There has been a lot of research into saturated fat and its link to heart disease. Some studies show that replacing saturated fat (e.g. butter) with unsaturated fat (e.g. olive oil) lowers the risk of heart disease, but others show no link between saturated fats and heart health at all. While the research is ongoing, health organizations such as the World Health Organization and the American Heart Association suggest cutting back on saturated fat and choosing unsaturated (good) fats first and foremost.

Bad fats: Trans fats found in ultra-processed foods such as prepackaged cookies and baked goods. They appear on ingredient lists as partially hydrogenated oil, margarine, or shortening and are bad for heart health and cholesterol levels. Canada banned trans fats back in 2018, and the US banned them in 2020.

DEEP DIVE: HEART DISEASE

When it comes to reducing heart disease risk, the types of foods that we eat and our overall dietary pattern are far more important than our total fat consumption.[10] So the old adage that dietary fat is "bad" is not really true at all. The types of fat—and more relevantly, the types of foods supplying this fat—are far more important than the total amount of fat consumed.

Omega-3 fat (particularly DHA and EPA)

WHY IS IT IMPORTANT?

Omega-3 is one of the "good" unsaturated fats mentioned above, but it's extra-important, which is why we have a whole special section here for it! Omega-3 fat is an umbrella term for a few different fatty acids, and these are essential for good health during pregnancy and in babies, kids, and adults. The most important types of omega-3 fat are called DHA and EPA, which are important for proper brain, eye, and nerve development.

SOURCES OF DHA/EPA

Omega-3 DHA and EPA are found mainly in oily fish and seafood such as salmon, low-mercury skipjack tuna, herring, Atlantic mackerel, and rainbow trout. Some eggs also contain DHA. See the chart on page 367. If you do not eat fish, you need to find DHA and EPA elsewhere. You can get them from fish oil or from algal oil supplements (there are toddler and child versions too!)—a vegan alternative to fish oil. Omega-3 ALA is found in plant-based foods such as walnuts, chia, flax, hemp, soy oil, and supplements, but ALA does not have the same health benefits for brain, eye, and nerve development as DHA and EPA do. While some of the ALA you consume is converted to DHA and EPA by the body, research suggests it is less than 1%.

> **DEEP DIVE: OMEGA-3 FATS**
>
> What do those acronyms stand for?
> - DHA: Docosahexaenoic acid
> - EPA: Eicosapentaenoic acid
> - ALA: Alpha-linolenic acid

Iron

WHY IS IT IMPORTANT?

Iron is essential for general health, growth, and development, and it carries oxygen to the body's tissues, keeping cells healthy and functioning optimally. It also helps the brain and nerves develop properly—obviously critical for our little ones! If iron levels dip low enough, it can lead to iron-deficient anemia, a condition in which the blood lacks adequate healthy red blood cells (these are the cells that carry oxygen throughout the body). Symptoms of iron-deficiency anemia develop slowly and may be mild, but include: dizziness, low energy, headaches, pale color, fussiness/irritability, slowed growth, shortness of breath and lack of concentration. It's important to see a doctor right away if you sense your child might have anemia, so that long-term health issues can be prevented.

Babies have a store of iron built up in their bodies from being in the womb. It keeps them going until they reach about 6 months, at which time they require additional food sources of iron to meet their requirements. This is why you'll notice us *reeeallly* driving home the message of the importance of iron when starting solids.

SOURCES OF IRON

Meat, poultry, fish, eggs, fortified cereals, legumes and pulses like beans and lentils, and leafy greens. See the chart on page 368.

DEEP DIVE: MAXIMIZE IRON ABSORPTION

Animal sources of iron are called *heme* iron and include all meats, poultry, and fish. Heme iron is well absorbed by the body. Plants such as beans, lentils, and grains, as well as eggs, dairy, and certain vegetables contain *non-heme* iron, which is not as well absorbed. Pairing non-heme sources with vitamin C helps boost iron absorption in the body. The chart below shows examples of non-heme iron sources and vitamin C sources you can pair together to maximize iron absorption—especially important if you eat a plant-based diet.

MATCH FOOD FROM HERE (NON-HEME IRON)	WITH FOOD FROM HERE (VITAMIN C)
Iron-fortified breads and cereals	Kale
Beans, peas, and lentils	Leafy greens: spinach, etc.
Blackstrap molasses	Tomatoes
Whole grains: oats, quinoa, millet	Broccoli
Nuts and seeds	Fruit: apples, oranges, lemons, kiwi,
Eggs	mango, papaya, strawberries
Dried apricots, figs, and raisins	Sweet peppers

Calcium

WHY IS IT IMPORTANT?

Calcium is important for building and maintaining healthy bones and teeth. It also helps with muscle function, nerve transmission, and hormonal balance. In babies and kids, it's extra-important because initial bone mass is being built to help support their bone health for life. It's also important in pregnancy and when breastfeeding because, well, you're supporting the calcium needs of another human!

SOURCES OF CALCIUM

Cow's milk, fortified plant-based milk beverages, yogurt, cheese, canned salmon with bones, sesame seeds, and almonds. See the chart on page 369.

Dietary fiber

WHY IS IT IMPORTANT?

There's no doubt you've heard that fiber is an important part of our diets. Fiber is a type of carbohydrate, but unlike other carbs (sugars and starches), it doesn't get broken down, digested, or absorbed by the body, nor does it provide us with a meaningful amount of calories or energy. But that's a good thing because it helps the body perform other essential jobs. Not to mention most fiber-rich foods are super nutritious! When eaten in the recommended quantities, fiber can:

- Prevent constipation and keep your digestive system healthy
- Lower your cholesterol
- Control your blood sugar
- Stabilize your appetite
- Help you maintain a healthy body weight
- Lower your risk of some cancers, like colon cancer

Getting enough fiber is particularly important during pregnancy and breastfeeding, as digestive issues such as constipation tend to creep in more (see pages 112 and 144). Pregnant and breastfeeding women need a few extra grams of fiber every day compared to other adults (see page 370). And kids need fiber every day too: it helps them to stay regular, feel full for longer, and stay properly nourished (higher-fiber foods tend to be more nutritious than lower-fiber foods). Many people get only about half the amount of fiber they need, so take a look at your diet and think if you should be trying to add more (see page 29 for ways to do it). But go slooow. If you are going to increase your or your child's fiber intake, do it slowly and make sure you are drinking enough fluids (fiber needs fluid to work properly!) and being physically active every day. If you introduce too much fiber too quickly, you could end up feeling bloated, constipated (or more constipated!), and uncomfortable.

SOURCES OF FIBER

Vegetables, fruits, whole grains, legumes like beans, lentils, and peas, and nuts and seeds. See the chart on the opposite page.

DEEP DIVE: SOLUBLE AND INSOLUBLE FIBER

There are 2 distinct types of fiber—soluble and insoluble—and they differ in their physical structure and impact on health. We need both, for different reasons. Foods can contain one or both types in varying amounts.

Soluble fiber is found in oats, barley, legumes, some fruits, chia seeds, hemp hearts, flax seeds, and psyllium husks. When it's combined with water, it forms a gel-like substance, which can help to prevent bowel irregularity (diarrhea and constipation) and has been shown to improve blood sugar control by slowing down the release of glucose into the bloodstream. It can also help to lower "bad" cholesterol (LDL) and make you feel full. This explains why a bowl of oatmeal is often more filling than a slice of white toast with jam—it's the fiber! Some forms of soluble fiber are also known as "prebiotics" (the food that the beneficial probiotics thrive off of). Cool, huh?

Insoluble fiber is found in most fruits, vegetables, and whole grains, especially wheat bran. It doesn't form a gel in the digestive tract, but instead provides bulk and structure to your stool, helping it to pass. For this reason, insoluble fiber also helps to keep you regular (remember when we said you needed both?). Diets with adequate insoluble fiber will help to prevent and manage constipation and hemorrhoids.

How to Increase Fiber in Your Family's Diet

FRUITS & VEGETABLES:

- Serve whole, fresh or frozen, and as often as possible. Try adding frozen veggies to a stir-fry or casserole, or add fresh, or dried fruits to cereal, oatmeal, yogurt, and smoothies.
- Don't peel apples, pears, peaches, etc. The peels of fruits and vegetables often contain fiber, so wash the skins rather than peeling. (But, yep, still peel bananas, oranges and pineapples!)
- Serve fruit instead of fruit juice as the juicing process removes all of the fiber goodness from the fruit.

GRAINS:

- Try serving grains for breakfast, like oatmeal or high-fiber cereal (at least 4 grams of fiber per 30-gram serving).
- Choose whole grains rather than refined grains. Try brown rice instead of white rice and choose whole grain rather than white bread and pasta options (at least 2 grams of fiber per 30-gram serving).
- Use whole grain wheat flour, barley flour, or oat flour rather than white when baking bread, muffins, and loaves.
- Add bran cereal to pancakes, muffins, and breads.

LEGUMES:

- Add lentils, edamame, or beans to soups, casseroles, chili, and salads.
- Spread hummus on whole grain flatbread, naan, or roti, or use as a dip for crackers or vegetables.

NUTS & SEEDS:

- Add ground flaxseeds, hemp hearts, or chia seeds to cereal or yogurt, or to dough when baking.
- Use nuts and seeds in salads, smoothies, or atop grain dishes.
- Try a small handful of mixed nuts and seeds as a great snack.

Vitamin D

WHY IS IT IMPORTANT?

We love vitamin D. A lot. This very important vitamin helps your body put to use the minerals that are a part of bones and teeth, including calcium and phosphrous. It may also help to reduce the risk of chronic diseases such as multiple sclerosis and cancer, and it is linked to a stronger overall immune system.

SOURCES OF VITAMIN D

Milk, fish, and eggs, are all sources of vitamin D (see the chart on page 317), and of course, sunshine! Read more about this in the Deep Dive opposite. But it's hard (likely impossible) to get all the vitamin D you need from food and sunshine alone, so we recommend everyone (babies, toddlers, children and adults) take a vitamin D supplement daily.

The current recommended Dietary Reference Intakes (DRI) for vitamin D is 400 IU for babies aged 0 to 12 months, and 600 IU for toddlers, children and adults. Our supplement recommendations meet this and then some: 400 IU for babies, toddlers

DEEP DIVE: SUN EXPOSURE

Vitamin D is made by the body after exposure to the sun. It's really cool, actually. The sun's rays hit cholesterol in the skin cells, providing the energy for vitamin D synthesis to occur. This happens quite quickly (in about 10 minutes), particularly in the summer. That means you don't need to tan or burn your skin to get your vitamin D dose. You only need to expose your skin for only about half the time it takes for your skin to begin to burn. Suncreen blocks some vitamin D–producing UV rays. So if you live in a cool climate (do you see snow for half of the year like we do?) or are really careful about sunscreen, you may not naturally get enough vitamin D. Keep wearing your sunscreen and add a vitamin D supplement. See opposite for more advice on these.

and children, and at least 1000 IU for adults. Why? Because the research on vitamin D is constantly evolving, and there are new benefits emerging all the time. It's very easy to become deficient in vitamin D, but, on the flip side, the health benefits are numerous when you're getting enough. Taking a supplement provides you with a healthy buffer to ensure that you're meeting your needs, plus more. And, don't worry, the tolerable upper limit for babies is 1000 IU per day, and 4000 IU per day for adults—so it's very difficult to overdo it.

Vitamin D supplements are available in dropper, liquid, and pill format. When breast-feeding, simply drop the vitamin D onto your nipple and the baby will ingest it while they feed. Note that formula-fed babies who are consuming more than 32 ounces a day will receive vitamin D through their formula, so a supplement isn't necessary for them.

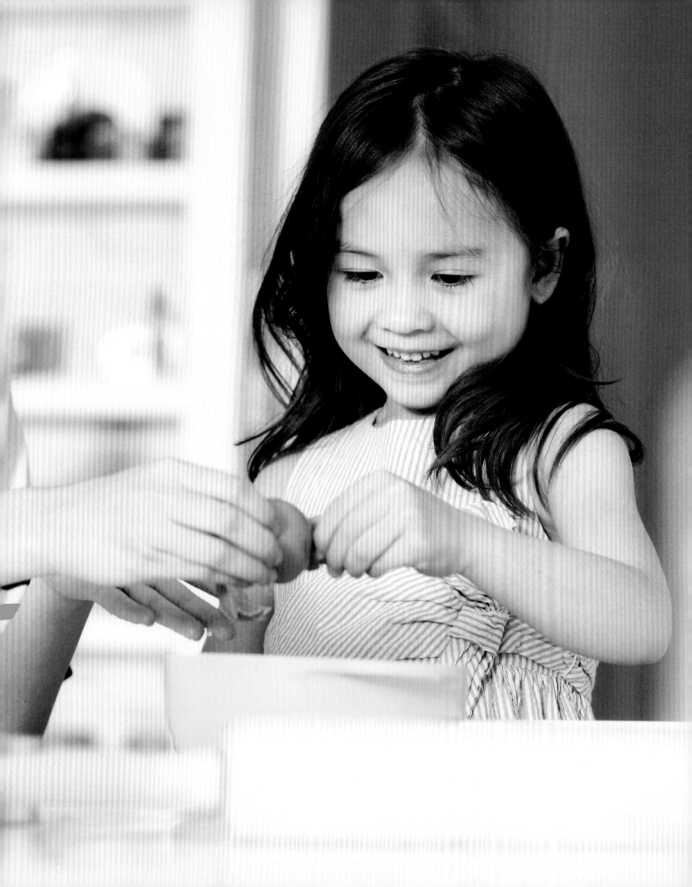

Carbohydrate, Sugar, and Salt

There's so much misinformation out there about carbohydrates, sugar, and salt (hello, Dr. Google), so we've decided to pay special attention to those nutrients here.

Carbohydrates

What is a carbohydrate? It's a nutrient found in many foods. Despite their reputation, carbs are NOT all bad. In fact, carbohydrates are our body's and brain's preferred source of energy and fuel. We need them. And so do our kids! All vegetables, fruits, whole grains, legumes, and milk contain carbs. And those are all super-nutritious foods that contain important things like fiber, vitamins, minerals, protein, iron, antioxidants, and phytochemicals. You may hear the term "bad" carbs; this usually refers to refined carbs that don't have lots of fiber, vitamins, and minerals—things like soft drinks, candy, cake, etc.

Focus on the carbohydrates found in nutrient-rich foods, and you're on the right track. If all of the carbs that you're eating (or feeding your child) are coming from ultra-processed foods, and it's time for a menu makeover. Too much of these foods can lead to health issues (see page 11) and can fill precious tummy space that should be reserved for more nutrient-dense foods.

BALANCING CARBOHYDRATE INTAKE

We don't advise eating carb-rich foods on their own—especially refined, white starchy carbs—instead, include them in balanced meals that also have protein and fat. Why? Because refined carbs are digested quickly and can spike blood sugar levels (see

Nutritious versus Less Nutritious Carbs
Nutritious carbs (whole)
• Whole grains • Beans • Lentils • Vegetables • Fruit
Less nutritious carbs (refined)
• Sugar, syrup and jam • Candy and chocolate • Baked goods • Ice cream • Chips, tortillas, and pretzels • French fries

below). But when protein, carbs (which contain fiber), and fat are part of the same meal, the blood sugar spike is minimized and food is digested more evenly and slowly—keeping you fuller for longer and decreasing the volume of food that you may eat throughout the day. Regularly consuming high-carbohydrate foods in excess or on their own (especially those refined ones that we mentioned) can potentially lead to overeating, excess weight gain (which, during pregnancy, is associated with a high-weight baby), and an increased risk of gestational diabetes (see page 98).

Blood sugar spikes

Huh? Blood sugar spikes? Okay, imagine this: You wake up on an empty stomach and choose a bagel (full of carbs from refined white flour, low in fat, and not a ton of protein) with jam (100% sugar carbs, no fat, and no protein) for breakfast. You eat your bagel and jam and your blood sugar level spikes because of the carbs (and lack of protein, fat, and fiber to regulate their impact). You feel

Balanced Meals & Snacks

Family meals should contain vegetables and/or fruits, whole grains, and protein-rich foods such as meat, low-mercury fish, poultry, dairy, beans, lentils, nuts, and seeds. These foods will give you the most nutrition bang for your buck and help to keep your appetite and blood sugar levels steady throughout the day. Here are some suggestions:

BREAKFAST:
- Eggs + fruit + whole grain toast
- Greek yogurt + nuts + berries + muesli

LUNCH/DINNER:
- Chicken + broccoli + quinoa
- Fish + salad + brown rice

SNACKS:
- Whole grain banana muffin + cheese
- Carrots + cucumber + hummus
- Apple + peanut butter

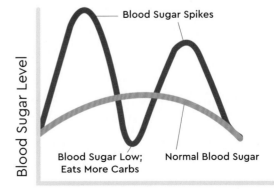

a quick burst of energy and feel full for a little while, but then you lose that in about an hour and feel hungry again. So you crave more carbs, and your day can easily turn into a blood sugar rollercoaster.

Scenario 2: You wake up and choose oatmeal (whole grain, high-fiber carbs) with Greek yogurt (protein), berries (fiber), and nuts (protein and fat) for breakfast. Your blood sugar level rises slowly and slightly and then stays stable, because the protein, fat, and fiber that are present in these foods are digested slowly. These nutrients also help you stay full for longer, so you're not hungry an hour later and craving more carbs.

REALITY CHECK: DIETS

FOR THE LOVE OF GOOD BREAD, DO NOT PUT YOUR CHILD ON A LOW-CARB DIET FOR WEIGHT LOSS. We strongly believe that healthy children should not be put on any sort of weight-loss diet (read more about this on page 342). Kids need nutrients to grow and develop properly. And nutrients come from all sorts of different foods, including carbs.

LOW-CARB DIETS

Low-carb plans have been popular for decades—they are known by names such as Atkins, South Beach, Dukan, paleo, or keto. These diets can help with weight loss, and some people find them to be helpful, while others find them overly restrictive and difficult to follow.

Studies show that while people may lose weight quickly on a low-carb diet, there is no difference in weight loss at the end of a year between a low-carb and a regular low-fat diet.[5] The truth is, the best diet is one you can stick to for the long term, because it contains foods you enjoy. Or better yet—no diet at all. Because most evidence shows that diets just don't work long term (see more about Intuitive Eating on page 44). And when it comes to pregnancy, low-carb diets are generally not recommended (read more on page 85). You should not be depriving your body of important nutrients (like carbohydrates) when you're growing a human and trying to stay healthy yourself.

Sugar

Many of us have a "sweet tooth" or a desire to eat sugary foods. It's not a surprise, really, since many sweet foods taste so good. Think about it: chocolate, ice cream, cake, cookies—yum, yum, yum, and yum. And our taste for sugar starts early, because even breastmilk tastes sweet! While a small intake of sugar is fine for our overall health, problems can start when we consume too much—which is linked to an increased risk of cardiovascular disease, stroke, type 2 diabetes, dental cavities, some types of cancer, and possibly other health conditions. So that raises 2 questions: what counts as "sugar" and how much of it is safe to eat?

WHAT IS SUGAR?

The sugar category is huge and goes way beyond the white stuff you add to your morning coffee. Sugar is split into 2 categories: added and natural. The World Health Organization defines added sugars as those that are "added to foods and beverages by the manufacturer, cook or consumer, and sugars naturally present in honey, syrups, fruit juices and fruit juice concentrates."[6] Natural sugars, on the other hand, are found in whole foods like fruits, sweet vegetables, and milk.

There are many more names for sugar than those included in the chart above, but you get the idea. Basically, anything else with the word "sugar" or "syrup" is an added sugar. Some product manufacturers try to sugarcoat these names (ha ha—pun intended) to make them sound healthier, but don't fall for it. For example, "organic coconut sap syrup" sounds SO healthy, right? Yeah . . . but it's just sugar.

Types of Sugars

Added sugars

- Sugar: white, brown, icing, demerara, caster, turbinado, coconut, date, cane, granulated, confectioners, muscovado, etc.
- Syrup: brown rice, coconut sap, maple, corn, golden, refiners, etc.
- Other: honey, agave, evaporated cane juice, fruit concentrate, molasses, etc.

Natural sugars

- Fruits
- Vegetables
- Milk

(REALITY CHECK)

Fruit juice is the one outlier in these added versus natural sugar categories. Technically, it's a "natural" sugar because it's made from fruit, but the World Health Organization doesn't classify it as such. Fruit juice falls into the added sugar category—yep, just like soda, candy, or ice cream. Did you know that ounce for ounce, soda and fruit juice (100% unsweetened fruit juice at that!) contain the same amount of sugar—about 1 teaspoon per ounce? So that 12-ounce juice bottle contains 12 teaspoons of sugar! With a sugar avalanche such as that, it doesn't matter where the sugar comes from—too much is too much, regardless of the source.

Packaged foods come with Nutrition Facts tables, which always list sugar content in grams. It's often more meaningful–and a better visual–to think about sugar in terms of teaspoons. So if you read a Nutrition Facts panel with sugar listed in grams, how can you figure out teaspoons? It's simple math! 1 teaspoon of sugar = 4 grams of sugar. Translate grams of sugar into teaspoons by dividing by 4:

> 1 bottle of soda = 56 grams of sugar
>
> 56 ÷ 4 = 14 teaspoons of sugar

HOW MUCH IS TOO MUCH?

When you read guidelines about how much sugar is safe to eat, they're usually referring to added sugars, not natural sugars. For both adults and children, the World Health Organization recommends that added sugars make up no more than 10% of our total daily calories.[7] This means the maximum amount of added sugar we should consume is:

- **Adult:** 12 teaspoons
- **Child:** 6 teaspoons

These are just estimates, as no one really knows exactly how many calories they eat in a day (nor do we suggest counting them!). But it should help you figure out how much sugar is too much. And remember, the limits are for added sugars only, not natural sugars. That means milk, vegetables, and fruits are fine to eat without counting the sugar content.

How much sugar is in that?

Studies show that about 68% of the packaged products sold in grocery stores contain added sugar, so it's found in a LOT of foods and beverages. Here's just a small list of how much sugar is in certain foods:

Food/drink	Teaspoons	Grams
Sugary cereal (1 cup)	3	12
Oreo cookies (3)	3	12
Instant oatmeal (1 pouch)	3	12
Barbecue sauce (2 tbsp)	4	14
Strawberry yogurt (¾ cup)	5	20

Food/drink	Teaspoons	Grams
Chocolate bar (1½ oz)	5	20
Gummy bears (17)	5	20
Soda/cola (8 oz)	8	32
Apple juice (8 oz)	8	32
Chocolate ice cream (1 cup)	9	36
Iced tea (16 oz)	11	44
Frappuccino (tall)	12	48
Cake with icing (3½ oz)	12	48
Soda (16 oz)	14	56

SUGAR AND BABIES AND TODDLERS

We don't recommend giving babies or toddlers sweet treats or desserts with added sugar until after they turn 2 (of course, special occasions and birthdays can be exceptions). There are a couple of reasons for this:

Nutrients should come first: Foods with a lot of added sugar tend to be calorie-rich but nutrient-poor. Babies' and young toddlers' nutrient requirements are so high (and tummies so small) that it's important to focus on nutrient-dense whole foods instead of filling tummy space with nutrient-poor sugary foods.

The more they taste, the more they want: Babies, toddlers, and kids are biologically driven towards sweet tastes and foods. They experience a pleasure response in their brain, which includes the release of "happy hormones" (like dopamine), and, not surprisingly, they'll crave that same feeling again and again. Who wouldn't?! If your baby is exposed to only naturally and subtly sweet foods like fruits and sweet vegetables, their taste buds will know only this subtle sweetness (not the intense sweetness of cookies or cake) until they're a bit older.

Salt

We all need a small amount of sodium for our bodies to function normally. Sodium is a vital part of nerve signal transmission, muscle contraction, and fluid balance. Consumed in excess though, it may put you at higher risk of stroke, kidney disease, and high blood pressure. Here are the actual numbers for adequate salt intake per day:

Age	Salt per day (milligrams)
0 to 6 months	110
7 to 12 months	370
1 to 3 years	800
4 to 8 years	1,000
9 to 13 years	1,200
14+	1,500
Adults (even if pregnant or breastfeeding)	1,500

WHERE'S THE SALT?

When you hear the words "salt" and "sodium," you may immediately think about the salt shaker on your table. So it may surprise you to learn that just 11% of your sodium intake comes from the salt you cook with or add at the table. Most of the sodium that kids and adults consume—a whopping 71%—comes from ultra-processed, packaged, and restaurant food.[8] Salt is in pizza, bread, burgers, deli meat, chips, pretzels, pickles, and condiments, to name a few. These foods are high in sodium because it's used for many reasons—to prevent spoilage, stop the growth of pathogens, improve appearance, and enhance flavor or texture. And sodium levels add up quickly when you're using bottled dressings and sauces. Sodium shown in the chart opposite is only for one teaspoon, so levels may be even higher depending on how much you use!

Condiment	Salt per 1 teaspoon (milligrams)
Vinegar	0
Mayonnaise	32
Ketchup	47
Yellow mustard	55
Sriracha hot sauce	75
Djion mustard	150
Reduced-sodium soy sauce	250
Soy sauce	330
Fish Sauce	400

WHICH SALT IS BEST?

The health halo over fancy salt is undeserved. Although pretty packages of pink Himalayan sea salt, fleur de sel, sea salt, or smoky gray salt are marketed for their health benefits (trace minerals! all natural!), it's just hype. Trace minerals are found in such tiny quantities that they contribute very little to overall health—plus, we get enough of these nutrients from the foods we eat daily. We don't need more from salt! The truth is that fancy salt and regular table salt contain the same amount of sodium by weight, and that's the nutrient of most concern.

From a culinary point of view, however, the type of salt matters. Different varieties will change the flavor profile and texture of a dish. For example, flaky Maldon salt adds a terrific crunch, while Hawaiian sea salt imparts an earthy flavor. So choose your salt for its culinary characteristics, not because you're sprinkling health onto your meals.

Top 10 Sources of Sodium[9]

1. Breads and rolls
2. Pizza
3. Sandwiches
4. Cold cuts and cured meats
5. Soups
6. Burritos and tacos
7. Savory snacks such as chips, popcorn, pretzels, snack mixes, and crackers
8. Chicken
9. Cheese
10. Eggs and omelets

REALITY CHECK

Babies and young toddlers don't need added salt. In fact, it's not healthy for them to have it. With the salt found in foods they already eat, such as bread, cheese, and milk, they will get the amount they need without you adding salt to their foods, and hold the salty condiments too. If you share family meals, or practice baby-led weaning, portion out your child's meal separately and avoid adding extra salt.

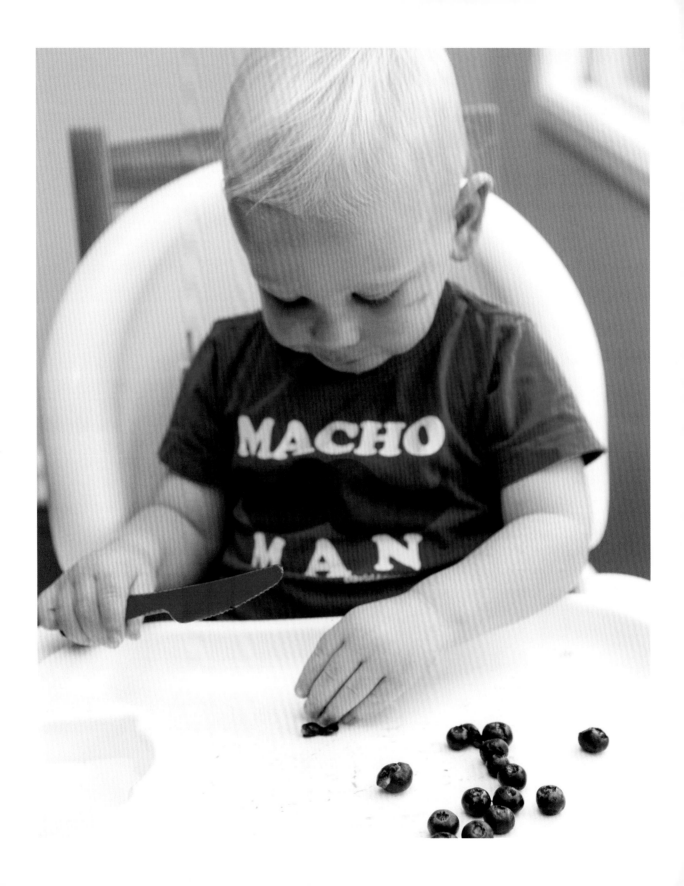

Approaches to Food and Feeding

We all know that what we eat is important, but you'll see in this book that we're equally passionate about *how* we eat, and how we encourage our children to eat. We know from experience—both personal and professional—and from doing a lot of research that *how* you feed children is critical to their long-term health and their relationship with food. By "how" we mean how food is talked about, how meals are served, how babies are fed, how snacks are offered, and how you model healthy eating with your own habits for your child.

Satter's Division of Responsibility

You will read about Satter's Division of Responsibility (sDOR) again and again in this book. It's something we're truly passionate about, and we also know that it works! When dietitians learn about childhood nutrition, we learn about Ellyn Satter's work. Satter herself is a registered dietitian, social worker, and family therapist who runs the non-profit Ellyn Satter Institute in the US. You can learn more at www.ellynsatterinstitute.org.

Satter's work is based on the fact that children have an innate sense of their own appetite, and their own likes and dislikes when it comes to food. Kids are naturally good eaters; left to their own devices, children will eat as much as they need, grow in the way that is right for them, and will learn to eat the food their parents eat—that is, if parents allow this to happen! The sDOR lays out distinct roles for parents and children, so that when you do your job of feeding, your children will do their job of eating:

Parents are responsible for	Children are responsible for
Infants	
• *What* is served to eat • Helping baby feel calm • Paying attention to baby's feeding cues	• *How much* to eat
Babies, toddlers, and school-age children	
• *What* is served to eat • *When* it is served • *Where* it is served	• *If* they want to eat • *How much* to eat

We all have the goal of raising healthy, confident eaters, and we want our kids to feel capable at the table, able to choose from the foods provided, and to pace themselves and feed themselves independently. Despite good intentions, when parents tell their children exactly what and how much to eat, they disrupt their child's ability to self-regulate. That's not a parent's job! Your job is to peel away any preconceived notions you may have about the right way to feed your child and to learn to *trust* your child and their body. We want their inner dialogue to be:

- "I can feed myself at meals."
- "I know how much food my body needs, and I'll eat until my tummy feels satisfied."
- "I know how much time I have to eat, so I'll pace myself according to that."

Unfortunately, when parents micromanage food intake, or regularly pressure their babies, toddlers or kids to eat (or not to eat), it translates into one or more of these messages in the child's mind:

- "I am not capable of feeding myself."
- "I am not eating enough/fast enough."
- "I should not trust my body."

Many parents have trouble believing that a child can or should choose *how much* or *if* they want to eat—we're part of a culture that tells kids to "clear your plate" or take "just one more bite." Too often, well-meaning parents don't recognize the signs that a child is full, or choose to ignore

WE GOT YOU!

We've seen the sDOR work time and time again—in fact, thousands of times!—in nutrition counseling practices and with our own kids. Please try it. And trust it. And be patient. It may take weeks or months for an older child to grow accustomed to it, but we promise it does work!

them, because they want to make sure that their child receives enough nutrition. On the other hand, parents can sometimes take food away too quickly if you're rushing through to get to the next task or if you're worried that your baby is eating too much. But the basis of the sDOR is that our kids are born intuitive eaters—they know how much they need and when to stop—so we need to trust this and not pressure them to eat more. By offering 5 to 6 eating opportunities a day (meals and snacks), with lots of variety, we can rest assured that our little ones will meet their nutrition needs over the period of a week, rather than focusing on any 1 specific meal. This makes for a much more pleasant eating experience and nurtures your child's natural ability to eat intuitively (read more about Intuitive Eating on page 44).

We are asked so many questions about mealtimes, and have found most of those can be answered by referring back to the sDOR. For example:

"My son likes to graze on snacks all day long. Is that okay instead of eating 3 meals?"
- In the sDOR, it's the adult's job to choose *when* to eat. If the child is making those decisions instead (and grazing all day at their discretion), the parent is not following the sDOR.
- **Solution:** Set designated meal and snack times to eliminate all-day grazing.

"My daughter gets distracted at mealtime, so I try to spoon-feed her or tell her she can't leave the table until she takes 3 more bites. If I didn't do that, she wouldn't eat! That's okay, right?"
- In the sDOR, it's the child's job to decide *if* and *how much* to eat. If the parent is making those decisions instead (and forcing the child to eat more), the parent is not following the sDOR.
- **Solution:** Offer food in a pleasant environment at regular intervals (consistently), and the child will do their job and eat what they need. This is called self-regulation. Don't spoon feed your child; they should be able to self-feed independently. And make sure mealtimes screen- and distraction-free.

Satter's Division of Responsibility

Parents feeding jobs:	Child eating jobs:
• Provide regular meals and snacks	• Decide if they will eat
• Choose and prepare food	• Eat the amount they need
• Be considerate about foods served, without catering to likes and dislikes	• Learn to eat the food their parents eat and serve
• Set mealtime boundaries	• Learn to behave well at mealtime
• Make eating times pleasant and positive	• Grow predictably
• Show by example how to behave at mealtime	
• Let children grow into the bodies that are right for them	

Responsive feeding

Responsive feeding and the sDOR go hand-in-hand. Think of it as another layer to the sDOR. Responsive feeding is a way of describing the two-way feeding relationship between parent and child, when parents pay close attention to their child's hunger and fullness cues (verbal or nonverbal), and then respond accordingly. For young babies who are feeding on demand, this means responding to cues that tell you they want to start, slow down, or stop feeding. For older babies v toddlers, who have a more established routine of solid food meals and snacks, this means responding to signs of hunger or fullness—offering more when they cue for more, and slowing down or stopping when they indicate fullness. Paying attention to hunger cues will help to avoid overfeeding and underfeeding, and may help to positively influence a child's ability to self-regulate their food intake long-term. Responding to your child quickly, communicates to them that you love them, support them and trust them. And this helps build their emotional health—and a foundation of trust between you—for years to come.

To play your part in responsive feeding, you need to be present and engaged in feeding times—not on the phone and doing laundry, too! Trust us, we're all too familiar with multi-tasking as a mom, but it's important that during feeding time you're dedicated to being present and focusing on your child.

Intuitive eating

We are also big fans of intuitive eating, the evidence-based, mind-body approach to eating created by dietitians Evelyn Tribole and Elyse Resch in 1995. This is our third layer to feeding children (and eating well as adults, too). Intuitive eating encourages people (usually adults who have forgotten!) to truly listen to their physical hunger cues; it is essentially about eating when you feel hungry and stopping when you're comfortably full. Intuitive Eating now has more than 90 studies[10] linking it to greater self-esteem, more enjoyment from eating, increased health and well-being, and better body appreciation and acceptance.

INTUITIVE EATING FOR KIDS

As with the sDOR, intuitive eating is based on the fact that babies are born intuitive eaters. What that means is that babies naturally eat when they feel hungry and stop when full. As we grow older, we start to develop eating habits more influenced by external factors (like craving cinnamon buns when we pass that stand in the mall, even if we don't feel hungry) which can become ingrained in us over the years. By the time we become parents, we can forget that for babies and kids eating is intuitive. Instead of trusting our children, we can become food micromanagers. And our interference—although well-meaning—disrupts our kids' natural tendency toward intuitive eating. If parents intervene too much, kids stop trusting their bodies when it comes to hunger and fullness, and instead rely more and more on external cues for eating, potentially resulting in dysfunctional eating habits, like overeating, sneaking food, or eating when not hungry. That's not great for building a long-term healthy relationship with food!

The first step in nurturing your intuitive eater is—to be blunt—to back off. The fact that children are naturally intuitive eaters is a really GOOD thing. Then look again at the sDOR (see page 41), which outlines our roles (for parents and kids) when it comes to feeding and eating, and encourages intuitive eating.

Top 5 tips for nurturing intuitive eating in kids

1. **Respect fluctuations in child's appetite.** Just like your appetite changes from day to day and meal to meal, so does theirs. Regardless of how they ate the day before, or the day before that, respect your child's feeding and eating cues and respond appropriately.

2. **Establish a routine.** Setting a fairly consistent and predictable meal and snack schedule will help your child learn to expect when eating opportunities are, and self-regulate their eating to be hungry at meals, but not starving. Don't let eating be a free-for-all; it will exhaust you, and your child will have a hard time figuring out their natural hunger and fullness cycles.

3. **Let your child explore new foods, pressure-free.** Part of becoming comfortable with a particular food is exploring it. When you see your toddler playing with or mushing up food, consider it a way of them learning more about the food and becoming comfortable enough with it to put it in their mouth; it's one step closer to them accepting it. Here's the thing: you don't want to pressure your toddler into eating something that they are not yet totally comfortable with. This will backfire. Allow a warming-up period.

4. **Stay neutral**. Resist rewarding your child with certain foods, or praising them for eating other foods, or you start to teach them that certain foods are "good" and others are "bad." If you praise your child for eating broccoli, they're going to start to wonder what the big deal is—and then if you reward them with a

cookie (after they've finished their broccoli), they will come to regard cookies as the sought-after "yummy" food and broccoli as not so great. Keep foods emotionally neutral.

5. **Check your own "stuff."** Many of us have our own long-standing food issues (ahem . . . yo-yo dieting), and this can spill over into parenting and feeding children. We want to avoid passing down any dysfunctional food habits, so make sure that you deal with your food issues in a healthy way. We recommend seeking help from a registered dietitian who has special training in intuitive eating.

SARAH SAYS: I adopted intuitive eating about 15 years ago, then quickly incorporated it into my practice as a dietitian because it worked so well for me personally. I found I was no longer restricted or deprived of foods, or on a dieting rollercoaster, but able to fully trust my body to tell me how much and what to eat. As my practice evolved to focus more on kids, I started teaching parents how to raise intuitive eaters and nurture their kids' relationships with food long-term to avoid things like weight issues and disordered eating down the road.

INTUITIVE EATING FOR ADULTS

Becoming an intuitive eater as an adult takes time, dedication, and reflection, and it comes with the sacrifice of throwing any weight-loss goal out the window (which will be freeing for some, and uncomfortable for others). It is not a diet or food plan (cue: sigh of relief!), which means there's no counting calories, carbs, points, or macros. If you truly become an intuitive eater, your weight will land where it's naturally supposed to, and that may not be what you originally thought it should be. You have to be prepared to let that go. As a place to start, look at the hunger scale Sarah developed (pictured opposite), inspired by the one in Evelyn Tribole and Elyse Resch's book Intuitive Eating. The goal is to eat when you reach a 2 and stop when you reach a 4 (indicated by the green arrow on the hunger scale opposite). If you can stay within the 2-to-4 range throughout the day, you can avoid getting too hungry at a 1 (which almost always leads to getting too full at a 5!). This takes time and patience and, honestly, it's not for everyone, although we are big advocates. Want to know more? Visit intuitiveeating.org or contact a Certified Intuitive Eating Counselor.

WE GOT YOU!

Intuitive eating is perfect if you are pregnant or breastfeeding, when dieting is not recommended and your appetite shifts with different nutrition and energy needs.

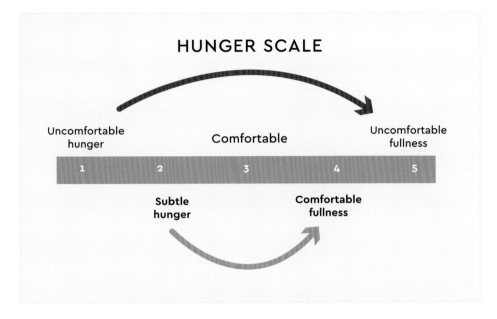

HUNGER SCALE

Uncomfortable hunger

Comfortable

Uncomfortable fullness

| 1 | 2 | 3 | 4 | 5 |

Subtle hunger

Comfortable fullness

CARA SAYS: *I grew up in a household with a full-on diet mentality. When I put on a few pounds, my mom would start serving more cottage cheese and cantaloupe (classic childhood diet foods) instead of pasta and pizza. As a loving mom, she thought she was doing the best thing for me, but had no idea (nor did I) that I was internalizing a message that my value had to do with a number on the scale. IT DOESN'T—and we know that now.*

Fast-forward to the present day, and now I'm the mom. My children have learned to eat a wide variety of foods—including cottage cheese, cantaloupe, pasta, and pizza. They eat when they're hungry and stop when full. They both know that their self-worth is not based on what they weigh. Positive body messaging can help ensure that your children don't base their self-worth on their appearance. Teach them to love themselves—regardless of size or shape.

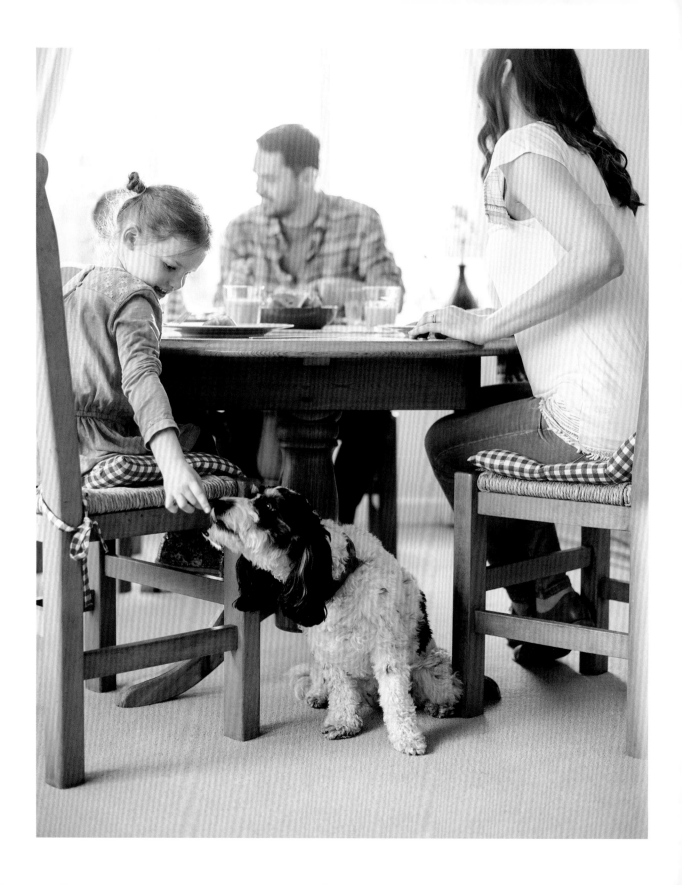

Picky Eating

Picky eating might be the most common and frustrating feeding challenge that parents face. Most "picky eating" behaviors are actually completely normal and most kids will go through some form of this phase. But to parents, picky eating can seem worrisome (we'll help calm your worry)—and quite honestly, be very annoying! In this section, we'll describe typical picky eating by toddlers and young children, and give you strategies on how to deal with them in a loving, productive, and healthy way. We will also describe how to recognize extreme forms of picky eating (page 61) and direct you to credible resources that can help.

One important thing to remember, is that every child learns at their own pace. Whether it's riding a bike, tying shoes, reading, or eating new foods, we as parents need to respect the pace at which our child takes to learn, and practice lots of patience in the process. The good news with eating is that the majority of the time, kids get all of the food and nutrients they need, even if it looks like they are not eating very much on any given day. And most picky eaters grow out of it, and go on to accept and enjoy a variety of foods.

WHEN DOES PICKY EATING START?

Babies are typically open to exploring new foods and textures from about 6 to 18 months—we call this the "honeymoon stage of feeding." And yes, it ends. Somewhere between 18 and 24 months, your toddler's cognition matures and they're able to analyze and process details like color, texture, and taste more than they were able to as a baby. That's why a previously loved food might be rejected suddenly—your little one is finally realizing the food they are eating is bitter and green and that they don't like it as much as they thought they did! This doesn't mean that they won't go back to it eventually—because they likely will—and it's important to remember your toddler isn't necessarily rejecting these foods, but rather being newly skeptical of them. Toddlers have no context for new foods, which means some foods are scary to taste and nearly impossible to swallow at first. Rather than diving right in as they would as a baby, they might observe *you* eat it first, then perhaps welcome it on their plate or tray, and then later bring it to their mouth, only to then take it out. Again and again. And again!

Toddlers and preschoolers crave control. Eating (or not eating) is one way they can feel as though they are in control. Control struggles between a parent and a toddler are normal—toddlers love watching parents become desperate when they refuse to eat something—after all, they're getting a reaction! But it's the *way* that *you* react to their behavior that is key—it can either create bigger, more serious eating issues down the road, or it can help a child grow their relationship with food in a healthy way, and minimize picky eating behavior in the future.

It can also be difficult for toddlers to accept that they are expected to follow a family mealtime schedule. After all, trucks! toys! TV! These are all more exciting activities than eating. And if they have been breastfed or formula-fed on demand since infancy, they have gotten used to it! The adjustment can be hard at first—and trust us—your toddler will make that known. But it's essential that they become accustomed to mealtime boundaries in order to learn self-regulation and manage their hunger and fullness throughout the day.

IS PICKY EATING NORMAL?

Up to 50% of parents classify their child as a picky eater.[11] That's HALF of us, which leads us to believe that what most parents classify as "picky" might actually be completely normal. Quite honestly, it would be unusual if your child wasn't a picky eater at some point! So, breathe easy and know that it's normal for kids to:

- Like a particular food one day but not the next
- Spit out foods they don't like
- Eat more one day than the next
- Eat small portions
- Eat shockingly large portions
- Have phases of only liking a handful of foods
- Not like foods because of their color, texture, etc.
- Vary in their love of eating
- Become hungry when meal time is over
- Not be able to sit still at mealtime
- Need to try a food up to 20 times before they accept it

WE GOT YOU!

It can take up to 15 to 20 tries (or more) for a toddler to accept a food. As frustrating as it is, continue to offer foods that your child hasn't accepted yet (without pressure). Mix it up with different forms, textures, temperatures, and shapes. You'll get there.

SO WHAT CAN YOU DO?

Typical picky eating stems from (or is perpetuated by) the same well-meaning but detrimental mistake parents often make: trying to control whether and how much their child eats. But successful feeding doesn't mean that your child comes to the table and happily munches away on every food item offered; successful feeding is when your child has a positive experience, and feels safe and confident enough to taste and eat foods in amounts that feel right for them. So the first thing to do is refer back to the sDOR (page 41) and familiarize yourself with the different feeding roles of kids and parents—hint: deciding *whether* to eat and *how much* to eat is 100% your child's job—and this may go a long way to help with your mealtime battleground. Bottom line: It's not your job to get your child to eat.

Prevention starts early: Even though picky eating typically starts around that 18-to-24-month window, you can be proactive right from the beginning. For babies 6 months and up, try not to become forceful or domineering when feeding, or feed in a way that doesn't respond to your baby's natural cues (see page 160). Also, avoid starting solids much later than 6 months (unless advised by baby's pediatrician) as this might make the transition to solid food more challenging and create picky eating issues.

Structure is key: A food free-for-all (grazing all day) will only lead to mealtime battles and potential picky eating habits. Structure may be harder to achieve at first, but it will make eating easier in the long run. It may seem cruel to turn down their random requests for a snack, but as long as you're providing scheduled meals and planned snacks in between, your little one won't go hungry—there are plenty of opportunities to eat!

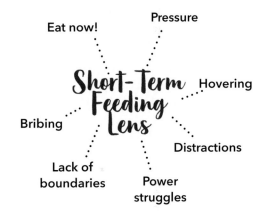

Focus on the long term: Next up: ditch your "short-term feeding lens" and replace it with your "long-term feeding lens." Many parents put on their short-term lens when it comes to feeding kids—especially if we are worried that a child is not getting enough to eat. It's tempting to turn to quick-fix solutions like pressured spoon-feeding, the airplane trick, coaxing, or bribing to address the problem. Instead, try to think of the long term and take the pressure off. Sit for mealtimes as a family and focus on your own eating instead of your child's—this will have a more powerful and positive impact on long-term eating habits than

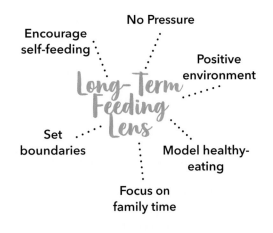

any kind of quick fix. When we start to feel frustrated and defeated in the face of picky eating, we can often resort to techniques such as:

- **Bribing:** "If you eat 3 more bites of broccoli you can have dessert"
- **Shaming:** "Your brother always eats his vegetables, so why can't you?!"
- **Punishing:** "No TV tonight for you because you didn't eat all of your dinner"
- **Forcing:** "You cannot get down from the table until you have had 2 more bites"
- **Distracting:** "You can watch your favorite show while you eat your dinner"

These may act as short-term solutions, but they can negatively affect our kids' eating and nutrition long term. Although these tactics are extremely tempting, especially when you've witnessed your little one *finally* eat a decent portion of his meal as a result, looking through your "short-term feeding lens" ("I just want him to eat his meal!") actually sets your child up for failure later on.

Try a food diary: Most toddlers and young kids won't let themselves go hungry. If they fall short at one meal, they will likely make up for it at the next. Throughout the course of a day, you may worry that your child isn't meeting his nutritional requirements, but we want to assure you that over the course of a week, your little one will usually get what they need. If you're really concerned about your child's nutritional intake, keep a one-week food diary to see if they are getting some vegetables or fruit; whole grains; calcium-rich foods, and protein-rich foods. Take time to look over it or, even better, you can hire a dietitian to review it! And if you're concerned about your child's growth or development, consult your doctor or a pediatric dietitian to explore further.

Resist demands and don't become a short order cook! We want our kids to eat at meals. But setting up the dynamic of letting them say no to a meal you've prepared, and then making them something else, is not the answer: this enables picky eaters. It tells them they never have to eat what's served, and makes them less adventurous eaters. Why should they try what's on the table if they can eat their favorite noodles instead? If children are encouraged to choose from the food that's served (and not given an alternative), they will eventually learn to be more flexible at mealtime and learn to embrace a wider range of foods. It takes time. It takes patience. But this is a healthy mealtime boundary.

CARA SAYS: *As a toddler, my son could never find his socks or the toy he needed, but somehow he could always find the tiny green herb in any meal he ate. He was only off green for a little while, but then it was anything orange–particularly squash. If I had met his demands with separate meals catered to his approved color palette of the week, I would have been saying to him, "You're right! Green herbs are yucky!" Not the message I wanted to send. Instead, I made sure the meal always had a few foods he did like, so even if he avoided one food, he could still have a balanced plate in front of him. And you know what? Now he LOVES green herbs!*

SARAH SAYS: *I will never forget the day that I happily dished up my son James's favorite spaghetti and meatballs, only to have it pushed away as he disappointingly said, "Ucky." Previously, he loved and devoured it every time I served it, and I always got excited to see the joy on his face when it was in front of him! That was a sad, sad day. I reminded myself that it was just a normal part of toddlerhood, but it goes to show that all kids can have picky moments, even when their mom is a pediatric dietitian!*

PROBLEM SOLVED: PICKY EATING

Anna's first child, Spencer, was the best eater, right from 6 months of age. Anything she put in front of him, he devoured–everything from infant cereal to cooked fish! But as soon as he turned 2, she noticed that he wasn't eating as well. He turned his nose up to foods he would normally gobble up.

He started accepting only a small list of foods, and Anna started getting worried. She unknowingly pressured Spencer to eat by spoon-feeding him (even when he turned his head), pushing foods closer to him on his tray, and doing the airplane trick. Things seemed to get worse and worse–the preferred food list got shorter, and mealtimes became increasingly stressful.

When Anna went for nutrition counseling, she was anxious that Spencer wasn't getting the proper nutrition that he needed and that he was now a "picky eater." With some reassurance and guidance, Anna took a deep breath, took the pressure off completely at mealtime, continued to reintroduce a variety of foods at meals and snacks, and made mealtimes positive. Within a few weeks, Spencer began to widen his palate again and accept a wider variety of foods. Anna mentioned that from time to time, he goes through another "food jag", but for the most part, he's still a good little eater! And taking the pressure off of him and herself has made feeding and mealtimes pleasant and happy again.

Top 17 tips to tackle picky eating

1. **Serve something for everyone.** Plan a meal that has at least one food that each person at the table enjoys. That way, even if your child (or spouse!) doesn't enjoy some things that are being served, there is at least one item that they love.
   - Doesn't like meat? Add some cubed cheese or chickpeas to the table.
   - Not a fan of lettuce-based salads? Have some carrots or cucumbers too.

   By doing this, you are setting parameters and providing much-needed structure, but also giving your child some control. It's being courteous, without catering!

2. **Serve meals family-style.** Break meals down into components, and let your child choose what they want out of those components and serve themselves. For example:
   - Spaghetti and meatballs night: Serve separate bowls of pasta, broccoli, meatballs, and sauce.
   - Taco night: Let your child choose their fillings from a tray of options—lettuce, tomato, cheese, avocado, herbs, etc. (instead of you assembling the taco you want them to eat).

   This way, you're giving your child some control to choose the ingredients that they prefer, which actually builds their eating competency.

3. **Stop hovering.** Toddlers feel pressure at the table in many ways. Sometimes it's direct, like when you do the airplane trick or physically put food into your child's mouth. Sometimes it's indirect, like when you watch your child or hover over them constantly throughout the meal. Instead, let your child breathe. Back off, keep things positive, and let them self-feed as much food as they want.

4. **Let your child explore new foods, pressure-free.** Part of becoming comfortable with a particular food is exploring it. When you see your child is playing with, mushing up, or smearing food all over her plate, consider it a way for them to learn more about the food and become comfortable enough to put it in their mouth. It's all right for children to try food with their other senses—they can smell it, examine it, and touch it before they decide if they want to taste it. Eating is a sensory experience, so you can encourage that. They don't have to try it the first time they are exposed to it. That's okay.

5. **Pair new foods with familiar foods.** It's scary for a child to sit down to a meal of many unfamiliar foods. It's overwhelming and intimidating. A better idea is to introduce a new food during a meal when you're serving a bunch of old favorites. So the pasta and cheese (which is a standard favorite) can be

accompanied by a new vegetable. That way, your child still has something to eat that will fill their tummy, and they don't feel forced to try something new.

6. **Keep serving new and previously rejected foods.** We know that it's tempting to skip right to the accepted and safe foods at meal times—trust us—but your child is not going to learn to accept a new or previously rejected food unless it's introduced many (many!) times in a pressure-free environment. It's frustrating and may feel like a waste, but it's key to molding a balanced healthy eater. So if asparagus is not a hit the first time your child tries it, it doesn't mean they will never eat it. You may just have to introduce it 10 times. Or 15 times. Or 20 times. Or more!

7. **Ditch the "one-bite" rule.** Although the idea of taking one bite of a new food might work with more adventurous eaters, it can increase fear and anxiety of new foods in apprehensive eaters. Instead, take the pressure off. When parents do this, kids often become more open to exploring and sampling new foods on their own. If your child *does* show interest or curiosity about a new food, you can gently encourage them to explore it or sample a small bite. Be prepared to accept "No, thank you" as an answer, and reply by saying "That's okay! Maybe next time you'll feel ready to try it."

8. **Switch up serving styles.** Something as simple as changing the shape or texture of food can make a difference to a child. If raw cauliflower, carrots, or celery are too crunchy, steam them. Mix cucumber "coins" with strips, or try sweet potato "fries" instead of roasted sweet potato, or butternut squash soup instead of baked butternut squash! Experiment to see what they like best. Read more ideas for this on page 282 and 283.

9. **Have a tester plate.** Try introducing a tester plate to sit next to your child's real plate or bowl. This is reserved for those foods that are unfamiliar, scary, or "yucky." Kids don't have to eat or even taste the foods on this plate, but they can touch them, smell them, mush them, stack them, lick them, or even taste and politely spit them out. It's a safe and fun way to explore the food without actually eating it. And it brings kids one step closer to eventually accepting them later on!

SARAH SAYS: When I instituted the tester plate, I found that my toddler at the time started to eat more at his meals, simply because the "yucky," new, or unfamiliar food was no longer touching the foods that he loved. In other words, those favorite foods weren't being "contaminated!" Separating the foods that your toddler loves from the ones they're scared or hesitant about might really make a difference. It's worth a try!

10. **Minimize distractions.** No toys at the table and no eating in front of the TV (that goes for the parent too—no cell phones at the table!). Many well-meaning parents depend on screens or toys to distract their child into eating 2 or 3 more bites, but this is counterproductive and can make the problem worse (and create a pesky, hard-to-break habit!). Screens and other distractions interfere with a child's ability to self-regulate and tune in to their appetite.

11. **Give them some power.** Include your children in planning, shopping, and cooking. Let them have input into the day's menu by asking them "Would you like hamburgers or chicken tonight?" Avoid the vague "What do you want for dinner?" question, as it's too broad. Give them 2 to 3 choices. Take kids to the grocery store and have them choose a fruit or vegetable that they want to try. Find a recipe and prepare it together. Or, visit a farmer's market or pick-your own farm. Nothing entices kids to eat apples as much as picking them themselves! If you have a green thumb, plant a garden and let your kids watch the fruits and vegetables grow, be harvested, and turned into dinner! Picky eaters are more likely to try foods that they've had a hand in choosing and preparing. See page 357 for more ideas on this.

12. **Acknowledge their bravery.** Parents often praise their kids for trying new foods or eating certain amounts. Although well intentioned, overpraising at meals sends the wrong message. We want our kids to eat *intuitively* and to learn to love a variety of foods in their own time. Instead of praising, notice and acknowledge your child's bravery when trying something new by saying something like, "That was so brave of you to try something new tonight!" It will boost their confidence and increase the likelihood of your child being more adventurous with other foods too.

13. **Be a good listener.** Ask your child to explain why she dislikes certain foods. You might be surprised to learn that it is the color, texture, temperature, flavor, or some other factor that you can alter. Just make sure that when you have the conversation about food, it's NOT in the kitchen or at the dinner table—that can be stressful for your little one. Raise the topic when you're playing a game or out for a walk. Sometimes asking the question when you don't have eye contact with your child is a great mode to obtain answers.

14. **Don't give them the "picky eater" label.** Try not to refer to your child as a "picky eater," especially when they are listening or around friends and family. Even at this very young age, this label can enable the behavior and decrease their self-confidence when it comes to eating. It can also create assumptions

and limit their exposure to new or unfamiliar foods. For example, if a caregiver or grandparent is told, "Oh, she doesn't like green vegetables," or "He won't eat meat, so don't bother serving it," it will decrease the chances of your toddler learning to love those foods because they won't be exposed to them regularly! Drop the label and keep reintroducing foods in a low-pressure setting.

15. **Be an adventurous eater yourself.** Make a point of trying something new at family meals. When your child sees this, as well as your positive reaction, they will feel more open and relaxed about trying new foods themselves.

16. **Be careful with milk.** Sometimes parents (and children) rely too heavily on milk for nourishment during the day, and this can lead to under-nutrition and picky eating (displacing precious tummy space that could be filled with other nutritious foods). For this reason, stick to milk at mealtimes only (water in between) and limit it to a maximum of 2 cups per day.

17. **And remember, sometimes they just don't like it.** Sometimes your child won't like a certain food even after multiple exposures, and that's okay! We've gotten to the point of, "Okay, I've tried it over 20 times, and I just don't like it!" Fair enough. You probably have a few foods you don't enjoy either, right?

CARA SAYS: *My daughter, Kasey, is an open-minded eater and is willing to try anything. She hated avocado when I first introduced it to her (shocking, right? It's the most creamy and delicious food ever!), and I figured she just needed multiple exposures until she learned to love it. I gave it to her on salads, to replace butter on breads, in vegetarian sushi rolls, and even in a chocolate-avocado pudding. Consistently, she would say, "Is there avocado in this?" To this day, my now-teenager has a very short list of foods she does not like: liver and avocado.*

Physical or medical concerns

If you suspect that there is a real, physical, or medical concern affecting your child's ability to eat, consult with your child's doctor and request a referral to a qualified speech language pathologist and pediatric registered dietitian who specialize in feeding issues. Here are some of the possible medical or psychological reasons for picky eating:

Eating is uncomfortable: Eating may actually hurt your child, if there is an underlying medical concern. This could be caused by food allergies, reflux, a tongue tie, eosinophilic esophagitis (painful erosions in the esophagus), or severe constipation. Other non-food related conditions that affect comfortable eating are breathing or muscle movement conditions (congenital heart defects, severe asthma, or muscular dystrophy).

Eating feels weird: Kids with sensory integration issues may be more sensitive to tastes, textures, smells, and even the sight of food (they just feel more intense!). Sometimes, they simply can't feel food in their mouth (this is where food pocketing may come in) or they only feel comfortable eating foods with a uniform texture (only crunchy or only smooth).

Eating is just TOO hard: When oral motor control and function are compromised, such as with a cleft palate or with malformations of digestive or oral muscles (trachea, esophagus, or tongue), eating can be really really tough and painful. Not to mention severe dental issues, or enlarged adenoids and tonsils. Ouch! In some of these cases, it is worth seeking professional help from a qualified speech language pathologist, especially if your child can't chew or swallow solid foods comfortably by about 15 months.

Eating is scary: Kids who experience trauma while eating—even with no history of picky eating—may refuse to eat (especially the particular food culprit). Think choking, or maybe an experience where a child was forced to eat. Or maybe they got sick (vomited), felt extremely nauseous afterward, or inhaled (aspirated) a food. All of these experiences can make food "scary."

WHAT'S YOUR BEST PICKY EATER STORY?

My son decided that he no longer liked peanut butter on his toast. So I told him it was peanut butter frosting and he ate 2 slices! –Emma

I once asked my son what he wanted for dinner, and he said, "Salt." When I replied that he may still be hungry after he eats his salt, he replied, "Fine, I'll have some butter too." –Grant

My daughter refused to eat oatmeal with a red spoon. It had to be a blue spoon. Apparently the red spoon was for ice cream only. –Carla

We were out for dinner and ordered noodles and Parmesan for our 3-year-old. The dish came with a sprinkling of parsley. Now for him, anything green was a disaster. A meltdown was seconds away. I turned to him and said, "OMG, you're so lucky! They put Hulk dust on your pasta! I thought that was only for superheroes!" He ate the whole bowl. –Robin

My daughter, who used to love mushrooms, now won't eat them, citing them as "slimy." Unless they are crispy, they are a huge no-go. –Mary Luz

When I was a kid, I would only eat the green "leaves" off of the "broccoli trees." I finally told my mom it was because I didn't think I could chew through the wooden trunk (aka the stalk!). –Angie

Our kids won't eat meat unless it is called chicken. So our "chicken" just sometimes happens to taste like beef or fish. –Janelle

My kids call lox "pink turkey." We think they know it's fish, but we're not sure. –Stacey

My son used to slowly peel hotdogs. On our way to Disney World, we stopped for a "quick" snack because he was hungry. An hour later he was still peeling the hotdog! His big sister wanted to kill him. –Angela

When I was a toddler, my mom made me a grilled cheese sandwich. As we know, it turns brown when you pan-fry it, but I said it looked dirty and INSISTED my mom wash it. Needless to say, my soggy grilled cheese was a bit of a disappointment. —Abbey

My son was so picky, he couldn't have bits of dill or parsley in chicken soup, and his loving grandma would strain it out just for him. Now he's 29 years old and during his travels ate barbecued scorpion! —Barbara

My kids loved quiche. Once, I lovingly made crust from scratch and filled muffin tins (instead of a pie plate) with ingredients for individual quiches. They were exactly like the quiches I always made, just smaller. Each kid took a bite, spit it out, and said they were disgusting. I promptly burst into tears! —Devorah

My kids were giving me a hard time about eating grown-up food for dinner, so I made them chicken Parmesan and told them it was "pizza chicken" (i.e. chicken with tomato sauce and melted cheese on top). Pizza chicken was a favorite for years to come! Amazing what a little marketing creativity can do. —Cheryl

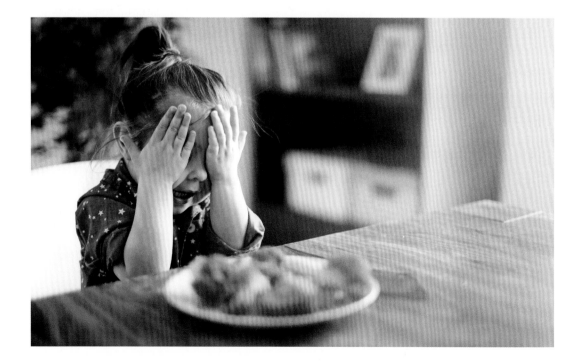

Extreme picky eating

When picky eating tendencies cross the borders of what's considered "typical" and start affecting your child's growth, weight, mood, and family mealtimes in a drastic way, it's time to seek help. Dealing with extreme forms of picky eating can feel hopeless and isolating. It also causes worry, stress, and sometimes panic for parents, as well as anxiety, fear, and social isolation for the child.

It's important for you to know that you're not alone, and more importantly, it's not your fault. Although there are many factors that can contribute to extreme picky eating, the most important step towards resolving them is the interaction between you and your child at mealtimes. Of course, dietitians, therapists, or other feeding specialists play active roles in the management of extreme picky eating, but the dynamic between parent and child is by far the most important. As the parent, it's important to arm yourself with the proper tools to help your child, and avoid advice and strategies that will make matters worse.

HOW DOES EXTREME PICKY EATING DIFFER FROM TYPICAL PICKY EATING?

The difference between extreme or severe picky eating vs. typical picky eating is that children are not eating enough food (quantity or variety) to support sufficient physical, social, or emotional development OR they have eating patterns that that cause significant conflict or worry. Picky eating isn't a one size fits all. Your child may have been labeled a "problem feeder" or "selective eater" and you may not know exactly what that means or whether it's accurate. Unfortunately, there isn't an official classification system for extreme feeding difficulties in kids, but these labels help parents to better understand their child:

Problem feeder: A child who eats fewer than 20 foods, drops food without adding others, eats different foods than the rest of the family, avoids entire food groups (like meat and vegetables), or becomes upset around new foods.

Selective eating disorder: Similar definition to problem feeder. Not officially a diagnosis in adults or children, but increasingly used to describe a limited range of accepted foods and refusal of unfamiliar foods.

Food aversion: May emerge after an unpleasant experience including illness, trauma, or choking; also generalized fear or anxiety around food. Often occurs with selective eating disorder or among problem feeders.

Neophobia: Fear of new things. Toddlers typically experience a phase of suspicion with new and even familiar foods, but this is an extreme negative reaction to new foods.

ARFID: Avoidant/restrictive food intake disorder, previously called infantile anorexia. The Diagnostic and Statistical Manual of Mental Disorders (DSM-5) defines it as starting before 6, lasting longer than one month, and characterized by an inability to take in enough nutrition orally for optimal growth, with a negative impact on weight and or psychological functioning.[12] There are three ARFID subgroups: sensory, little to no appetite, and aversion.

Failure to thrive: Inadequate physical growth. Often defined as weight below the fifth percentile; however, clinicians have used cutoffs at the tenth, fifth, or first percentile, or when growth slows significantly.

Feeding disorder: According to the American Speech Language-Hearing Association, this describes problems gathering food in the mouth and sucking, chewing, or swallowing for appropriate intake.[13]

HOW DOES EXTREME PICKY EATING AFFECT MY CHILD?

Children who experience extreme forms of picky eating are affected not only physically, but emotionally and socially as well. Emotionally, a child may become upset, or cry at the sight of food, feel bad or self-conscious about their eating habits, and feel inadequate or that something is wrong with them as compared to their peers or siblings. They may feel socially isolated and not want to participate in play-dates or go to friends' houses, or they may avoid sleep-overs. They may be ridiculed by peers or friends, and are often over-observed and hovered over by well-meaning adults (parents, teachers, etc.). Not fun.

Extreme picky eaters aren't trying to be "bad" or misbehave—they genuinely cannot eat in a typical way, for one reason or another—sometimes this reason will never surface, and that's okay. You can still help your child without a clear diagnosis as to why they struggle with extreme picky eating.

Temperament and mood can affect the eating of extreme picky eaters. In their book *Helping Your Child With Extreme Picky Eating*, Katja Rowell, MD, and Jenny McGlothlin, MS CCC-SLP, describe that many of their patients feel, and express, intense emotions while eating, becoming easily upset and frustrated. They also have a strong desire to figure things out in their own time and in their own way. Many neurologically typical children with extreme picky eating are often very independent, strong-willed, and determined; they are very attuned to the pressure that their parents put on them and may experience anxiety because of this. Food refusal can be seen in kids who are shy, emotional, and irritable, among other traits (see page 57 for possible physical and medical reasons for extreme picky eating).

Rowell and McGlothlin mention that parents should be aware of a syndrome called Pediatric Acute onset Neuropsychiatric Syndrome (PANS or PANDAS), which is a "rapid-onset brain-based illness occasionally triggered by infection"[14] if their child all of a sudden stops eating, becomes fearful of food, or starts experiencing obsessive compulsive thinking around food. They stress that it's important to rule out PANS as well as any underlying medical condition, eating disorder, or aversive food experience.

WHAT YOU CAN DO IF YOU THINK YOUR CHILD IS AN EXTREME PICKY EATER?
We suggest consulting with a pediatrician and requesting a referral to a qualified speech therapist who specializes in feeding issues as well as a dietitian who has specialty training in pediatric feeding, feeding disorders, and picky eating.

DEEP DIVE

A study in *Pediatrics* showed that (after screening caregivers of over 900 children aged 2 to 5), children with severe forms of picky eating were much more likely to experience elevated symptoms of social anxiety, general anxiety, and depression.[15] It was also found that moderate forms of picky eating were associated with symptoms of separation anxiety and ADHD. Although these findings likely aren't terribly surprising—especially to parents of extreme picky eaters—they will hopefully create more awareness and perhaps pave the way for more appropriate screening tools and intervention strategies for those kids who struggle with picky eating.

Food Allergies and Intolerances

A food allergy is an immune system response to a substance in food, usually a protein. The substance that a person is allergic to is called an "allergen." When an allergen is consumed it can cause an allergic reaction, which can cause symptoms such as wheezing or breathing difficulties, vomiting, diarrhea, skin rashes, or hives. Severe reactions can cause anaphylaxis, described below. It's good to be aware of the information on allergies, but please do know that food allergies only affect between 6% to 8% of kids.

Signs of an allergic reaction

There are different types and severities of allergic reactions, and many possible symptoms. An allergic reaction will often have more than one of these symptoms:

- Hives
- Rash
- Red or itchy skin
- Trouble breathing
- Difficulty swallowing
- Swelling of the eyes, lips, or tongue
- Diarrhea
- Vomiting
- Fainting
- Weakness

Most Common Food Allergens

- Peanuts
- Tree nuts (e.g., walnuts, almonds, hazelnuts, cashews)
- Cow's milk
- Eggs
- Fish
- Shellfish (e.g., shrimp, crab, lobster, mussels)
- Soy
- Sesame seeds
- Wheat

Any of these symptoms can appear within a few minutes of baby eating a food, but could also take up to 2 days to appear. If you are concerned that a food is causing your baby to have an allergic reaction, stop giving the food and talk to your baby's doctor.

WHAT IS AN ANAPHYLACTIC REACTION?

Anaphylaxis is the most severe type of allergic reaction and can be really scary, especially when it involves a little one. It is sudden, severe, and potentially life-threatening. Between 1.6% and 5.1% of Americans are estimated to have experienced anaphylaxis,[16] and reactions can be caused by a food allergy, an insect sting, or medication. Almost any food can cause an anaphylactic reaction, but the most common are peanuts, tree nuts, shellfish, fish, cow's milk, eggs, sesame seeds, and soy. People with asthma and food allergies are at greater risk of having an anaphylactic reaction to foods. Individuals who are at high risk for anaphylactic reactions must be especially careful to avoid allergy-causing foods and should carry an epinephrine auto injector (i.e., EpiPen or Twinject) with them at all times.

> **REALITY CHECK**
>
> 911: Symptoms of an anaphylactic reaction require attention right away. Call your local emergency number immediately if you see any of the following:
>
> - Difficulty talking
> - Difficulty swallowing
> - Difficulty breathing
> - Drop in blood pressure
> - Rapid heartbeat
> - Unconsciousness

Food intolerances

A food intolerance (also called a food sensitivity) is a reaction to food that involves the digestive system, not the immune system. Symptoms include gas, bloating, cramping, diarrhea, and nausea. Lactose intolerance is an example of a food intolerance to the carbohydrate in milk. It's when the body cannot break down lactose sugar in milk and causes gas and/or diarrhea. This is different than a milk allergy, which is caused by an immune response to the protein in cow's milk.

DEEP DIVE: PEA PROTEIN

Some research shows that pea protein may be an under-recognized food allergen that is potentially harmful for those with peanut allergies. It is estimated that 95% of patients with peanut allergies can tolerate peas, but for the remaining 5%, the exposure can be life-threatening.[17] Pea protein, a highly concentrated pea product, is often found in meat alternatives as a way to increase the overall protein of the food, but can also be found in other foods as an added protein source. If you're worried about a pea protein allergy, talk with your doctor about getting a referral to an allergist for testing.

What to do if you suspect a food allergy or intolerance

Discuss your concerns with your family doctor. They can refer you for tests or to an allergy specialist. Getting a proper diagnosis is important as some food allergies can be severe and life-threatening. The most important action for people with food allergies is to avoid foods that cause a reaction. It's important to read food labels and check with food manufacturers and restaurants to know which foods to avoid.

If you have a food intolerance, you may still be able to eat small amounts of that food. For example, if you have a lactose intolerance, you may not be able to drink regular cow's milk but can eat small amounts of yogurt and/or cheese (many are low in lactose or enjoy lactose-free milk). Everybody with an intolerance reacts differently, and you will have to figure out what works for you or your child.

CAN A CHILD OUTGROW AN ALLERGY?

Many children outgrow food allergies to milk, soy, and eggs within a few years. Allergies to peanuts, tree nuts, fish, and shellfish are more likely to last to adulthood, although about 20% of children can outgrow their peanut allergy by school-age.

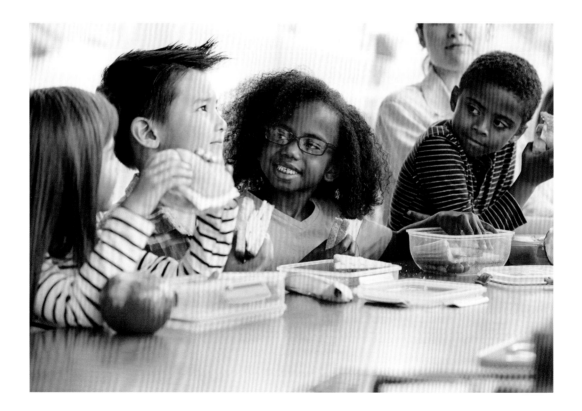

Food Safety

We're not talking about slipping and falling on a banana peel here; we're talking about bacteria and toxins that can grow on your food and cause food poisoning, something that often gets passed off as the stomach flu. And the reason that we're including this up front is because food poisoning is more likely to affect those with weaker immune systems, like pregnant women and babies. Here are some tips to help protect your family from food poisoning:

Keep it clean

- Wash hands, utensils, and cooking surfaces with soap and hot water before and after you handle food (especially meat or poultry).
- Use paper towels or dishcloths to wipe counters to avoid the spread of bacteria. Avoid using sponges to clean surfaces since they're harder to keep clean.
- Wash cutting boards with hot, soapy water after each use. Acrylic, plastic, or glass boards can be washed in a dishwasher.
- Once cutting boards become excessively worn or develop deep grooves, replace them. Wooden cutting boards are more likely to become contaminated as they have more grooves and are harder to clean.

Prep food with care

- Wash fresh vegetables and fruits with cool running water to remove dirt and residue. Before cutting, scrub fruits and vegetables that have firm surfaces or rinds, such as carrots, oranges, melons, and potatoes. And be sure to cut away damaged or bruised areas on produce–bacteria love these places.
- Use separate cutting boards and utensils for raw meats and vegetables. Never put cooked food on a dish that previously held raw food.
- Keep raw meat, poultry, and seafood separate from other foods in the refrigerator. Store in plastic bags or sealed containers on the lowest rack in the fridge to prevent juices from leaking onto other foods.

Cook it right

- Keep hot foods hot and cold foods cold! Prepare foods quickly, cook them thoroughly, and serve them soon after cooking. Don't let foods linger at temperatures where bacteria can multiply (39°F to 140°F).
- Use a digital or instant-read meat thermometer to ensure foods are cooked to a safe temperature (see chart opposite). Take the temperature from the thickest part of the meat, away from any bones.
- Do not pour sauce that's been used to marinate raw meat, poultry, or seafood onto cooked foods. Boil leftover marinade for at least 1 minute, prepare extra for basting cooked food, or use another sauce that has not come into contact with the raw food.

(REALITY CHECK)

Did you know flour is actually a raw ingredient? Recipes made with wheat flour need to be baked or cooked before eaten, as raw flour can be contaminated with harmful bacteria such as *E. coli*. Yup, that means it's not safe to eat raw cookie dough.

Safely chill your food

- Refrigerate or freeze prepared food and leftovers within 1 hour in hot weather (90°F), and up to 2 hours when temperatures aren't quite hot. If you are unsure, throw the leftovers out.
- When you cook ahead of time, divide large portions of hot food into small, shallow containers to ensure safe, rapid cooling. If you don't think that you will be able to eat the leftovers within a couple of days, freeze them.
- To keep foods safe in the fridge or freezer, make sure your fridge is set at 40°F or colder and the freezer at 0°F.
- Don't overstuff your fridge. Cold air needs to circulate above and beneath food to keep it properly chilled.
- Thaw foods in the refrigerator or in cold water. Use the defrost button on the microwave if you plan to cook the food immediately after thawing.

Take precautions when eating outdoors

- Pack foods in a well-insulated cooler with plenty of ice or frozen gel packs. Pack foods first that you think you will use last. Take 2 coolers—one for cold drinks and another for perishable foods so that warm air won't get into the perishables every time someone reaches for a drink.
- Transport the cooler in the back seat of an air-conditioned car, not the hot trunk. At the picnic or campsite, make sure the cooler is out of the sun—place it under the shade of a tree or keep it under a blanket or tarp.
- Bring hand soap and water to wash your hands before preparing foods and eating. If soap and water aren't available, pack disposable wipes or hand sanitizer.
- Drink bottled water or tap water from a safe source. Try not to drink water from lakes or streams even if the water looks clean. If necessary, buy water purification tablets or water filters at stores that sell camping gear and outdoor sporting goods to purify lake or stream water prior to drinking it.

SAFE INTERNAL COOKING TEMPERATURES[18]

Food	Temperature
Beef, lamb, and veal	
Medium-rare	145°F
Medium	160°F
Well-done	170°F
Game meats: venison, deer, elk, etc.	165°F
Pork	160°F
Poultry: chicken, turkey, duck, goose, etc.	
Whole	180°F
Pieces (breast, drumstick, thigh, wing)	165°F
Ground meat	165°F

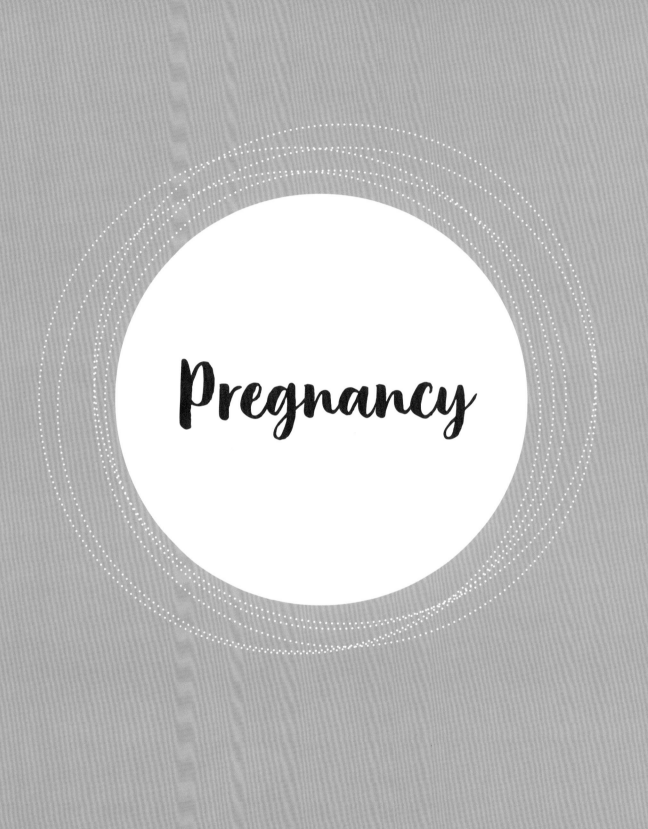

Pregnancy

Introduction

Congratulations momma-to-be! You're expecting a baby, which is one of the most exciting times of your life. You're likely feeling many different emotions: excited, overwhelmed, happy, nervous, and maybe a bit afraid! Trust us—we've been there a total of 5 times between the 2 of us—we know just *how emotional* the whole process is.

As soon as you know a baby is on the way, you might start to wonder about things like: "Have I been eating the proper foods and nutrients up until this point?!" or "I really need to start thinking about my nutrition now!" And you're right to—nutrition is key during pregnancy (you're growing a little human, after all!) making sure that you're getting the proper nutrients and enough energy is important. In this chapter, you'll learn everything from which foods you should eat more of, to which supplements you should be taking during pregnancy, to how to manage pregnancy-related digestive issues—and much more! Of course, you may have cravings, aversions, intolerances, or changing likes and dislikes along the way—it's all part of the joy of pregnancy! We know that you have many, many questions, and we're here to help.

Pregnancy terms can be confusing, so here are some quick definitions:

- **Prenatal:** while you are pregnant, before the birth of the baby
- **Perinatal:** a few weeks just before and after giving birth
- **Postnatal:** the period after the baby is born (when referring to the baby)
- **Postpartum:** the period after the baby is born (when referring to the mom)

WE GOT YOU!

There is so much conflicting and confusing information out there when it comes to prenatal nutrition that it's hard to know what to follow and what to ignore. *Everyone* has an opinion and *really* wants to share it with you. Your friends and family mean well; they want you to have a healthy pregnancy, learn from their mistakes, and grow the healthiest baby possible. And some of their advice and guidance may be spot-on and super-helpful! But sometimes, as well-meaning as their advice is, it's just not credible or based on science. So . . . enter us!

Food choices

When you're expecting, it's important to eat a nutritious diet and listen to your body's hunger cues. Your appetite might be different when you're pregnant—and for good reason—so it's important to pay attention to your own body rather than be blinded by "guidelines." Read more about eating intuitively on page 44.

During the first trimester, there's no need to consume any additional calories, which is something many people don't know. During this early stage, you can eat the same amount as you usually do. That whole "eating for 2" thing? Well, you do need to eat a *bit* more as your pregnancy progresses, but certainly not double! Flip to page 102 to learn more.

Nutrients

During pregnancy, there are certain nutrients that you should pay closer attention to—these are the ones that help to grow healthy babies and keep you healthy in the process. Nutrients such as folate, iron, vitamin D, calcium, and omega-3 are all extra important during pregnancy and will be explained in detail in this chapter (turn to page 74). Read on, momma-to-be!

Prenatal vitamins

Aside from eating nutritiously, it's important to take a prenatal multivitamin daily. We recommend starting before you begin trying to conceive (because you often don't know you're pregnant until several weeks after conception!), but don't worry if you haven't yet—just start today. And nothing fancy needed here. Just make sure that it contains 0.4 milligrams (400 micrograms) of folic acid, 15 to 27 milligrams of iron, and a minimum of 400 IU of vitamin D. It should also have less than 5,000 IU of vitamin A, which can be harmful at higher doses. Full information on page 78.

Weight gain

Most likely, you'll gain about 2 to 4 pounds in the first trimester. But you may not gain any weight, or you may gain 5 pounds or more—every pregnancy is different. During the second and third trimesters, your weight gain target is about 1 pound per week. But, again, everybody is different. Learn more on page 102.

There aren't really any magical pregnancy foods that you absolutely must eat more of, but there are certainly some nutritious foods that you can focus on. Here are the nutrients (and foods that contain these nutrients) to pay attention to while pregnant. We'll explain why they are good choices and offer alternatives in case you are having an aversion (see page 111) to something on the list.

Nutrient: Protein

How much do you need? About 71 grams per day or ¼ of your plate at meals. Protein helps build and maintain structural components of your body (and your baby's body!), such as muscle, skin, and hair. Protein also helps to support a healthy placenta, which is the important structure that supplies your baby's nutrition during pregnancy and prevents harmful substances from passing to your baby's bloodstream.

Many protein-rich foods also supply other important nutrients for pregnancy. For example, fish is a fantastic source of vitamin B_{12}, omega-3 fat, and in some cases—like salmon, trout, and snapper—even vitamin D. Which foods contain protein? See the chart on page 364.

Nutrient: Omega-3 fat—particularly DHA and EPA

How much do you need? At least 300 milligrams DHA per day. Omega-3 fatty acids are essential for good health in both babies and adults, so it's really important to get enough during pregnancy. These health-promoting fatty acids travel through the placenta to your baby to help grow their brain and tissues in the womb. Official recommended amounts have not been established yet, but we do know that an omega-3 fat called DHA is important for proper brain, eye, and nerve development in your growing baby. So experts (like us!) suggest at least 300 milligrams of DHA and EPA combined per day.

> **REALITY CHECK**
>
> You may be wondering, "If I need omega-3 fat for my baby's health, can't I just eat a handful of flaxseeds and walnuts?" Well, no. Plant-based omega-3 fat does not contain DHA and EPA, which are the special fatty acids that are best for baby's brain, eye, and nerve development. Walnuts, flax, hemp, and chia seeds contain ALA instead, which can be converted by the body to DHA and EPA, but in very small amounts (read more on page 25).

A review of 70 studies showed that consuming 500 mg DHA per day (from food or supplements) showed a lower incidence of preterm births with less risk of having a low birthweight baby or needing neonatal intensive care admission.[19] So, aim for that 300 to 500 mg/day range of DHA from food or supplements.

REALITY CHECK

It's important to avoid eating a lot of high-mercury fish such as shark, albacore tuna, swordfish, king mackerel, and tilefish during pregnancy (see page 13). Fish oil supplements contain little to no mercury, but fish liver oil supplements (such as cod liver oil) contain high (potentially toxic) levels of vitamin A and D and are NOT recommended for pregnant or breastfeeding women.

When it comes to omega-3, oily fish is the gold standard—it's by far the best way to ensure that you're getting enough. We recommend you consume 2 to 3 servings (3 ounces per serving) of fatty, low-mercury fish (like salmon or trout) per week. Which other foods contain omega-3s? See the chart on page 367. If you're not a fish fan, you can take a daily omega-3 fish oil supplement during pregnancy (with 300 to 500 milligrams of DHA).

It's important to make sure you don't overdo it if you're taking a supplement. Make sure your daily dose of fish oil supplement contains no more than 3 grams (3,000 milligrams) of DHA and EPA per day. This amount has been studied and is safe for pregnant women.[20] Fish *liver* oil supplements are not recommended during pregnancy (see Reality Check). If you are vegetarian or vegan, look for DHA and EPA supplements made from algal oil, which comes from algae (a plant from the sea, like seaweed). Cool fact: fish are high in DHA and EPA because they eat algae! So you can skip the fish and go right to their source.

If you're one of the unlucky people who experience "fish burps" after taking an omega-3 fish oil supplement (yuck!), try choosing pharmaceutical-grade fish oil that's enterically coated. That means the pills have a coating around them so they don't dissolve in the stomach. Instead, they stay intact until they reach the intestines, and you can't burp them back up from way down there. Phew.

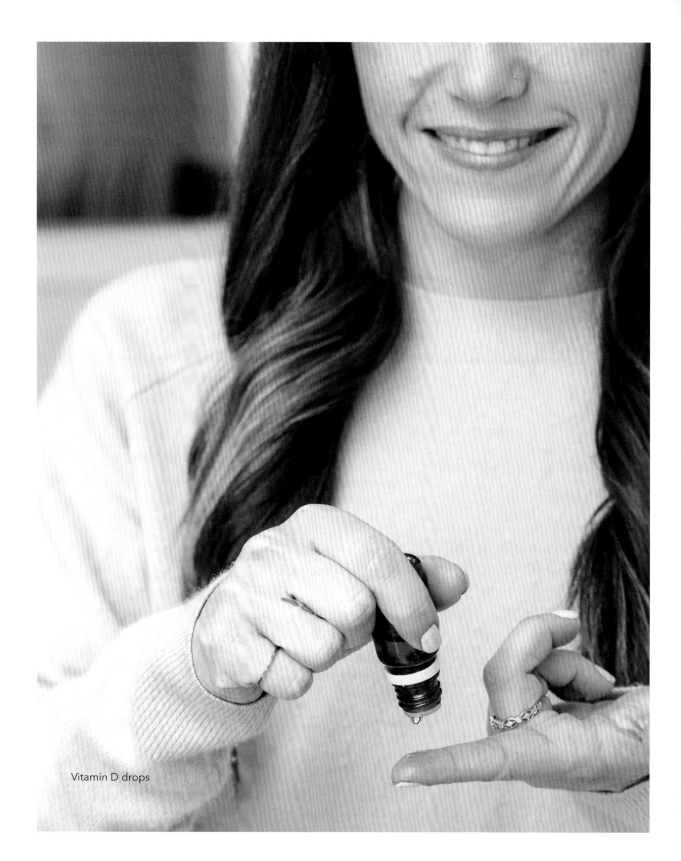

Vitamin D drops

Nutrient: Iron

How much do you need? 27 milligrams per day.

During pregnancy, you need about twice the amount of iron you did before because your body uses iron to make extra blood for your baby (which is essential for growth and development). Your body also uses iron to make extra blood (hemoglobin) for you (the one growing that baby!). Iron also helps move oxygen from your lungs to the rest of your body, and to your baby's. Getting enough iron can prevent a condition of too few red blood cells, called iron deficiency anemia, which can make you feel tired and low in energy. Having anemia can cause your baby to be born too small or too early.

Iron needs are higher when you are pregnant (when not pregnant, you need only 18 milligrams per day), so it's important that you consume foods that are high in iron every day. It's hard to get the extra iron required from diet alone, so your prenatal multivitamin should include some iron, and ideally the full 27 milligrams. If you become anemic during pregnancy, your doctor, dietitian, or midwife may recommend an additional iron supplement. And if you experience constipation related to your iron supplement, skip to page 112 where we help navigate that little gem.

Nutrient: Calcium

How much do you need? 1,000 milligrams per day (1,300 milligrams per day if you're under age 19).

Calcium is important for building and maintaining healthy bones and teeth, as well as for proper muscle function, nerve transmission, and hormonal balance. It's especially important during pregnancy because you are not only maintaining your own bone health and mass, but also supporting your baby's needs.

You can get calcium from many foods (see page 369), and your prenatal multivitamin will likely contain another 200 to 300 milligrams of it.

Nutrient: Folic acid

How much do you need? 600 milligrams per day.

Folic acid is required in the first days and weeks after conception—a time when many women are not aware that they're pregnant yet—as it is critical to help protect your baby against neural tube defects such as spina bifida. That's why it's important to take folic acid when you're even considering the idea of getting pregnant. Every woman of childbearing age who *may* become pregnant should take it daily. Most folic acid supplements are 400 micrograms, which is enough if you get the other

200 micrograms from food (see the chart on page 372). Folate is the naturally derived form of the vitamin found in foods, whereas folic acid is the form found in supplements.

If you're at a higher risk of delivering a baby with neural tube defects (for example, if you've previously delivered a baby with a neural tube defect or you have a family history of neural tube defects), your doctor may recommend that you take additional folic acid prior to and during pregnancy. On the other hand, for otherwise healthy pregnancies, *too much* folic acid can be a concern, with possible side effects such as impaired fetal growth and increased risk of childhood asthma. Short story: Avoid 1000 microgram folic acid supplements and stick with 400 micrograms only.

Nutrient: Vitamin D
How much do you need? 600 IU per day but we recommend at least 1000 IU (see page 30).
During pregnancy, it's very important to get enough vitamin D. There are very few food sources of vitamin D, so we recommend you take a supplement (see below).

What should I look for in a prenatal multivitamin?

Even if you are a superstar healthy eater, it's nearly impossible to meet all of your body's pregnancy requirements with food alone. Now this doesn't mean that you need to go out and spend your life savings on expensive vitamins! One good-quality prenatal multivitamin will suffice. Your health-care provider may suggest a certain brand that they prefer or trust. Here are some things to consider across the board:

Does it contain folic acid? It should have 400 micrograms of folic acid (see page 77); avoid supplements with 1000 micrograms or more. It's important that it also has vitamin B_{12} (most prenatal multivitamins will contain about 2.6 micrograms) because high doses of folic acid can hide a vitamin B_{12} deficiency.

How much vitamin D does it have? Most prenatal supplements have 400 to 600 IU. We recommend taking a vitamin D supplement of 1,000 IU per day in addition to this for a few reasons. Read about them on page 30.

What's the iron content? You need extra iron when you're pregnant—27 milligrams per day total (see page 25). It's hard to get this extra iron from diet alone, so most prenatal vitamins have the full 27 milligrams. Too much iron (or certain types of iron) can lead to an upset stomach or constipation (which is the last thing you need when you're pregnant!). We find that it helps if you take your prenatal vitamin with meals or at night before you go to sleep. If you're still having trouble with stomach upset, you can split the multivitamin dose in half (some in the morning, some at night), choose one that divides the morning and evening dose (ask your doctor for a brand recommendation), or try a chewable or liquid vitamin instead of a capsule or tablet, which may help ease symptoms.

CARA SAYS: *I mostly follow a vegetarian diet (plus fish), so my iron intake was low during pregnancy. My pharmacist recommended a polysaccharide iron supplement (such as FeraMAX, iFerex, Ferrex, or Niferex), which is super-high in iron. But . . . it also has the amazing superpower of NOT causing constipation. It helped keep my iron levels high, and I wasn't exhausted all of the time. Win! If you tend to be low in iron, are anemic, or are vegetarian, check with your doctor to see if this type of supplement could help.*

Is there enough calcium? Most prenatal multivitamins contain about 300 milligrams of calcium. A prenatal supplement will not support all of your calcium needs (see page 26), so it's important that you're also including calcium-rich foods in your diet.

Bonus: DHA! Omega-3 DHA is crucial for the developing baby's nervous system, so experts recommend at least 300 to 500 milligrams per day. Some prenatal multivitamin and mineral supplements now contain DHA. If you can find one, great! If not, read page 74 for how to ensure you're getting enough DHA during pregnancy.

(REALITY CHECK)

No other crap please. Some fancy (often unregulated) prenatal multi-vitamins sold in health-food stores or specialty clinics contain a bunch of fancy herbs and hard-to-pronounce ingredients. No. Just no. Unless you are going to take the time to independently look up and verify that each and every additional ingredient is safe to take during pregnancy, don't buy that supplement. And please don't think, "Oh, it says the word 'prenatal' on it, so it's safe for me and my baby." Do your homework and don't take any supple-ment that isn't 100% safe.

Be careful of vitamin A: You also want to make sure that you're not getting TOO much of any nutrient. More specifically, you don't want to overdose on vitamin A, because it may cause birth defects in your baby. Limit your vitamin A supplementation to no more than 5,000 IU per day. Most regulated prenatal multivitamins will not exceed this amount.

Once you have chosen your prenatal supplement, follow these tips for safety and effectiveness:

- Take your supplement daily (but don't panic if you miss one now and then), following the directions of your health-care provider or the directions on the label. There's no need to double up one day if you missed the previous day.
- If you have other kids (or nieces, nephews, friends, etc.), store ALL of your supplements out of reach of children. When taken inappropriately, supplements (especially iron) can be fatal to little ones.

PROBLEM SOLVED: TOO MANY SUPPLEMENTS

Carmen went to a dietitian for nutrition counseling when she was 4 months pregnant. It was her first pregnancy and she was experiencing some nausea and low energy. She had recently seen a holistic health practitioner because of the same concerns. The dietitian reviewed Carmen's food journal and blood work, and asked questions. She learned that Carmen was eating a well-balanced diet for pregnancy and was gaining weight at a healthy rate (and her blood work showed she wasn't deficient in any nutrients).

The dietitian reassured Carmen that she was doing a great job, and that unfortunately nausea and low energy are common symptoms during pregnancy and that they would likely lessen in time. When the dietitian asked Carmen about what supplements she was taking, her eyes lit up as she brought out a big bag of pills that she had just purchased based on recommendations from the holistic health practitioner. The dietitian was surprised and rather worried when she saw the high doses of vitamins and minerals that were being suggested, and urged Carmen not to take them. The doses that were recommended put Carmen at risk for vitamin and mineral toxicity and could harm her baby (there were extremely high doses of B vitamins, iron, and vitamin A).

The dietitian then gave Carmen tips and guidance on how to manage nausea (see page 106) and boost energy without high-dose supplements.

It's important to make sure that the foods and supplements you consume are safe. When in doubt, talk to a registered dietitian, doctor, or pharmacist.

Should I be taking any additional nutritional supplements?

In short, probably *yes*. Here are some other supplements you could consider taking during pregnancy:

Omega-3: Prenatal multivitamins typically do not include omega-3 fatty acids, but it's important to make sure that you're getting enough prior to and during pregnancy, as your requirements are higher (see page 74).

Vitamin D: Turn back to page 78 for the details.

Anything else? Okay, there is a TON of information out there about herbs, teas, tinctures, powders, and every other form of supplement that you could possibly take. Our advice is please be careful! Do not take anything (no matter how "natural" it is) unless it has been vetted and approved by your doctor, dietitian, and/or pharmacist. It's easy to think, "Oh, it's just an herbal supplement, it will be fine . . ." But something "natural" doesn't mean it's safe for the baby growing inside you. Think about it. Plants are "natural," but some of them, like poison ivy and hemlock, can cause harm. It's not worth the risk when there is a baby involved.

SHADES OF GRAY: PROBIOTICS

Probiotics are likely safe during pregnancy, but we can't be sure they are 100% safe, because they have not been fully tested yet. Research is limited, but there's promising hope that probiotics reduce the risk of yeast infections and digestive complaints, allergy prevention, and even boost immunity![21] And studies also show that probiotic supplements during late pregnancy and breastfeeding may reduce risk of eczema in your baby.[22]

The tricky part is, scientific findings for one probiotic strain cannot be applied to other probiotic strains (they're all different and act in different ways). That's why so much more research is needed in this area before we can confidently make recommendations. Tighter regulations around probiotic supplements (government regulation is seriously lacking now) also needs to happen as well as more stringent quality control.

If you *do* choose to take a probiotic supplement, make sure to speak to a dietitian or other trusted healthcare provider prior to purchasing.

Most foods are completely safe for you to enjoy without worry. However, there are some foods that should be avoided during pregnancy (or even when you're TRYING to get pregnant). These foods can be *potentially* harmful to a developing baby as well as a pregnant mom. The risk isn't the food itself, but the potential for the food to contain harmful bacteria that can lead to food poisoning—think salmonella, *E. coli,* or listeria. Foods that are raw and unpasteurized are often a risk. You *so do not* want food poisoning while you are pregnant, so it's better to skip these foods. It's not forever—just 40 weeks (give or take)! Play it safe by avoiding these foods while pregnant:

AVOID CERTAIN FISH AND SHELLFISH
- High-mercury fish (see page 84)
- Smoked seafood like smoked salmon (lox) or smoked trout
- Raw fish or shellfish: Yes, this includes sushi. Try a dynamite roll (cooked shrimp) or a California roll (imitation crab), or stick with vegetable rolls for a while. Many people believe that consuming flash-frozen raw fish from reputable sushi restaurants is low-risk. But low-risk isn't no-risk, and ultimately, it's up to you. If you do eat sushi, make sure it's low-mercury fish (see page 84).

AVOID SOME MEATS
- Deli meats and hotdogs: Only eat them if you cook them thoroughly until steaming.
- Raw meat: This includes raw chicken, beef, pork, lamb, etc. And by raw, we mean both really raw (like steak tartare) and sorta

DEEP DIVE: LISTERIA

When you are pregnant, your immunity to certain foodborne pathogens decreases, so you and your unborn babe are at higher risk for food poisoning. Take listeria, for example: studies show that the incidence of listeria among pregnant women remains about 20 times higher compared with the general population.[23] And it's not just dealing with some mild diarrhea. Listeria can cause miscarriage. The good news is that food manufacturers take measures to reduce things like listeria, so it's rare that you'd get sick from eating any of these foods. But mistakes still happen. Better to be safe, right?

raw, as in you didn't cook it well enough. For $10, invest in a meat thermometer to ensure you are cooking your meat and poultry to a safe internal temperature. Use the chart on page 69 as your guide.

AVOID UNDERCOOKED EGGS AND CERTAIN DAIRY FOODS

- Raw eggs: Certain sauces, spreads, and drinks, such as Caesar salad dressing, hollandaise sauce, unpasteurized eggnog, custard, and homemade ice cream, may contain raw eggs, so it's important to ask questions. Commercially manufactured ice cream, dressings, mayonnaise, and eggnog are made with pasteurized eggs and do not increase the risk of salmonella.
- Unpasteurized dairy products: Milk or cheese made with unpasteurized milk should be avoided due to the risk of listeria. Experts disagree about the safety of soft cheeses like Brie, feta, and goat. Some say they are fine if they are pasteurized, and some say not to consume them in any format. If you want to play it 100% safe, avoid soft cheese altogether during pregnancy (including feta and goat). If you can't live without feta cheese (hello, Greek salad), make sure that the cheese is pasteurized by checking on the label or calling the manufacturer.

AVOID UNPASTEURIZED JUICES

- Was the fruit washed before it was juiced? Was the equipment properly sanitized? Was it kept refrigerated? Not sure? Skip it. Washing and then juicing at home should be fine as long as fruits and vegetables are washed properly and equipment is sanitized properly.

WE GOT YOU!

Okay, so raise your hand if you read that list and freaked out because you totally ate Brie, Caesar salad, or sushi before you knew you were pregnant? Take a deep breath. You are fine. Your baby is fine. The risk from eating foods on this list is getting food poisoning from salmonella or listeria or other bacteria. But you didn't get food poisoning—and you're fine. Food poisoning is not going to happen now if you ate the sushi 3 months ago. You're good to go!

Which fish should I eat or avoid during pregnancy?

Fish primer: Omega-3 fat = good, mercury = bad. You want a fish that is high in omega-3 fat (see page 367), but low in mercury (see page 13). Your best bets are salmon, trout, low mercury skipjack tuna, anchovies, herring, and sardines. Avoid high intake of fish species that are high in mercury, including king mackerel, marlin, orange roughy, shark, swordfish, tilefish, and bigeye tuna, because mercury has been linked to an increased risk of birth defects and learning disabilities in children. Larger predatory fish (e.g., Chilean sea bass, grouper, swordfish) end up absorbing larger quantities of mercury, and as larger fish eat smaller ones, toxins build up and become concentrated. Unfortunately, cooking doesn't lessen the amount of mercury in these. The fish you can eat changes as environmental conditions evolve, so as a safeguard, download an app that's up to date.

(REALITY CHECK)

What about tuna? Well, there are several varieties of tuna, and some have more mercury than others (1 serving = 4 oz.).

- **Best choice** (2 to 3 servings per week): canned, fresh, or frozen skipjack tuna. If buying canned tuna, look for "light" instead of "white" tuna, and ensure the ingredient list says "skipjack."
- **Good choice** (1 serving per week): canned, fresh, or frozen yellowfin or albacore tuna. Canned albacore tuna is called "white" tuna.
- **Choices to avoid:** bigeye tuna (not available canned—usually used as steaks, sushi, or sashimi).

What about ahi tuna? Be careful here. Ahi may refer to yellowfina tuna, which is safe to consume, but it may also refer to bigeye tuna, which you should avoid. If you are offered ahi tuna, find out which species it really is.

Now that I'm pregnant, should I eat only organic?

We are no strangers to the question "should I buy organic foods?" especially from our pregnant momma friends, clients, and readers. Ultimately, the choice is yours. Check page 18 for our overview on organics. You will see that organic food has lower pesticide residues than conventionally grown food. What's uncertain is whether the trace amounts of pesticides in conventionally grown foods are clinically relevant. What we mean by that is that no definitive study has actually linked consumption of specific pesticides with adverse long-term health effects for you or your baby.

Organic foods are more expensive than conventionally grown foods. If you can ably afford them and they are easily accessible, it's fine to choose organic foods while you're pregnant. If the price tag or availability of organic foods are issues, please don't worry! There is no definitive science that says pregnant women must eat organic food.

Is it true that I should eat fewer carbs while pregnant?

DEEP DIVE: FOLIC ACID AND GRAINS

Pregnant women on low-carb diets have a higher chance (30% higher) of giving birth to a baby with neural tube defects, such as spina bifida.[24] Why is that? Well, Canada and the US add folic acid to grains (in Canada, folic acid is added to wheat and cornmeal; in the US, it's added to wheat, rice, grits, and cornmeal). Women on low-carb diets cut down on wheat, corn, and rice, so they don't get the folic acid that helps prevent neural tube defects. They may be taking folic acid in supplements, but the quantity may still not be high enough.

Some people find that they feel better when they follow a low-carb diet (see page 32 for more on this), but this type of diet can also be restricting and lack important nutrients that are crucial for pregnancy. If you're focusing on nutrient-rich foods that contain carbohydrates, like vegetables, fruits, grains, legumes, and milk, you're on the right track. If all of your carbs are coming from super-refined store-bought foods like crackers, cookies, refined breads, chips, soft drinks, donuts, and pies, your diet is not very balanced (read more on page 33).

So YES—it's good to minimize sugary and starchy carbs (pastries and pop) during pregnancy, but you do NOT need to minimize nutritious carb-containing foods (vegetables, fruits, whole grains, beans). It's all about balance. Your main meals should contain whole grains (oats, brown rice, quinoa, etc.) or enriched grains (enriched wheat flour contains folic acid) in reasonable portions—about a ¼ of your plate. If you're eating 6 cups of spaghetti per meal and it fills your entire plate, it is time to cut back a bit and maybe replace some of it with more vegetables or a little more protein. Check out the plate on page 11 and use it as a model for your own meals.

If you've been on a low-carb diet for years and it's your way of life, it doesn't need to end. Just be sure to check with your doctor or dietitian to see how much additional folic acid you need (from supplements). And make an appointment with a dietitian to ensure you are getting enough carbs to feed your growing baby's need. Yes, that little baby inside of you requires carbs for normal growth and development.

Also, if you are not currently on a low-carb diet, DON'T START DURING PREGNANCY. (Yes, we just yelled at you. Sorry.) Pregnancy is not the time for drastic dietary changes or for trying to lose weight (which is the premise of low-carb diets). See a dietitian after your baby is born if you want to discuss weight-control options (and read pages 139 to 143).

Give me all of the sugar!!! How do I control my sugar cravings?

Are you a sugar craver? Some of us crave carbohydrate-rich, starchy, or sweet foods during pregnancy such as baked goods, bread, and pasta. We can attest to this! Cara's cravings for Cinnamon Toast Crunch cereal are legendary (that is NOT an endorsement—it's just a fact). And Sarah's pining for chocolate was off the charts while she was pregnant.

Although it's completely fine to indulge now and then—even once or twice a day on small portions (not the whole box of cereal, Cara)—it's important to fill up on nutrient-dense foods first. Pregnancy is not a license to go crazy on junk food. It's not good in the short term or the long term. Permission to eat some sugar? Granted! Suggestion to limit it? Yes, please.

A good rule of thumb—and one that is endorsed by the World Health Organization—is to have 10% or less of your diet coming from ADDED sugar, per day.[25] That equates to about 48 grams or 12 teaspoons (if your diet is around 1,800 to 2,000 calories per day) from sources including white sugar, brown sugar, honey, corn syrup, maple syrup, agave, molasses, evaporated cane juice, date sugar, coconut sugar, or any other sweetener. A teaspoon of sugar in your coffee is fine. A ½ cup of ice cream is a lovely treat. Those are your sweet treats and will put you close to your sugar limit for the day. Whether on its own, added to foods, or used in food processing, sugar adds up quickly.

This 12-teaspoon value does NOT include natural sugars found in fruit and milk. Those foods are nutrient-dense and their sugar comes alongside a host of nutrients like calcium, fiber, and vitamin C. That beats the sugar from candy every time. Read more about sugar on page 35.

(REALITY CHECK)

There is no "better sugar" when you are consuming too much of it. We don't care if it's organic evaporated cane juice or unrefined raw coconut sugar or sugar cubes from your grandma's sugar bowl. We call bullshit on any "natural sugar" (agave, honey, coconut sugar, etc.) that claims to be healthier because of silly things like "trace minerals" or a "low glycemic index." Remember: they are ALL sugar and ALL can be harmful if consumed in excess.

Is it okay to have caffeine while pregnant? How much is safe?

News we love to share: you can enjoy coffee during pregnancy! In moderation, of course.

You'll hear contradicting advice on this subject from various health experts (and even non-health experts—thanks, mother-in-law), but most authorities agree that up to 300 milligrams per day of caffeine is safe during pregnancy (although, just FYI, the American Pregnancy Association recommends avoiding caffeine altogether). We recommend being cautious. Limit your caffeine intake to about 200 milligrams per day, which is the equivalent of about 1½ cups of coffee or 3 cups of strong brewed tea, if you are already a caffeine drinker. Obviously, we don't recommend starting to drink it during pregnancy if you did not previously. Keep in mind that soft drinks and certain foods like chocolate (Sarah's favorite) also contain caffeine.

If you plan to cut back on caffeine during pregnancy, don't quit cold turkey—you may experience withdrawal symptoms such as headaches. Instead, gently and slowly decrease your consumption over several days or weeks.

HOW MUCH CAFFEINE IS IN MY FOOD AND DRINK?

Food/drink	Milligrams
Decaf tea, 1 cup	0
Herbal tea, 1 cup	0
Decaf coffee, 1 cup	3
Hot cocoa mix, per 8 ounces	5
Milk chocolate, per 1 ounce	7
Dark chocolate, per 1 ounce	25 to 28
Green tea, 1 cup	30
Cola, per 12 ounces	36 to 46
Matcha green tea, 1 cup	40 to 70
Black tea, 1 cup	40 to 80
Instant coffee, 1 cup	76 to 106
Espresso, per 1 ounce	64
Percolated coffee, 1 cup	118
Brewed coffee, 1 cup	135
Filter drip coffee, 1 cup	179

Energy drinks: Some energy drinks contain about as much or more caffeine per serving as 1 cup of brewed coffee. Some of this caffeine can come from herbs such as guarana or yerba mate (which wouldn't necessarily be listed or accounted for on the label). This means that you may unintentionally be consuming more caffeine than what is safe. Not to mention that some of these herbs may also not be safe during pregnancy (see page 83). We advise that you stay away from energy drinks during pregnancy.

Kombucha: With less caffeine than coffee, green and black teas are also fine to consume in moderation. One caution is with home-brewed kombucha tea, which runs the risk of being contaminated with harmful bacteria if it's not prepared properly. Kombucha also contains a small amount of alcohol (created during fermentation). Better to avoid it. Yes, some people do safely sip kombucha throughout pregnancy. But why risk it?

Can I drink herbal tea during pregnancy?

The impact of consuming most herbal teas during pregnancy and while breastfeeding has not been studied, so there's not a ton of information available on this topic. We do know that certain herbs and herbal products can act like drugs in your body, and some are considered unsafe during pregnancy.

If you do choose to consume herbal teas, make sure that you're not having more than 1 to 2 cups per day, that the tea lists all of the ingredients, and that none of the ingredients are considered unsafe or potentially unsafe. It's best to alternate the types of tea you drink, and avoid steeping for long periods. You can also try making tea out of your favorite fruits by steeping minced apples, oranges, lemons, raspberries, blueberries, or strawberries. Turn the page for 2 herbal tea recipes to make at home.

Herbal Teas & Pregnancy

CONSIDERED SAFE: Ginger, Lemon balm, Orange peel, Peppermint

CONSIDERED UNSAFE: Aloe, Buckthorn bark, Chamomile, Chicory root, Coltsfoot, Comfrey, Dock root, Hibiscus, Labrador, Lobelia, Pennyroyal, Sassafras, Senna

INSUFFICIENT EVIDENCE TO CONFIRM: Burdock, Echinacea, Evening primrose, Fennel, Ginkgo, Hops, Japanese mint, Linden, Red bush (rooibos), Rosehip, Saint-John's-wort, Tea tree, Valerian, Wild yam

GINGER MINT HERBAL TEA

If you are looking for a soothing herbal beverage that's safe to sip while pregnant, try this blend.

Makes 1 serving

2 tbsp fresh mint leaves
½-inch piece fresh ginger, cut into strips
1 lemon wedge
1 to 1¼ cups boiling water

1. In a large mug, place the mint and ginger. Squeeze the lemon juice into the mug, then add the whole lemon wedge.
2. Add water and steep for 5 minutes to allow flavors to develop. Enjoy.

CARA SAYS: *Make it easy for yourself to prepare this tea daily! Cut ginger strips and store them in the freezer, and cut your lemon into 8 wedges and store it in an airtight container in the fridge. That's a week's worth of tea at the ready.*

APPLE-CINNAMON HERBAL TEA

This soothing blend has a hint of apple cider flavor and is delicious hot or cold. Make a double batch and refrigerate leftovers for a refreshing iced tea. It's ideal during pregnancy and breastfeeding, when thirst increases.

Makes 1 serving

1 apple peel
1 cinnamon stick
1 lemon wedge
1 to 1¼ cups water
1 tsp honey (optional)

1. In a small pot, place the apple peel and cinnamon stick. Squeeze the juice from the lemon over top, and toss in the lemon wedge too. Cover with water.
2. Simmer over medium heat for 10 minutes. Remove from heat and steep the tea for another 5 to 10 minutes for best flavor.
3. Pour tea through a sieve into a mug. Stir in the honey (if using), and enjoy.

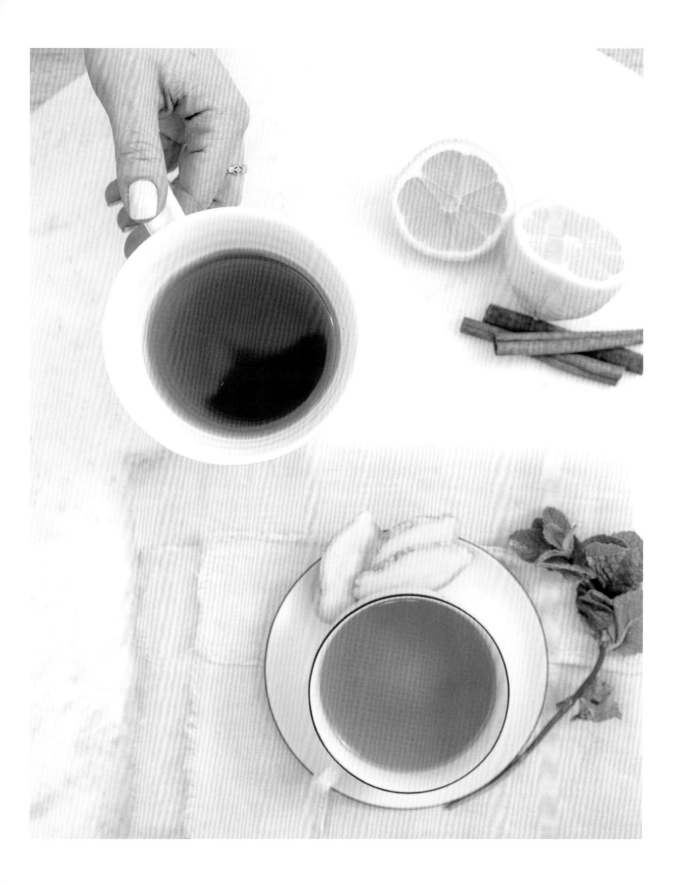

?

DID YOU DRINK CAFFEINATED BEVERAGES WHILE PREGNANT?

I'm not a coffee drinker by habit, but I love tea. I usually have one Earl Grey tea a day, and that habit didn't change when I was pregnant. —Kelly

I worked right up until the week my baby was due, and my weekdays are always fueled by coffee. I cut back when I was pregnant and had 1 to 2 medium-sized coffees daily. —Sabrina

Latte in the morning. I always have it with milk or almond milk, so it's got my calcium too! —Shawna

Red Bull. Nah, kidding. I'm a coffee drinker. One to wake me up in the morning. One to keep me awake in the afternoon. —Christina

I switched to decaf when I was pregnant. Maybe that was overly cautious. But it was fine. —Lenore

Coffees and lattes. Maybe 2 to 3 cups per day. —Renee

Those frozen milkshake drinks with coffee in them. My baby was born in August of a very hot summer and I probably had one of those every day. —Mickey

One latte every day. I had to stay awake somehow! —Tabitha

I eliminated all caffeinated beverages. None at all when I was pregnant or nursing. —Nazima

With 2 pregnancies, I immediately had an aversion to hot drinks. I added coffee back in after about 28 weeks, and it was mostly decaf. —Ann

I actually started drinking coffee when I was pregnant because I was so tired! —Jill

Can I drink alcohol while pregnant?

We like to think of ourselves as realists as well as dietitians, and we pride ourselves on finding a healthy balance with most foods and indulgences. But when it comes to alcohol and pregnancy, we're going to be direct and to the point: No. Just no.

No one knows how much alcohol it takes to harm a developing baby. When you consume alcohol during pregnancy, it quickly reaches baby through your bloodstream, and the effects on baby can vary depending on your health, your size, the amount consumed, and the timing of the consumption. We know that binge drinking is especially harmful for the developing baby, but we suggest avoiding alcohol altogether during pregnancy, because we just don't know what amount is safe (if any). That was an easy question to answer.

REALITY CHECK

If you drink alcohol while you're pregnant, you're putting yourself at risk of having a baby with fetal alcohol spectrum disorder (FASD). FASD encompasses a range of disabilities (physical, social, mental/emotional) that may affect people with mothers who drank alcohol while pregnant. FASD may include problems with learning and behavior, doing math, thinking things through, learning from experience, understanding the consequences of one's actions, and memory.

Is it safe to consume artificial sweeteners while pregnant?

You may wonder if it's okay to use sweetener in your coffee or to drink diet cola, and no doubt you've encountered conflicting advice. Although more research is required to fully determine the effects of artificial sweeteners in pregnancy (which is ethically almost impossible to conduct), research up until now doesn't suggest adverse effects.

However, we recommend that sugar substitutes be consumed in limited to moderate amounts, and that you stick to the acceptable daily intake standards set by regulatory agencies. Generally speaking, common sugar substitutes such as aspartame (Equal or NutraSweet), sucralose (Splenda), acesulfame potassium (Sunett Ace-K), and stevia are safe in moderate doses. Cyclamates (Sucaryl, Sugar Twin, and Sweet'N Low in Canada) are not recommended in pregnancy. Saccharin (Sweet'N Low in the US) is not safe during pregnancy.

SO WHAT'S CONSIDERED A "MODERATE DOSE?"

The safe amount of aspartame to consume per day is 2400 milligrams. One coffee-shop sized packet of artificial sweetener contains 15 milligrams aspartame, and a can of diet soda contains 185 milligrams aspartame. So, drinking a can of diet soda or adding a packet of Equal to your coffee is well within the safety guidelines. The safe amount of sucralose to consume per day is 540 milligrams. Each packet contains 12 milligrams. You can do the math!

Should I avoid allergens like eggs and peanuts?

Oh, how times have changed. When Cara was pregnant with her first baby in 2006, the practical advice was to avoid allergens to help prevent your baby from having food allergies. So if your doctor told you not to eat peanuts, that information was correct . . . A LONG TIME AGO. It's not the case today.

Guidelines used to recommend that pregnant women with a history of allergies, eczema, or asthma should avoid peanuts. This advice changed in 2009 because of the lack of evidence that eating them increased a baby's risk of allergy. Then science began to emerge showing that eating peanuts during pregnancy was actually PROTECTIVE against your baby developing an allergy (see the Deep Dive on page 96). We now know that there's no evidence to support the avoidance of any single high allergenic food—peanuts, milk, eggs, fish—to prevent allergies from developing in an infant. The top allergenic foods are also highly nutritious: peanuts, tree nuts, fish, milk, eggs, soy, and wheat are filled with vitamins, minerals, fiber, and protein. So don't cut them from your diet—there's no reason to! Of course, if YOU are allergic to a certain food, continue to avoid it.

Is it safe to drink the orange liquid for the gestational diabetes test?

Let's get the most important point out of the way quickly: this drink is NOT toxic—despite what you may have read on a Facebook forum. Why would your doctor recommend something toxic?? The drink—often called Glucola—is given before a blood test to check if you have gestational diabetes. It's important to know this diagnosis as it changes your self-care and medical care; having gestational diabetes can affect your baby, and it needs to be monitored and treated.

The concerns that people have about the drink are the artificial colors, corn syrup (made from genetically modified corn), and brominated vegetable oil it contains. We get it—it's not health food. But it's also not something you will be consuming daily. You only have to drink it ONCE in your whole pregnancy. If you currently drink pop or soda, you are consuming artificial color, corn syrup, and brominated vegetable oil (see the Deep Dive below) regularly, which is way more problematic than this one-time medical drink.

If you have an intolerance to artificial colors or you are trying to avoid genetically modified foods, you can skip the drink, BUT DON'T SKIP THE TEST. The most important part of the drink is the 50 grams of glucose sugar it contains, which is required to test your glucose tolerance. Talk to your doctor about a glucose-rich substitute. One study back in 1999 looked at the use of 50 grams of jelly beans instead of Glucola for diabetes testing, and found that women had accurate results with either method (yup, just ONE study).[26] Of course, if you're skipping artificial color and GMOs, you'll have to buy dye-free, organic jelly beans at a health-food store.

If you are diagnosed with gestational diabetes turn to page 98.

DEEP DIVE: BROMINATED VEGETABLE OIL

What is brominated vegetable oil? It is a food additive mostly used in the soft drink industry, primarily to help keep citrus-flavor oils suspended in beverages so they don't float around and form a yucky film at the top of the drink. Basically, it's vegetable oil bonded with atoms of the element bromine, which can be unsafe at high doses. What's a high dose? Drinking 15 to 20 cups of orange pop a day, every single day. So, don't do that. But that ONE-TIME DOSE of Glucola? It's not toxic and is no more a concern than a can of orange pop during pregnancy.

ONE-POT PEANUT BUTTER NOODLES

This crowd-pleaser is quick to prepare and great as leftovers too!

Makes 4 to 6 servings

Peanut sauce

⅓ cup natural peanut butter

2 tbsp sodium-reduced soy sauce
  or tamari

1 tbsp toasted sesame oil

1 tbsp rice vinegar

2 tsp minced garlic

1 tsp minced fresh ginger

8 oz whole grain spaghetti or
  other pasta

½ tbsp olive oil

2 raw chicken breasts, cubed

¾ cup water

3 cups your favorite diced veggies
  (try carrots, red peppers, purple
  cabbage, celery, broccoli, snow
  peas, mushrooms, etc.)

Peanuts (optional)

Chopped cilantro (optional)

1. In a medium-size bowl, whisk together all of the peanut sauce ingredients, and set aside. It will be thick! Once it's in the pan with the rest of the ingredients, it will "melt" a little and incorporate nicely.

2. Cook the pasta according to the package directions until slightly undercooked—you want it to be al dente! Set aside.

3. Set a large pan or wok over medium heat. Add the oil and chicken, and stir-fry until about two-thirds of the way cooked. Transfer to a bowl, cover with foil, and set aside.

4. Add the water and raw veggies to the pan. Cover and steam for about 3 to 4 minutes, until tender-crisp and bright in color.

5. Return the chicken to the pan, plus the pasta and the peanut sauce. Mix gently until the sauce is dispersed evenly. Decrease heat to medium, cover, and cook until the chicken is cooked through (about 3 to 5 minutes).

6. Serve family-style in a large bowl, topped with fresh peanuts and cilantro.

DEEP DIVE: ALLERGEN EXPOSURE

A 2015 study published in the *JAMA Pediatrics*[27] looked at over 10,900 births and compared incidence of peanut allergy with mothers' diets. The babies were monitored over time to see if they tested positive for food allergies as they grew. The researchers found 140 cases of peanut or tree nut allergy among the kids, and this number was significantly lower in kids whose mothers consumed more peanuts or tree nuts in their pregnancy diet (5 or more times per month). The researchers concluded that early allergen exposure increases tolerance and lowers risk of childhood food allergy. So mom's peanut or tree nut consumption does not appear to increase the risk of nut allergy in her offspring . . . it actually is protective against it.

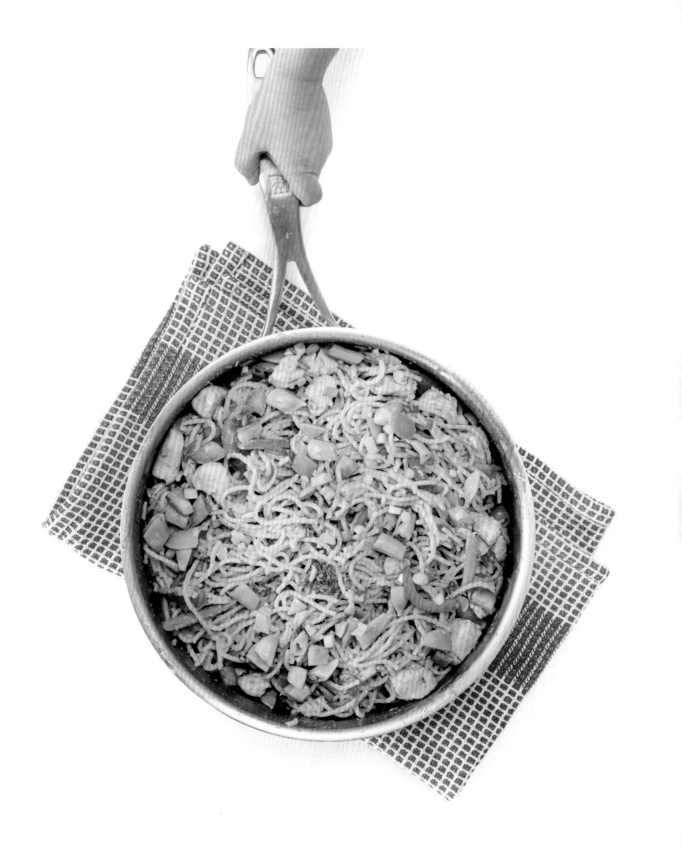

What Should I Know About Gestational Diabetes?

Gestational diabetes (GD) is a condition that can develop during pregnancy causing high blood sugar. Any pregnant woman can develop GD, so it's recommended that you be tested between 24 and 28 weeks of pregnancy using the oral glucose tolerance test (that sugary orange drink we talk about on page 94). If you're at higher risk (see below) you may be tested earlier than this.

WE GOT YOU!

Between 2% and 20% of pregnant women develop GD each year—so you're not alone! It's normal to feel scared, overwhelmed, and a bit anxious at first (naturally). But remember that GD will most likely disappear after your baby is born. *Phew*.

WHO IS AT RISK OF GD?

All pregnant women. You can decrease your risk of developing GD by staying active, eating well, and not gaining more weight than is recommended throughout your pregnancy (see page 102). But please know, even if you're doing "all the right things" the following factors can still play a role:

- Family history and genetics
- Personal history of:
  - Gestational diabetes, prediabetes, or other problems with insulin or blood sugar
  - Polycystic ovary syndrome or another health condition linked to problems with insulin
  - High blood pressure, high cholesterol, or heart disease
  - Previously having a stillbirth or miscarriage
  - Previously giving birth to a large baby (weighing more than 9 pounds)
- If you are:
  - Black, indigenous, and a person of color
  - Overweight
  - Over age 25

WHAT ARE THE SYMPTOMS OF GD?

Chances are you may not have any symptoms (and that's why it's so important to take the test). If you do experience them, they may include: fatigue, increased hunger, thirst or urination, nausea, frequent vaginal, bladder or skin infections, and blurred vision. The tricky part here is that many of these symptoms are common in ANY pregnancy—and that's another reason why you should get the proper testing.

WHAT ARE THE RISKS OF GD?

If GD is left untreated, there are risks to you and your baby. High blood sugar can cause preeclampsia (i.e. very high blood pressure during pregnancy) and this can potentially damage organs, such as your kidneys or liver. GD can also result in a very large baby, which may lead to a more difficult birth. Moreover, GD can translate into a higher risk of health problems—for both you and your baby—down the road, including an increased risk of type 2 diabetes and heart disease.

The good news? There are many strategies to manage your blood sugar levels. With the proper support, you'll be able to have a healthy pregnancy and a healthy baby. Your doctor or midwife should refer you to a dietitian or certified diabetes educator who can walk you through the recommended dietary, medical, or lifestyle changes.

HOW IS GD TREATED?

Every case is different. What works for one woman might not work for another. So, it's crucial to seek guidance from a health professional who is trained in diabetes management. You may be asked to monitor your blood sugar levels throughout the day. Some women are able to control their blood sugar levels by changing their eating habits and increasing physical activity; others may need to inject insulin for better control.

One thing that we DO NOT want you to do is go on a very restrictive or limiting diet. There are simple, nutritious, and realistic changes you can make without depriving yourself of foods. You'll notice that what we recommend for those diagnosed with GD is very similar to what we recommend for any pregnant woman: no crazy restrictions, no dieting, no unnecessary removal of food groups. The basics are laid out here:

Stick to regular, balanced meals and snacks: Enjoy three evenly spaced balanced meals each day, with snacks in between. Follow the plate model on page 11, so each of your meals contains vegetables, proteins, and some grains. Time one of your snacks for bedtime as this will help to control blood sugar levels overnight.

Manage carbohydrate intake: The carbohydrates found in nutrient-rich foods, such as vegetables, beans, and whole grains, provide energy and important nutrients for pregnancy and overall health. If you have GD (even if you are taking insulin), you don't need to avoid these nutrient-rich carbs outright. However, you will need to know how best to manage your carbohydrate intake, and your healthcare provider will guide you. Always keep in mind that:

- **Not all carbs are the same!** Choose fiber- and nutrient-rich carb sources such as vegetables, fruits, whole grains, beans, and lentils.
- **Limit refined carbs:** Avoid those carbs from high-sugar foods such as candy, soda, baked goods, chocolate etc. (read more about this on page 32).
- **Space out your carb intake:** Do this in a way that is personalized for you (depending on your diet, blood sugar level, and insulin (if taking)). We highly suggest working with a dietitian on this.

DEEP DIVE: INSULIN

The role of insulin in our body is to lower blood sugar levels after eating and keep blood sugar within a healthy range. Think of insulin as little vehicles that trap sugar molecules in your blood and then carry them to your body's tissues to give you energy and help you function. GD may occur because of insulin resistance (which means the tissues in your body aren't accepting the insulin, or the insulin isn't trapping the sugar properly) or due to a reduced production of insulin. Usually, insulin keeps your blood sugar levels stable. During pregnancy, hormone levels change and it's harder for your body to process blood sugar efficiently. This can make blood sugar levels rise, and if insulin isn't working properly (to lower blood sugar levels) then they stay high. The GD test shows how much sugar is in your blood and whether you are processing it efficiently.

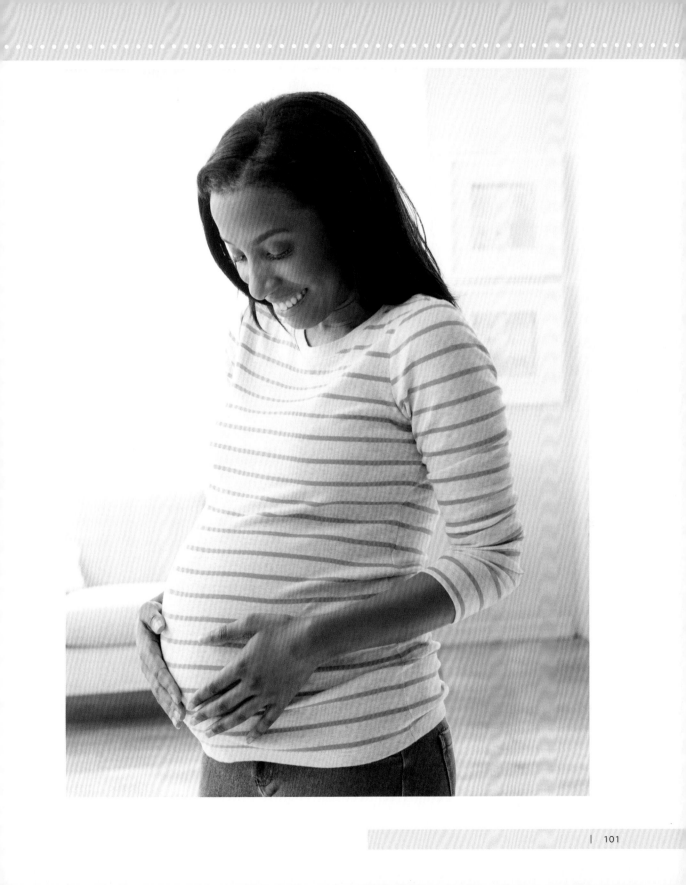

How much weight should I gain during pregnancy?

Guidelines from The Centers for Disease Control and Prevention and other health authorities say most women should gain 25 to 40 pounds during pregnancy (or 35 to 45 pounds if you're expecting twins), using this estimate you can anticipate:

- 2 to 4 pounds gained during the first 3 months you're pregnant
- 1 pound a week gained during the rest of your pregnancy (or 1.5 lbs per week with twins)

Of course, you may gain more or less weight than what these numbers show because every woman is different. Gaining weight during pregnancy is normal and healthy—trust us, this is not a good time to diet or intentionally lose weight. Women who don't gain enough weight during pregnancy may be at an increased risk of having a low-birthweight baby and/or preterm delivery, while women who gain excess weight run a high risk of requiring a C-section.

SHADES OF GRAY: WEIGHT GAIN GUIDELINES

How much women should eat—and how much weight they should gain—during pregnancy isn't agreed upon by national health authorities around the world. For example, Health Canada recommends that women increase their calorie intake by 340 calories per day in the second trimester and 450 calories in the third trimester, but England's National Health Service and the National Institute of Health Care Excellence in the UK recommend only increasing calories in the third trimester, and then only by about 200 calories per day. We're not fans of calorie counting in this way, as prescribing a specific amount of extra calories to adhere to doesn't align with the well-researched Intuitive Eating model (see page 44) and encourages women to ignore their physical hunger cues. So, this whole field is filled with differing opinions. Some women like to follow the medical guidelines and others eat intuitively. Ultimately, it's up to you.

How much food should I eat throughout my pregnancy?

There's a lot of confusion about how much to eat while pregnant—as in, if you're "eating for 2," do you need to eat double the amount? Um, no. Your baby is tiny and doesn't need 1800 extra calories a day. But nice try! Your first priority should be to eat a well-balanced and nutrient-rich diet—after all, you're growing a little human! Pregnancy is not the time to lose weight or restrict your intake, but it's also not a license to eat as much as you want or overindulge regularly.

Here's what's most important: if you're eating balanced, nutritious meals and snacks every 3 to 4 hours (depending on your appetite) and stopping before you become overfull, then you're on the right track. Read more about intuitive eating on page 44. You may notice that some days you're ravenous and other days you're not very hungry at all, and that's okay. Eat according to your physical hunger cues, and know that it's not going to be the same every day. You might also find that you have to eat more frequently (and not as much at each sitting) because there's not as much room in your stomach, or because eating too much at one time makes you nauseated.

However, if eating intuitively doesn't work with your personality type and you prefer concrete numbers, here's a general idea of what your body may require:

- **First trimester:** It's not necessary to eat any more than normal. Just eat like you normally would!
- **Second trimester:** You'll likely feel hungrier than normal because your energy and nutrient needs are rising. You'll probably need 300 to 350 more calories per day. That's like an apple with 2 tablespoons of peanut butter; or a cup of yogurt with some fruit. But follow your appetite.
- **Third trimester:** As your baby grows, your appetite may increase a bit more. You'll probably need 400 to 450 more calories per day. That's like a small sandwich or some crackers with cheese and fruit.

Extra calories should come from nutrient-dense foods such as lean proteins, vegetables, fruits, and whole grains. Limit foods that are overly processed with a lot of added sugar, salt, or saturated fat. But, do give yourself permission to indulge once in a while on something that you absolutely love and can't live without.

REALITY CHECK

The information we give in this book is for women pregnant with only one baby. If you are expecting twins or multiples, please talk to your doctor or a registered dietitian about how your nutritional needs may differ.

I'm gaining too much weight. How do I slow it down?

If you've noticed (or if your doctor or midwife has noticed) that your weight gain is too rapid, don't panic. You and your baby are likely totally fine. But there are a few things you can do to get back on track.

Eat filling foods: Make sure that you're eating foods that are nutrient-dense and filling at each meal and snack. Always include protein-rich foods such as meat, poultry, fish, dairy, beans, and lentils at each meal or snack, because they help to keep you fuller longer. Have vegetables and fruits at meals—fiber is also filling!

Choose better carbs: When you eat starchy carbohydrates or grains, make sure that they're whole grains (most of the time), such as quinoa, whole grain pasta, brown rice, or oats, instead of white, overly processed starchy foods. Whole grains provide a heck of a lot more nutrition and will keep you fuller longer.

Eat intuitively: Don't eat for the sake of eating. Eat when you start to feel subtle hunger (when you get that first feeling of emptiness in your stomach). Don't let yourself become ravenous before you sit down to a meal or snack, because chances are, you'll overeat. Trust us—you'll be much more comfortable and be able to eat more mindfully if you start eating at that first sign of hunger. Read more about Intuitive Eating on page 44.

Be a bit picky: When it comes to treats and desserts (or higher-calorie savory snacks, like chips), be picky—indulge in only those treats that you absolutely love and can't live without. Instead of eating something sweet just because it's there or just because you see it, decide which treats will bring you the most satisfaction and don't waste your time on the mediocre ones.

SARAH SAYS: *When it comes to sweets like candy, donuts, cake, or ice cream, I can take them or leave them (which means that I usually leave them). Chocolate, on the other hand, I can't live without. This is why I make room for it every day (and don't ever feel guilty about it).*

I'm not gaining enough weight. How do I do it?

There can be several reasons why you're not gaining enough weight during pregnancy—it could be due to excessive nausea, loss of appetite, food aversions, or other digestive concerns.

It's fine if you don't gain any weight in the first trimester. In fact, your growing baby is so tiny that it has minimal calorie needs. Lack of weight gain at this stage won't affect your baby. But as you get into the second trimester, weight gain should become steadier. Your calorie needs increase and so do the nutritional needs of your baby (and likely your appetite!). Here are some ideas for helping appropriate weight gain along:

Choose calorie-dense foods: If you have a small appetite, it's crucial to make every bite count! That means you want to get the most nutrition (protein, vitamins, minerals, etc.) in the foods you choose. Even if you get full quickly or have a small appetite, you will know you've taken in some great nutrition.

Try smaller, more frequent meals: You may be turned off of larger portions of foods, and eating might feel overwhelming if your plate is too full (which can actually decrease your appetite). Instead, try having 5 or 6 smaller (snack-size) meals. So, maybe this means eating every 2 to 3 hours versus every 3 to 4 hours. For example, instead of having a big spaghetti and meatball dinner, have 1 piece of French toast with Greek yogurt and berries. These snack-size meals can still pack a nutritional punch and provide the calories that you need, but might be less overwhelming and more appealing.

Rethink the salad: Wait, what? Did the 2 dietitians just advise you to rethink a salad? While vegetables are super-healthy, they are also low in calories and high in fiber. A big bowl of lettuce with cucumber can make you feel full quickly, but provides only 20 calories. That's not enough to meet your needs! If you really have a low appetite and can eat only a small amount, it's better to have more calories with every bite. For

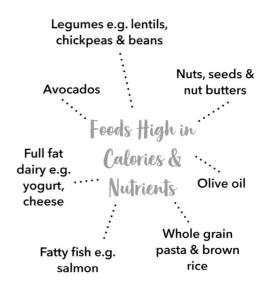

Legumes e.g. lentils, chickpeas & beans

Avocados

Nuts, seeds & nut butters

Full fat dairy e.g. yogurt, cheese

Foods High in Calories & Nutrients

Olive oil

Fatty fish e.g. salmon

Whole grain pasta & brown rice

example, try whole grain toast with peanut butter and banana slices (yes, you CAN and SHOULD eat peanuts when you're pregnant—see page 94), or a pasta salad with avocado, nuts, meat, and cooked veggies. Both of which would have more calories than a light green salad. Look at the numbers to see what we mean:

- Whole grain toast with 1 tablespoon peanut butter and a banana: 220 calories
- 1½ cups romaine lettuce and cucumbers: 20 calories
- 1½ cups romaine lettuce, cucumbers, and 1 teaspoon dressing: 60 calories

If you ARE craving salad, do it up right! Add at least a tablespoon of dressing to your lettuce, and top it with nuts, seeds, chickpeas, quinoa, avocado, or any other calorie-dense foods (see page 105).

Don't turn to junk food: We know what you're thinking: "I need to eat more calories! I can have all of the ice cream I've ever wanted!" Uh . . . no. If only it were that easy! Yes, you need more calories. BUT. You also don't need tons of sugar and fat. You want the calories to come from nutritious foods. Yes, you can certainly have a bowl of ice cream. But don't get your day's worth of calories from pint after pint.

Curb the nausea: Morning sickness? Yeah. Sucks. More than half of all pregnant women get it. The good news? It does pass—usually by 12 weeks, when weight gain really needs to ramp up as the second trimester begins (isn't Mother Nature brilliant?).

I have morning sickness. Why? Is there anything that helps?

Symptoms of morning sickness typically occur during the first trimester, and for many women, they are one of the first signs of pregnancy! Symptoms typically appear by the sixth week of pregnancy and generally disappear around the end of the twelfth week. More than half of women experience morning sickness, with the severity ranging from slight queasiness to excessive vomiting, known as hyperemesis gravidarum (see the Deep Dive on page 108).

Despite its name, morning sickness can happen during all hours of the day, and sometimes it can last a lot longer than the first trimester. Some women are ill only in the morning, some women feel sick all day long, and others may feel sick only in the evening. While you are feeling nauseous it can be difficult to eat enough food to get the calories and nutrients you need to gain weight for a healthy pregnancy. Here are some tips that may help reduce nausea:

Don't get too hungry: Having a healthy snack between meals can help your blood sugar levels stay stable and help you feel full. An empty stomach can trigger nausea. Try peanut butter on celery; chicken and vegetable soup; crackers with cheese; or hummus with raw vegetables. Even a quality protein shake or bar paired with vegetables can do the trick.

Eat more protein: The sight or smell of meat can trigger nausea in many pregnant women, but eating enough protein can help keep that queasiness away. Luckily, there are many non-meat sources of protein to help you meet your needs. Things like nuts (including nut butters), seeds, beans, eggs, cheese, and Greek yogurt are good sources of protein that are less likely to cause nausea. Having a high-protein snack before bed can also prevent the queasy feeling associated with an empty stomach in the morning.

Eat what you crave–within reason: If you crave a certain food, chances are it will sit well with you. Eating a small serving can help alleviate the queasiness long enough to eat a nutritious meal.

Change your prenatal vitamin: Many women find that the supplemental iron and folate in their prenatal vitamin make them nauseous. If you are unable to tolerate the prenatal vitamin your doctor has prescribed, try a different brand or for a chewable alternative. Take your supplements with food and not on an empty stomach, or try taking them at bedtime.

Keep a light snack on your night table: Have a nibble before you get out of the bed in the morning. Soda crackers are a popular option. They don't go bad (no refrigeration required) and are neutral in flavor.

Try ginger: It's an age-old remedy, but this one is backed by science too, especially during the first trimester.[28] Ginger really can reduce nausea and vomiting in pregnancy. Slice some fresh ginger into a mug and pour boiling water over it–you've just made ginger tea. Not a fan of warm drinks? Try gingersnaps, candies, or crystallized ginger. You can also use ginger in your cooking and baking—stir-fries, muffins, fruit salad, etc. Or try our Ginger Mint Tea on page 90.

Drink fluids before or after meals, instead of with meals: Sip throughout the day so you don't get dehydrated, especially when you are vomiting a lot.

If none of these tips help, you may have hyperemesis gravidarum (see Deep Dive below) and should discuss it with your doctor.

I'm having weird food cravings. What's that all about?

Ah yes, the famed pickles and ice cream diet for pregnant woman! About 75% of women say that they have some sort of craving, and scientists aren't really sure why. Some postulate that we crave foods that contain nutrients that our body is lacking—so if you're low in calcium, you may crave dairy foods. But there's no actual evidence for this. Some people crave really healthy foods (we have a friend who craved sautéed garlic kale—okay, it was Cara!), while others have more indulgent desires (Sarah couldn't live without salt and vinegar chips!). It's fine to give in to cravings as long as the foods are safe to eat while pregnant (e.g. no raw meat) and you are mindful of portions. You don't want to give into junk food cravings to the exclusion of healthy foods in your diet.

DEEP DIVE: HYPEREMESIS GRAVIDARUM

Hyperemesis gravidarum is severe nausea and vomiting during pregnancy. It can lead to weight loss, electrolyte imbalance and kidney problems. It occurs in about 2% of pregnancies in North America, and can impact the quality of life for mom and even your developing baby too. The cause is largely unknown, but it may be more common in women whose immediate family members (such as sisters) also experienced it. Talk to your doctor about treatment options, which may include switching your prenatal vitamins to folic acid only; using ginger supplements; trying acupressure wristbands; or using prescription medications. Drinks that contain electrolytes may be advised to prevent dehydration. In terms of nutrition, avoid foods that trigger nausea. Some women find that switching to smaller meals and snacks can help prevent mild cases of nausea and vomiting from getting worse. Some also find relief with meals containing more carbs and protein, but less fat.

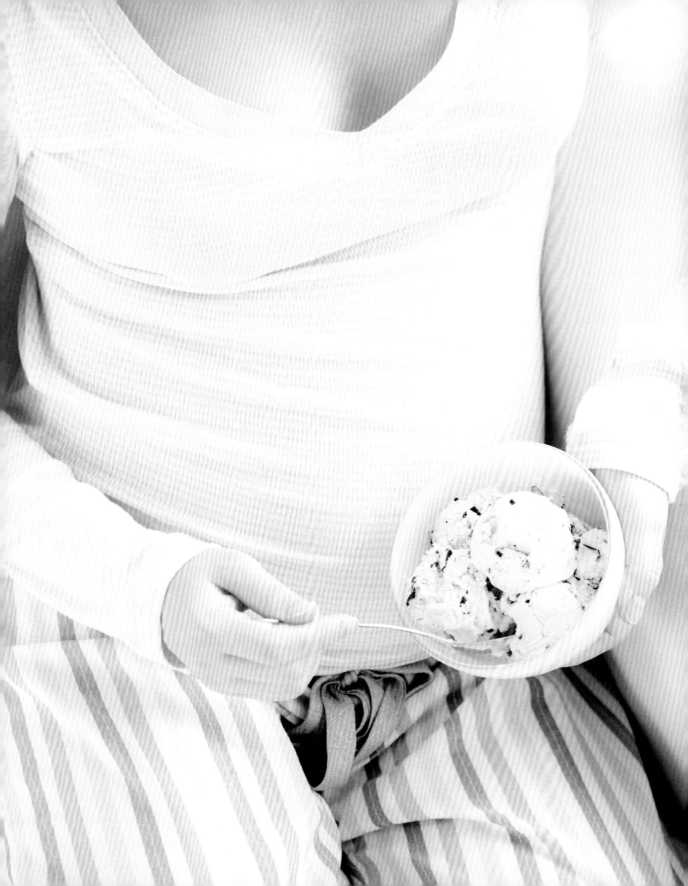

WHAT CRAVINGS DID YOU HAVE DURING PREGNANCY?

Sardines. Fishy, salty sardines. And I don't even like sardines. —Sabrina

I craved salty and crunchy foods, like pretzels, chips, and tortillas. And fried, not baked. —Alicia

Apples. Pears. Oranges. Apple juice. Grapes. I couldn't get enough of sweet fruits, but they had to be really cold. —Viv

I liked sweets more than usual. Cookies were a big one for me, and I'm not usually a dessert person. —Rupinder

I loved lemon-flavored things. Lemon in water helped ease my nausea, and I was really into lemon candy. —Larissa

Cheese, please. It had to be strong—like Asiago, extra-aged Cheddar, or Parmesan. —Gila

Ice cream. I had a bowl of it every evening and I looked forward to it. The coldness, the creaminess, the sweetness. Huge craving. —Jill

I craved sweet, but I tried to be healthy about it. I was obsessed with fresh dates, bananas (okay, banana bread), and cherries. —Xania

Peanut butter. By the spoonful. —Stephanie

Bread. —Leif

That baseball-park yellow mustard. On anything. —Fabiola

I craved sushi, but avoided raw fish. I was really craving the soy sauce! —Nina

Chocolate. —Eden, Eve, Kelly, Rebecca, Kym, Lee, Fauzia, Faye, Ramani, Kateryna, Judy, Danya, Callie, Tania, Christine . . .

What about food aversions during pregnancy?

There may be certain smells or flavors that turn your stomach when you're pregnant—and often they are foods you used to love. Common food aversions are to strong flavors, such as garlic, onions, spices, and coffee. If you can't stand the taste or smell of certain foods, simply avoid them. Know that it's totally normal, it's common, and it will pass!

So why do these things happen. The answer is, wait for it . . . hormones! Interestingly, both cravings and aversions tend to happen around the same time in the first trimester, along with hormonal shifts. Researchers examined the link between the first occurrences of nausea, vomiting, food cravings, and food aversions during pregnancy and found a significant positive correlation between them. Interestingly, 60% of women reporting both nausea and food aversions said that the first occurrence of each happened in the same week of pregnancy.[29] What does that mean? You may be turned off by foods that made you feel queasy. Makes sense!

How do I manage some of the other digestion-related side effects?

As magical and wonderful as pregnancy is, there are certain symptoms that you may deal with while pregnant that are less than . . . well . . . magical. Because of a combination of wacky hormonal fluctuations and the fact that a human is growing inside of you (making for less space to digest your food), you may notice that your once well-functioning digestive system is now causing you some serious discomfort and frustration. The symptoms stop once the baby is born (yay!!), but for now, it sucks.

You may feel bloated and gassy near the end of the day, or you may get that terrible burning sensation in your esophagus while you're lying in bed. That's heartburn. You also may not feel as "regular" as you once felt prior to pregnancy, which may cause cramping and painful bathroom breaks. Oh, and hemorrhoids—you could get those if you push too hard when you're constipated (note: don't do that, and read page 112). As unpleasant as these symptoms are, they are usually a normal part of pregnancy, and in most cases are manageable with certain changes to your diet and lifestyle.

BLOATED AND GASSY

Hormonal changes cause your body to digest food more slowly when you're pregnant. The longer food sits in your digestive tract, the more gas is produced. This unfortunately often translates into uncomfortable cramping, bloating, and excess gas.

We've been there. Fortunately, though, there are certain things that you can try nutrition/diet-wise that can help:

- Eat smaller meals and snacks.
- Be active regularly. Moving your body will help with the digestion process.
- Although healthy, go easy on gas-producing foods such as beans, lentils, raw cabbage, onions, and broccoli. If you do eat these gas-producing vegetables, it may help a little to eat them cooked instead of raw.
- Avoid carbonated beverages.
- Sip beverages from a cup instead of slurping through a straw, which makes you swallow more air (and burp).
- Avoid chewing gum (and any other foods, like candies) that contains sugar alcohols such as sorbitol, maltitol, and xylitol. These tend to produce excess gas. Also, you will swallow excess air while chewing gum.
- Avoid any food products that contain the ingredient "inulin." Inulin is a natural fiber coming from chicory root that is known to cause excess gas.
- If you are gassy after drinking milk, it may be from lactose. See if switching to plant-based milk like soy or almond milk helps in the short term.

CONSTIPATION

Constipation (i.e., infrequent bowel movements and hard-to-pass stools) affects more than half of all pregnant women. Inactivity, anxiety, and a lower-fiber diet can exacerbate constipation. And sometimes the iron found in prenatal supplements can make constipation worse or cause it in the first place. Try these tips to ease constipation:

- Drink plenty of fluids (mainly water) to help food travel down your digestive tract.
- Eat a higher-fiber diet including lots of vegetables and fruits, bran cereals, oats, and barley. If you increase the amount of fiber (you should be aiming for a total of 25 to 30 grams per day), make sure to increase your water consumption as well.
- Minimize white, low-fiber starchy foods when you can.
- Try prunes, which are nature's laxative. Start with 3 prunes and a glass of water. Try that for a few days to see if it loosens you up.
- Get some chia seeds. These marvelous little seeds absorb water and become gelatinous. Mix 2 teaspoons of chia with 2 teaspoons of water and wait 5 minutes

to see what happens. Little jelly seeds! So cool. Add that topping to oatmeal, yogurt, smoothies, etc. It works as a gentle laxative.

- Try a psyllium husk supplemental drink (such as Metamucil) every day. Start with using 1 teaspoon a day and increase as needed. Make sure to drink plenty of fluids.
- Move your body everyday. Go for a walk, do a light workout, or do a pre-natal yoga class. Movement can help with . . . movements (if you know what we're sayin').
- Make sure that you take time to go to the bathroom every day. As silly as this sounds, it's really important to establish a routine where you give yourself enough time to relax and go to the bathroom. Sometimes with busy schedules, kids, and work, it's hard to remember to take time to "go" (if you already have kids, you know that uttering the words "Mommy is in the bathroom!!!" doesn't keep any little ones out! It's like a magnet . . . why is that?!).

(REALITY CHECK)

When you feel the need to go, don't push too hard. If you do, you increase the risk of developing hemorrhoids, which are small (painful and itchy!) swollen blood vessels around the rectum. They are especially common in the third trimester. They can be caused by holding in your bowel movement for too long, pushing too hard, hormonal changes, and the added weight from the growing fetus. Lovely, right?!

Some practitioners say that doing Kegel exercises can help—these simple exercises increase circulation in the rectal area and strengthen the muscles around the anus, reducing the chance of hemorrhoids (see the We Got You! below).

If you notice that you are consistently constipated, make sure to talk to your doctor, dietitian, or midwife about possibly changing the amount or type of iron that you're taking, switching prenatal multivitamins, increasing fiber and fluids, or trying stool softeners that are safe during pregnancy.

(WE GOT YOU!)

What's a Kegel?? It's an exercise to tighten your pelvic floor muscles. Kegels help to strengthen the muscles that support the bladder, uterus, and bowel, muscles that are very important during labor and birth. Not sure where these muscles are? To identify them, stop urination in midstream. If you succeed, you've got the right muscles. Here's how to do your Kegels: while lying down, tighten the muscles for 5 seconds, then relax for 5 seconds, and repeat 5 times. Try to do this 3 times a day—start in bed in the morning, and do another set when you are going to sleep at night. The third time is up to you!

HEARTBURN

Heartburn is caused by acidic stomach contents creeping back up after eating. Many of us deal with heartburn during pregnancy, and it's more common during the second and third trimesters. It is most often due to hormonal changes during pregnancy, causing the muscles of the digestive tract and the opening of the esophagus to relax too much, allowing for stomach contents to splash back up. To manage heartburn during pregnancy, try these tips:

- Eat smaller, more frequent meals and snacks rather than 3 large meals. This prevents your stomach from becoming overfull and may help to stop acid reflux and allow for better digestion.
- Go easy on acidic foods such as citrus fruits and juices, vinegars, mustards, and tomatoes/tomato sauces.
- Avoid eating too much right before bedtime or a nap. You want to give your digestive system enough time to digest food and allow gravity to help with digestion before lying down.
- Eat slowly to allow yourself time to digest food properly and to avoid overeating.
- Avoid highly spiced or seasoned foods.
- Avoid high-fat, deep-fried foods.
- Minimize caffeine from coffee, tea, chocolate, and soda pop. Caffeine can relax the lower esophageal sphincter, allowing acid to creep back up the esophagus.

If your heartburn doesn't get better and is causing you pain, talk to your doctor about pregnancy-approved heartburn medications.

What about nutrition for labor and delivery?

Sometimes old guidelines hang around, regardless of whether they are still legit. Historically, it was recommended that women avoid eating while in labor. Lots of doctors still follow this, but many other doctors, nurses, midwives, dietitians, and anesthesiologists heavily debate it. It's one of the most common questions we hear from expectant moms.

There's no current, solid science to back up the notion that eating and drinking during labor causes negative outcomes for mom and baby. The whole "no eating during labor" guideline is based on really, REALLY old science—we're talking 80 years ago. In the 1940s, scientists found that women who consumed food or drinks (other than the standard ice chips) while in labor were at risk of gastric aspiration (inhaling stomach contents) when put under general anesthesia. That's because when you're put under, you're at a higher risk of vomiting due to muscle relaxation. But these days it's extremely rare for a woman to be put under general anesthesia when having a baby. It's more common to have a local anesthesia—like an epidural—so the recommendation to not eat doesn't really make sense anymore.[30]

One review of the topic looked at almost 400 studies on eating during labor and found only one case of aspiration between 2003 and 2015, in what was considered a high-risk delivery. So the risk of increasing bad outcomes by eating during labor is very low. In fact, there's actually a bit of research to show that eating could lessen the time in labor (one study says by 16 minutes).[31]

And the notion that eating too much during labor increases your chances of vomiting is not really backed up by science either and has been contradicted by other research, making the overall findings inconclusive.[32]

SO CAN I EAT DURING LABOR?

We say, most likely yes, but check with your healthcare team first. If you feel hungry during labor, try eating small portions of food, sticking to carbohydrate-rich choices such as fruits, grains, and low-fat dairy (since carbs are the body's preferred source of fuel). Foods that are higher in fat, protein or fiber may lead to an upset stomach or more cramping (which is not what you need during labor!) because those nutrients are slower to digest. It's important to stay hydrated too, so sipping water, eating ice chips, or even drinking a sports drink (which also contains electrolytes and carbohydrates) can help keep you hydrated and energized. A smoothie with frozen fruit and yogurt can be a good choice in early labor. Smoothies are great because you can pack a lot of nutrition into them—things like fruit, yogurt, milk, nut or seed butters, and hemp hearts or chia seeds! Drinking a smoothie with some slower-releasing carbohydrates like oats and berries (especially in the early stages) can help to extend the energy release during labor.

WE GOT YOU!

In a survey of mothers who gave birth in US hospitals, 80% reported that they did not eat during labor.[33] You may just not feel like it! Pack your hospital bag with easy-to-digest snacks like granola bars, fruits, homemade muffins, or any other light foods you may crave, just in case.

In reality, though, when you hit the throes of labor, eating might be the last thing on your mind—we know this from experience! Everyone is different and every labor is different. Listen to your body, eat when you feel like eating, and do a little planning. Our guess is that you may be like us and perhaps nibble in the early hours, then gradually decrease any food consumption as labor becomes more intense.

Please note: Our advice on eating during labor is for low-risk pregnancies. If you are having a planned C-section or are at high risk for an emergency one (e.g., you're having multiples, you have health problems, or you have had a prior C-section), check with your doctor about eating or drinking once labor has started. No studies have examined eating during labor for women who are at higher risk of needing C-sections with general anesthesia.

DEEP DIVE: KETOSIS IN LABOR

During labor, the abdominal muscles are contracting constantly, burning off a whole lot of calories. In fact, it's estimated that women need about the same amount of calories (energy) during labor as they would to run a marathon! Glucose, which comes from carbohydrate-containing foods, is the body's preferred source of fuel. And when the body's fuel stores are depleted (such as during extreme energy-burning, like in labor), other stored energy sources are used (i.e., glycogen—this is the body's stored version of fuel, which is used up when there's no available glucose from food). When glycogen stores run out, and there's no other incoming source of fuel, your body kicks into ketosis (the production of ketones, which increases the acidity in mom's and baby's blood). This happens often to women in labor. Being in a state of ketosis—especially if your body isn't used to it—could cause nausea and vomiting (this could explain why so many women get sick during labor and delivery), but otherwise, there's not much research on the effects of being in ketosis during labor.

SARAH SAYS: *I was in labor for a loooong time with my first baby, and cannot imagine not having food during it—that would have been 14 hours, and there's no way I had the stamina to endure that! Although I was told that it's a better idea not to eat too much, I made sure to have a filling meal when I started feeling contractions, and while I was still feeling okay in the first few hours, I had some nutritious snacks— homemade muffins, yogurt, and a fruit smoothie.*

Top 10 Tips
for pregnancy

1   **Take a prenatal supplement.**
Choose one with 0.4 milligram of folic acid, 27 milligrams of iron, and 400 to 600 IU of vitamin D.

2   **Remember folic acid is important.**
This essential vitamin helps reduce the risk of birth defects like spina bifida.

3   **Get enough protein.**
Aim for about 71 grams per day. Good sources are fish, meat, poultry, dairy, beans, eggs, nuts, and tofu.

4   **Remember omega-3 fat.**
Eat at least 2 servings per week of low-mercury fish such as salmon or take a fish oil supplement.

5   **Eat safely.**
Avoid foods that are raw (fish, meat, eggs) or unpasteurized (cheese, milk, juice).

6   **Enjoy vegetables and fruits.**
Whether organic or conventional, fill half your plate at every meal.

7   **See carbs as your friend.**
It's fine to cut back on sugar, but don't cut back good carbs like whole grains, beans, and vegetables.

8   **Drink coffee and tea if you want.**
Stay below 200 milligrams of caffeine per day. That's 1½ cups of coffee or 3 cups of strong-brewed tea.

9   **Don't eat for two.**
You need only 300 to 350 more calories daily in the 2nd trimester and 400 to 450 in the 3rd trimester.

10   **Go nuts!**
It's fine to eat peanuts and tree nuts during pregnancy (as long as you're not allergic to them!).

Postpartum

Introduction

Bringing a baby into the world can be one of the most wonderful, magical things you'll ever experience, and can trigger insanely intense feelings of love, adoration, and emotion. Some of us may also experience trauma and disappointment during labor and birth, and we don't want to discount those experiences either. The first few days with a baby are overwhelming, tiring, and amazing all at the same time.

> The first few days with a baby are overwhelming, tiring, and amazing all at the same time.

Your health is very important in the postpartum stage. You'll need lots of support from your partner, friends, family, and health professionals in the weeks after bringing baby home, to ensure that you can take care of not only your baby, but yourself too. If you have other children, you'll need help with childcare, and you may want to recruit friends or family members to help out with meals and household tasks like cleaning. You may also need help and support from a trained lactation consultant when it comes to feeding. Never be embarrassed or afraid to ask for help!

Proper nutrition and hydration are essential for healing, recovery, and staying healthy as you care for your newborn. If you're breastfeeding, you'll likely find that you're hungrier (and thirstier) than normal, and for good reason—you're expending hundreds of extra calories producing breastmilk! It's important to focus on nutrient-dense whole foods (see page 9), such as protein-rich options (poultry, fish, beans, eggs, dairy), fruits, vegetables, whole grains, and nuts, to ensure optimal healing and to stay healthy and nourished as you care for your new baby and return to your pre-pregnancy weight (gradually and healthfully).

You'll be happy to hear that you can enjoy some of your favorites such as sushi and alcohol now, but there are still a few limitations when it comes to the types of fish and amounts of caffeine and alcohol you should consume if you're nursing (see page 135).

Recovery

Your body has just been pushed (and literally stretched) to its limits to bring a new little human into the world. As miraculous and wonderful as it is, it's also slightly traumatizing (to your body at least) and requires some tender love and care during the healing process.

Most people refer to the "postpartum period" as the 6 weeks following the birth of your baby, which is misleading. At 6 weeks, you're still recovering from childbirth, and it could take up to 6 months or longer for your muscle tone and connective tissue to restore to their pre-pregnancy state, assuming no complications. So even if you look and feel "back to normal," you're still very much in recovery mode and still have a lot of healing to do.

> ♥ **WE GOT YOU!**
>
> Proper nutrition and hydration, gentle exercise, and lots of physical and emotional support are all key components to healing after birth. *Hello* spouse, partner, parents, siblings, friends, or hired help! As moms, we need to be patient and gentle with our bodies. Having support in any form you can get it is a big part of this.

Nutrients

When it comes to nutrition, pay special attention to some key nutrients that support healing and recovery post-birth.

CALCIUM

Calcium helps with many things—muscle relaxation, blood coagulation, transmission of nerve impulses, enzyme reactions—in addition to promoting tooth and bone health and lowering the risk of developing osteoporosis (see page 26). Calcium is found in food and your prenatal multivitamin, which we recommend you continue taking for 6 months after the birth or as long as you're breastfeeding. You need 1,000 milligrams of calcium per day, (see the list of calcium-rich foods on page 369), plus what's in your prenatal supplement (about 300 milligrams).

VITAMIN D

Vitamin D is important for so many reasons (see page 30)! Specific to postpartum healing, there's a link between pelvic floor muscle strength and higher vitamin D status. There's also a link between low vitamin D status and a higher probability of postpartum depression. Vitamin D also helps with calcium absorption and bone health. For these reasons, plus the fact that vitamin D deficiency affects up to 80% of women of reproductive age, we recommend that you take 1,000 IU vitamin D supplement daily in addition to what's in your prenatal vitamin. You can also get vitamin D from foods like salmon and milk, but most women should be supplementing, especially in the winter months if you live in a cold climate that doesn't get much sun.

IRON

Although dietary recommendations for iron return to prepregnancy levels in the post-partum period (18 milligrams per day), you may need iron supplements if you lost a lot of blood during delivery or if the interval between your pregnancies is less than 2 years—in this case, your doctor may recommend an iron supplement. See more about iron on page 25.

PROTEIN

Protein is important for building and repairing muscle tissue (see page 23) and for wound healing post-delivery or C-section. Aim for 20 to 30 grams of protein at each meal and 10 grams with each snack. That's about 65 to 120 grams per day. See the chart on page 364 to know how much protein is in foods.

VITAMIN C

Vitamin C helps immune system and with wound healing, including the synthesis of collagen, which is the main structural protein found in connective tissue. This can be beneficial postpartum because—whether you deliver vaginally or by C-section, fellow mommas—there will be wounds (*cringe*—we know). As humans, we can't store vitamin C in our body, so it's important to get adequate amounts in our daily diet. When it comes to feeding your baby, you need 120 milligrams of vitamin C per day if you're breastfeeding, or 75 milligrams per day if you're not breastfeeding (vitamin C is vital for tissue growth in the breastfed infant—and they get it from your breastmilk!). Some great options include oranges, strawberries, kale, and bell peppers. As long as you include a variety of fruits and vegetables in your day (at least 1 to 2 servings at each meal or snack), you should be covered!

DIETARY FAT

Dietary fat helps the body absorb vitamins A, D, and E, which are important for wound healing. Omega-3 fat, which is found in oily fish such as salmon and trout, can help prevent postpartum depression (see page 145). We recommend that you have at least 2 servings of low-mercury oily fish per week, or that you continue taking your omega-3 supplement (read more about this on pages 24 and 74).

Hydration

As a busy new mom, it's very easy to become dehydrated, especially when you're breastfeeding. Staying properly hydrated helps to keep your digestion, blood volume, body temperature, muscles, and joints in check, and helps with wound healing and breastmilk production. It's important that you're drinking enough water or other hydrating fluids throughout the day, especially post-delivery and while nursing. We recommend that you always keep a full water bottle on hand and drink *at least* 8 to 12 cups (if not more) of water or other hydrating drinks per day.

> **WE GOT YOU!**
>
> How do you know if you're drinking enough? Check the color of your urine when you pee. If it's dark yellow or golden, you may not be sipping enough throughout the day. Aim for pee to be clear and very light yellow, like lemonade.

Food choices

How you eat after delivery is not much different than how you ate during pregnancy. Listen to your appetite, eat when you begin to feel hungry, and stop when you feel comfortably full, but not stuffed (read more about eating intuitively on page 44). This often translates to eating every 3 to 4 hours, or 3 meals with snacks in between. Include protein-rich foods in every meal and snack (meat, poultry, fish, dairy foods, lentils, beans, eggs, etc.), as well as lots of vegetables and fruits. When you do include grains and starches, make sure they're whole grain choices most of the time, and be mindful of portions (we usually recommend filling your plate with half veggies and fruits, one-quarter protein-rich foods, and one-quarter whole grains; see page 11).

When friends and family members ask if there is anything they can do to support you, say YES! Request some groceries, nutritious snacks, or ready-made meals—they can provide much-needed relief and sustenance. When you are feeling motivated, whip up a batch of healthy muffins or energy bites and keep them stocked in the freezer for snack breaks. Make sure that you have nutritious grab-and-go items that will keep you fueled between meals—things like homemade granola bars (page 128), energy bites

> When friends and family members ask if there is anything they can do to support you, say YES! Request some groceries, nutritious snacks, or ready-made meals

(page 336), fruits, vegetables, cheese, etc. And if they can be eaten one-handed, even better!

Supplements

We recommend that you continue taking the nutritional supplements (prenatal multivitamin, mineral supplement, and vitamin D and omega-3 supplements) that you've been taking during pregnancy, until at least 6 months postpartum, if not longer (see pages 78 to 81 for more info on dosage). This is especially true if you:

- Are breastfeeding
- Don't eat dairy—you'll need additional calcium and vitamin D
- Don't eat animal products—you'll need additional calcium, vitamin B_{12}, vitamin D, zinc, and iron
- Tend to diet or habitually consume less than 1,800 calories a day

Your body is not only healing from delivery, but also producing breastmilk, which requires the additional nutrients present in these supplements, many of which help with healing too. We consider this a nice top-up for peace of mind as you transition into life with a new baby (even when you consume a fairly well-balanced diet). Talk to your doctor or dietitian about your personal supplement needs if you're unsure.

CARA SAYS: *It's easy to forget to eat every 3 to 4 hours in this postpartum period. Brain fog, utter exhaustion, lack of motivation, lack of hands, an empty fridge—these are all common scenarios. But you need to keep your energy level up, and food is human fuel!*

(WE GOT YOU!)

Every birth story is special, including those babies who come to us via adoption or surrogacy. And every new parent needs to care of themselves, whether you were the one to give birth or not. If you welcomed (or are preparing to welcome!) your baby though adoption or surrogacy, you may be wondering what the different options are for feeding your baby. The great news is you have a few, and all of them can promote closeness, bonding, and love. Feeding options for babies 0 to 6 months include: pumped breastmilk from birth mom, or from a milk bank or milk sharing service; formula (read more on page 156); and even breastfeeding yourself (yes, it can be possible!). Every family's situation is unique, so talk to your doctor about what's best for you and your baby. You've got this, momma!

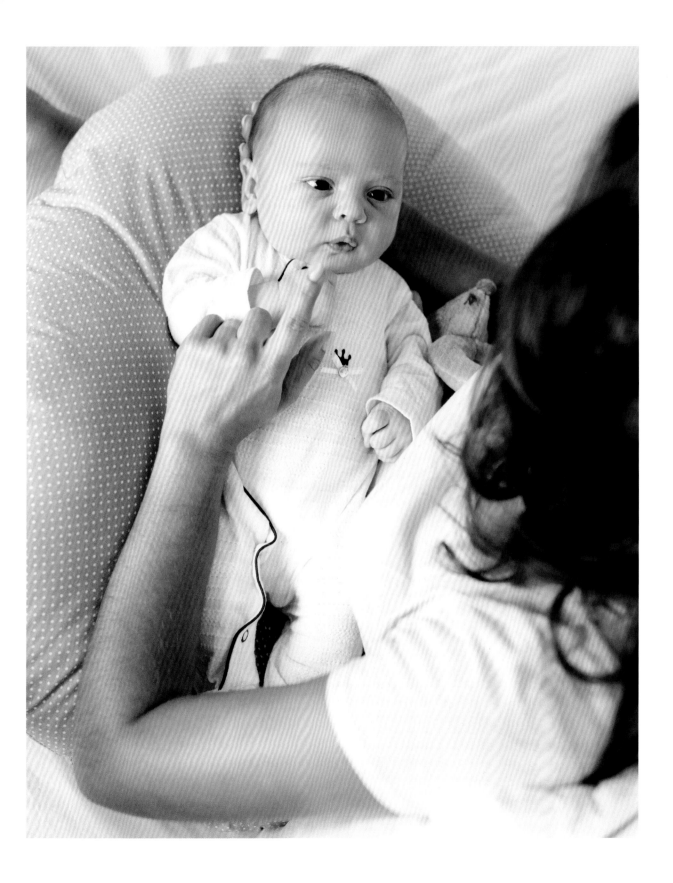

What should I be eating while breastfeeding?

Eating while breastfeeding shouldn't be complicated or stressful. There is no special "while-I'm-breastfeeding diet" that you need to be on. It's business as usual. Your breastmilk will provide the ideal source of nutrition to your baby even with a less-than-ideal diet of your own. It's your health, as the nursing mom, that will suffer if your nutrition is not up to par. We both found that the biggest challenge was making sure that we had easy and nutritious options on hand (and that we could eat one-handed!) while feeding or holding the baby.

When choosing foods to eat at meals and snacks, you should aim for lots of variety and focus on whole, nutrient-dense foods most of the time. Aim for at least 3 different foods at meals (see the table on page 13) and 2 at snacks, and always include something protein-rich and a vegetable or fruit. This isn't any different than the advice we would normally give, but keeping it in mind will be a good way to keep tabs on your nutritional intake. Continue to take your prenatal multivitamin, and eat a well-balanced diet overall.

(REALITY CHECK)

Drinking enough water is crucial for maintaining your milk supply, enjoying proper digestion, staying hydrated, and losing weight. Drink at least 8 to 12 cups per day, and more if you're really active or it's really hot outside.

SARAH SAYS: *The best, I mean THE BEST gift I received from friends and family was food. Casseroles, muffins, soups, pasta sauce, healthy homemade snacks . . . they were all wonderful. After having a baby, you just don't have the energy to cook or bake. If people ask what they can do to help, say "food please!"*

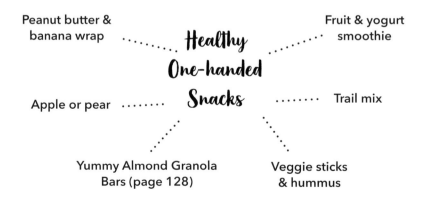

Peanut butter & banana wrap

Fruit & yogurt smoothie

Healthy One-handed Snacks

Apple or pear

Trail mix

Yummy Almond Granola Bars (page 128)

Veggie sticks & hummus

How much should I be eating while breastfeeding and/or pumping?

If you are exclusively breastfeeding, you may find that you're hungrier than normal and need to eat more often. And for good reason! You use 300 to 600 calories per day to make the full amount of milk most babies need from birth to 6 months. Think about it— it makes sense that you are hungry because you are feeding your baby food you are making with YOUR OWN BODY (it's pretty cool, huh?).

About two-thirds of those 650 calories will come from the nutrient-dense foods you eat, and the remaining will be drawn from the weight you gained during pregnancy.[34] This is how you can achieve gradual and healthy postpartum weight loss. So adding about 350 to 400 calories to your pre-pregnancy eating plan (if you're exclusively breastfeeding) should do it—that's like adding ¾ cup of Greek yogurt, some berries, and ¼ cup of nuts to your day.

But please don't stress about counting calories or keeping track of every morsel of food that you eat every day. Instead, just remember the plate model (see page 11) and aim to include protein, vegetables, and whole grains at meals, and make mini versions of this model for snacks. Eat when you feel subtle hunger and stop when you're comfortably full. This is what's called "intuitive eating" (see page 44). Your body is the best guide when it comes to amounts of food to eat.

(REALITY CHECK)

Don't decrease your calories too much—your milk supply may suffer! Breastfeeding moms who consume less than 1,800 calories per day (which could be the case if you're trying to lose weight rapidly) might produce less milk than they need for their baby. Supply issues can also be triggered by stress, anxiety, and fatigue. So take the time to eat nutritious meals and snacks, and drink enough fluids.

SARAH SAYS: *I remember waking up in the middle of the night starving, and making eggs and toast at 2 a.m. to satisfy my hunger when I was breastfeeding my son, Ben. I learned my lesson for my next 2 kids! I made sure to have lots of healthy foods on hand—either quick snacks or foods that I could reheat during the night if I woke up hungry. Things like homemade muffins, hard-boiled eggs, and energy bites.*

YUMMY ALMOND GRANOLA BARS

These are a great one-handed snack for while you're feeding baby with the other hand. And if they crumble a bit, add more almond butter, or enjoy it by the handful! Make a few batches for the freezer.

Makes 12 bars

2 cups rolled oats
½ cup roasted almonds, chopped
¾ cup chopped dried apricots
½ cup almond butter
3 tbsp honey

1. Line an 8-inch square baking pan with parchment paper.
2. In a large bowl, mix together the oats, almonds, apricots, almond butter, and honey until blended.
3. Transfer into the prepared pan and press in firmly, ensuring you reach all 4 corners.
4. Freeze for 30 minutes, or until firm.
5. Flip the square onto a cutting board, peel off the parchment paper, and slice into 12 equal-size bars.
6. Store bars in the freezer for up to 3 months. They can be enjoyed from frozen or at room temperature.

CARA SAYS: *If you're not a fan of apricots, try raisins, dates, prunes, or dried tart cherries for a change. I sometimes make these with ½ cup dried pineapple and ¼ cup shredded coconut. Tropical treats—yum!*

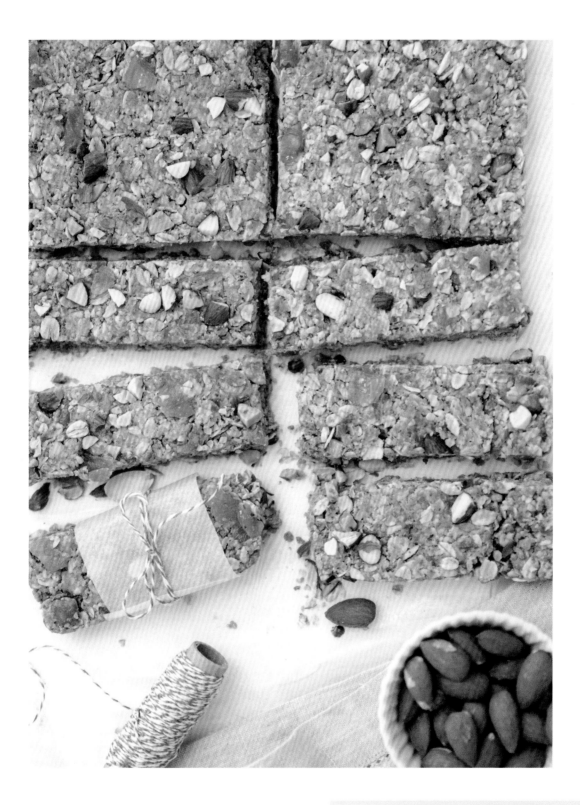

WHAT WAS YOUR GO-TO SNACK WHEN BREASTFEEDING?

I made or bought muffins and froze them so they'd always be available. —Gerri

I needed energy quickly. Often it would be trail mix—nuts, seeds, and dried fruit. —Alice

Smoothies. I would keep frozen vegetables and fruit on hand, add Greek yogurt, and whip up creations. —Hanna

Dim sum or any kind of little dumplings. Small bites! —Angie

Granola bars. Ones with lots of nuts and seeds. —Amelia

Anything I could hold in one hand! Sandwiches, apples, granola bars, bananas, protein bars, smoothies, energy bites, wraps, etc. —Lauren

Dosas stuffed with yummy ingredients like veggies or lentils. —Sue

Hard-boiled eggs. I would boil a dozen and they lasted all week in the fridge. —Allison

Homemade granola bars with lots of hemp and flax—often with peanut butter. —Carla

My mom is an amazing cook. She'd make containers of pasta salad, kale salad, lasagna, and other foods that tasted good cold so I could eat them quickly. She was my savior for the first few months! (Thanks, Mom.) —Lara

Handful of almonds. Or almond butter on toast. Quick and easy. —Monica

Cut-up veggies and hummus. —Ashley

Are there foods, drinks, or supplements to increase my breastmilk?

Many breastfeeding mommas turn to foods, herbal supplements, tinctures, and teas to increase their milk supply, despite the lack of regulations or good research in this area. Most resources have mixed reports and recommendations, which makes it super-confusing for moms during an already overwhelming time.

There are very few human studies on consuming herbs while breastfeeding because it's simply not ethical to conduct research on mothers and infants. So we just don't have enough solid research to say "yes, pop those herbal pills to boost your milk supply," because we don't know whether it's (a) going to work and (b) safe for you or your baby. Here is the information we *do* have on some foods, beverages, and herbs commonly mentioned in connection with breastfeeding. Talk to your doctor or a lactation consultant before taking any herbal supplements.

First, a cool new word for you: galactagogues. That's the word for foods, herbs, or medications that are said to increase or stimulate breastmilk production. See the table on the next page for a detailed breakdown of the potential effectiveness of these.

> **REALITY CHECK**
>
> Water is key (we know this for a fact), and an obvious one when it comes to breastmilk production. Stay well hydrated and keep a water bottle handy at all times.

DEEP DIVE: MOTHER'S MILK TEA

The safety of this popular tea blend meant to help increase milk supply, by US-based tea company Traditional Medicinals, was tested in 2019 in a clinical study. 60 breastfeeding women were randomized into 2 groups. The first group received the Mother's Milk tea (which contains fennel, anise, coriander, fenugreek seed, and other herbs) and the second group drank lemon verbena leaf tea. They kept track of any adverse effects for 30 days, then post-study calls also assessed any adverse effects for the infants until they were 12 months old.

The results? The tea was safe. There were no adverse effects reported and the tea was found to present no safety risk to moms or their infants.[35] This study did not test the effectiveness of the tea however, but some moms have found that it does increase milk supply. That's all anecdotal, of course. But you can go ahead and try it for yourself—it's safe.

GALACTAGOGUES: SAFETY & EFFECTIVENESS

Galactagogue	Safety	Effectiveness
Garlic	Research shows that a few days of taking oral garlic supplements causes no adverse effects in nursing mothers or infants. It's also safe to eat (with noted side effects being bad breath and body odor!).	When mom eats garlicky foods, studies show it increases infant sucking time because babies like the taste (see page 136). And when babies suck for longer, you may create more breastmilk.
Green tea	Safe when consumed as tea, 1 to 2 cups per day. Not recommended as a supplement due to high caffeine content.	No concrete studies have shown it to be effective.
Oats and barley	Safe to eat daily.	These whole grains contain fiber called beta-glucan, which can help increase prolactin—also known as the breastfeeding hormone—but there are no studies to tell us the amount necessary to be effective.
Fenugreek	The safe dose used in clinical studies is 6 to 7 ounces of tea, consumed up to 3 times per day, OR 600 milligrams capsules, taken 2 to 3 times per day. Higher doses may cause diarrhea, sweating, and worsening of asthma symptoms. Do not use when pregnant (it can cause contractions) or if you have a bleeding or clotting disorder.	Studies show that fenugreek may help increase breastmilk supply.[36]
Fennel	1 to 2 cups per day of fennel tea is likely safe. There's not enough research to guarantee the safety of fennel supplements or a recommended dose. Some sources recommend limiting the duration of treatment to 2 weeks.	Research shows fennel can boost milk supply, milk volume, and fat content (which helps support baby's weight gain). Fennel has been studied extensively, but it's still unknown as to why it may work for breastmilk supply.

Some doctors recommend taking the medication Domperidone to increase breastmilk supply. One of the main hormones that controls breastmilk production is called prolactin. When you take Domperidone, it raises your levels of prolactin, which helps increase the production of breastmilk. Many moms say that their breastmilk production improved within a week of starting the medication (some say it just takes a few days). Interestingly, Domperidone doesn't work for everyone (some moms notice no difference in their supply), and researchers aren't sure why.

Talk to your doctor about a prescription for the dosage that meets your needs. It usually starts at 10 milligrams 3 times a day, and some doctors suggest doubling the dose for greater effect. Also to note: in very rare cases (about 1 in 10,000 women), Domperidone causes a rapid heart rate[37] (observed in women who have previously had problems with a rapid heart rate), so always discuss the pros and cons with your doctor. If you know you have a heart condition or ventricular arrhythmia (rapid heart rate), this medication is likely not for you.

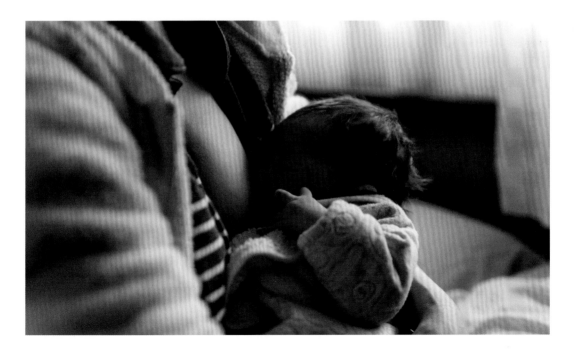

WHAT METHODS DID YOU USE TO TRY TO INCREASE YOUR BREASTMILK SUPPLY? DID THEY WORK?

I used Domperidone and saw a difference within 48 hours. —Jill

I saw a lactation consultant, and it helped so much! She suggested pumping between feeds, which signals the body to produce more milk. It was beneficial for sure. —Carol

Fenugreek tea worked well for me. But you will smell like fenugreek!! —Cameron

Before trying Domperidone, my lactation consultant suggested trying to rest more (sleep when the baby sleeps!), more skin-to-skin contact, breastfeeding more often, and pumping between feeds. Not sure which part helped, but it did increase my milk supply. —Melina

My doc said breastmilk is supply and demand—the more your baby nurses or you pump, the more milk is produced. I started pumping between feeds and it did boost my supply. —Andrea

I tried Domperidone at a high dose (3 tablets 3 times a day) and saw changes within the week. Maybe even in a few days. It did work. —Olga

I use fenugreek and blessed thistle. I think there's a small difference. I don't pump, so it's hard to measure for sure! —Sandra

I used Mother's Milk tea and did see a difference after a few days. —Shelly

Domperidone, but it didn't work for me. Turned out that my baby had a tongue tie, which was why he wasn't feeding well. —Orly

I got a prescription for Domperidone from my doctor and saw a difference within 2 days. —Alina

I tried teas, cookies, fenugreek, oatmeal, and smoothies before I finally exhausted all avenues and filled a prescription for Domperidone. It worked in a few days. —Paula

What should I avoid eating or drinking while breastfeeding?

Rejoice momma! You can go back to eating most of your favorite foods after you give birth. There are still a few that you have to be careful with, though, because what goes into your body is transferred to your breastmilk. You eat and drink it, and baby does too!

Avoid high-mercury fish: Steer clear of king mackerel, marlin, orange roughy, shark, swordfish, tilefish, and bigeye tuna. Turn to page 13 for low-mercury alternatives.

Limit caffeine: Okay. A cup of coffee is a necessity for many of us after having babies. So. Many. Sleepless. Nights. You can drink a moderate amount of caffeine—the equivalent of 2 to 3 cups of coffee—without it affecting your baby. Some newborns are a little more sensitive to caffeine than others, and can become fussy and have trouble sleeping even with small amounts, although this seems to lessen as they grow. We suggest no more than 300 milligrams or about 2 cups of regular coffee per day. Remember, caffeine is found not only in coffee but also in tea, soft drinks, energy drinks, and chocolate (see page 88 for the amount of caffeine in various drinks and foods).

Limit alcohol: It's fine to enjoy a glass of wine (or beer . . . or Scotch) after baby is born. But if you're breastfeeding, it's important to pay close attention to how much you're drinking and the timing of each drink to ensure that you keep your baby safe. The truth is, there's no level of alcohol in breastmilk that's considered safe for your baby. If you do decide to have a drink, you want to limit your consumption to no more than one standard alcoholic drink per day.

If you do choose to drink alcohol, have the drink right after breastfeeding, and avoid breastfeeding until the alcohol has completely cleared your breastmilk. You can pump to relieve pressure and tenderness while waiting for it to be safe to breastfeed (and you may even consider having

> (REALITY CHECK)
>
> Alcohol may blunt the flow of breastmilk and also hinder your baby's motor development if consumed in excess. Having the occasional glass of wine is okay, but do not go overboard.

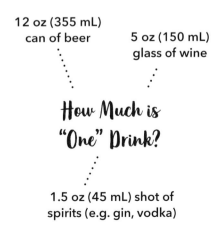

12 oz (355 mL) can of beer

5 oz (150 mL) glass of wine

How Much is "One" Drink?

1.5 oz (45 mL) shot of spirits (e.g. gin, vodka)

pumped milk ready for your baby's next feed before drinking alcohol). It takes about 2 to 3 hours for alcohol to clear from your breastmilk, depending on your body weight.

> **REALITY CHECK**
>
> Let's talk pumping and dumping: Despite what you might have heard, pumping and dumping doesn't speed the elimination of alcohol from your body. That would be great, right? But no. The only alcohol-related reason to pump and dump is to feel more comfortable (e.g., not become engorged) while you're waiting for the alcohol to clear your system. And for some, pumping at a time when you would normally breastfeed helps to keep milk supply up too.

Is it true that what I eat changes the taste of my breastmilk?

Many women wonder if the flavor of their breastmilk changes when they eat different foods. If you eat something garlicky, will your baby taste the garlic? The short answer is yes. A mother's diet really can affect the taste of her milk, and babies don't just notice these flavors, they respond to them too!

DEEP DIVE: IMPACT OF GARLIC

One study analyzed a group of breastfeeding moms, half of whom were given garlic pills and the other half were given a placebo pill. The moms took the pills and then were asked to feed their 3-month-old babies once garlic had made its way into their milk (it peaks around the 2-hour mark). The babies of the real garlic pill moms spent more time feeding, indicating that babies prefer garlic-tasting (or smelling) milk.[38, 39]

Breastmilk—similar to amniotic fluid during pregnancy—contains flavors that directly reflect the foods, spices, and beverages consumed by mom. Researchers have found that exposure to a flavor in amniotic fluid or breastmilk modifies an infant's acceptance and enjoyment of similarly flavored foods when they start solid foods. So make sure to consume a variety of foods, tastes, and cuisines while pregnant and breastfeeding if you'd like to increase the chances of raising a budding foodie!

But, of course, go by trial and error. If your breastfed baby seems uncomfortable or irritable after you eat a specific strongly flavored food, something super spicy for example, avoid that food while breastfeeding.

Brenda had been seeing a dietitian for about 6 months when she learned she was pregnant with her first baby. She was overjoyed! The counseling sessions turned from weight control to how to eat well during pregnancy, and she wanted to resume weight-control measures after baby was born. When her baby Jordan was 2 months old, she went back to see the dietitian. She was loving motherhood, but had a few struggles. Since the dietitian was also a mom, they talked about breastfeeding, sleep deprivation, and baby's fussiness.

Brenda said she always found that little Jordie was fussier on weekends, and she assumed it was because he was overstimulated from having so many visitors. Her husband was home from work, her nephews (3 of them!) often dropped by, and the pace was a bit more frantic. Made sense.

As part of the counseling, the dietitian wanted to see how Brenda's eating habits were shaping up, so she asked Brenda to keep a record of what she ate over a 3-day period. Brenda recorded her food on Thursday, Friday, and Saturday before she saw the dietitian on Monday. In going through the record, a lightbulb went on in the dietitian's head. She said, "I notice that you start each day with 1 cup of coffee. But on Saturday, it looks like you have 3 cups of coffee. Why is that?" Brenda explained that when her husband was home on the weekend, they leisurely walked to their local Starbucks and she ordered a Venti-size coffee for their stroll. The dietitian wondered if maybe the extra caffeine (2 more cups) could account for the fussiness that Jordie experienced on the weekend. She suggested that Brenda order a smaller coffee and see if it made a difference.

Four weeks later, Brenda was back to check in with the dietitian. And she had good news to report: the dietitian's suggestion had worked! Cutting back on her caffeine helped with the fussiness that Jordan exhibited on Saturdays, and the last 3 weekends had been much easier to handle. The dietitian explained that some babies are sensitive to caffeine, but it was likely to change as he continued to grow. Venti coffees were still in Brenda's future!

We all know that weight gain during pregnancy is normal, natural, and healthy, but many moms are still a bit anxious about shedding the "baby weight" once baby is born. It doesn't help that we're constantly surrounded by images of celebrities who "effortlessly" (with personal trainers, chefs, nannies, huge bank accounts, and Photoshop to help out!) bounce back to their prepregnancy weight in a few weeks. That's not realistic, and that's not the norm. It's really important to remember that it took 10 months to put on the weight necessary to support a healthy pregnancy, and it will take time to lose it. Patience, momma!

It's normal to want to reach your comfortable pre-pregnancy weight, but losing weight too fast can put you at risk for nutrient deficiencies, decreased metabolism, and issues with breastmilk supply and quality, so try to give yourself a break—be patient with postpartum weight loss and give yourself time to lose it healthfully. And know that it's okay if you don't get back to your prepregnancy weight. Try to embrace your new, beautiful post-baby bod—and remember that your value is not based on the number on the scale.

If you're breastfeeding, make sure that you wait until your supply has been established and is steady before attempting to lose any weight. You may have heard that breastfeeding can help with weight loss—it can for some women who breastfeed for at least 6 months, but it's not always the case. Regardless, breastfeeding has endless benefits for both mom and baby (read more on page 154), so we highly encourage it.

SARAH SAYS: *It wasn't until I was completely done breastfeeding (even a few months after) all 3 of my babies that I actually felt like I "had my body back" (and even then, it was never quite the same). Slowly but surely, I increased my activity level and tried my best to eat nutritious meals and snacks, and listen to my body when it came to how much I ate (which was more than typical), and eventually I reached a weight that I felt comfortable at. It was hard to wait, and tempting to push myself harder, but I'm glad I took a gradual approach because both helped to keep my milk supply up and helped me to reach my ideal weight in a healthy and sustainable way.*

After having a baby, how do I lose weight in a healthy way?

It's important to lose weight slowly—no more than about one pound per week—to avoid an impact on your milk supply. We suggest a more mindful, realistic, and long-term approach to losing baby weight rather than going on a "diet" with strategies that won't leave you feeling deprived or restricted. Here are our top strategies for healthy weight loss:

Stay properly hydrated

Drink more water: For weight loss? Yes! Thirst is often confused as hunger, which leads to mindless snacking when, really, all your body needs is a good drink of water. You will drink more water if you always carry a water bottle around with you, as seeing it will remind you to drink it. Sip all day.

Drink water instead of sweet drinks: Okay, how crazy is this: the top source of added sugar in our diets is sweetened drinks—soft drinks, juice, sweet coffee drinks, lemonade, iced tea . . . all of them! Unfortunately, they provide sugar and calories, but few nutrients.

Tasty Ways To Enjoy Water

MAKE IT FRUITY: Squeeze in some fresh orange, lemon, or lime for a refreshingly zesty taste; or infuse with watermelon, apple, or pineapple slices for fruity flavor.

SPICE IT UP: Add a whole cinnamon stick, or try flavor combinations like ginger-lemon-mint, or apple-cinnamon, or add ginger slices to sparkling water to make ginger ale.

FRESHEN WITH HERBS: Fresh mint leaves are awesome.

MAKE IT SPA WATER: Just add cucumber slices, close your eyes, and pretend you're at the spa!

TRY ICED TEA: Brew hot herbal tea then refrigerate.

So you end up drinking a ton of calories, and you don't compensate by eating any less! If you're trying to drop the baby weight, stick to water. You can jazz it up if you find plain water too boring.

SARAH SAYS: *I bought a pretty purple water bottle and it never left my side while I was nursing my little ones. Having it with me reminded me to sip all day—otherwise I would have forgotten to drink!*

Foods to choose

Eat breakfast: It may be 4:30 a.m. (good morning, baby!), but you have to start your day with some morning fuel. Eating a healthy breakfast containing protein can help you control your appetite and cravings all day, and prevents mindless snacking later on. It also gives your metabolism a kick-start first thing in the morning. We know how easy it is to get caught up in morning survival mode with babies (especially if you have other children at home too!), so having something quick and easy to grab may come in handy.

Healthy, Quick Breakfast Ideas

OVERNIGHT OATS: Toss equal amounts oats and yogurt in a jar with lid. Refrigerate overnight. Add fruit and nuts in the morning.

AVOCADO TOAST: Toast whole grain bread and top with mashed avocado, a fried egg, and hemp seeds.

QUICK PARFAIT: Layer Greek yogurt with fruit, nuts, seeds, and your favorite granola or whole grain cereal.

DRESSED UP BANANA: Slice a banana and top it with nut or seed butter and a sprinkle of nuts, seeds, or coconut.

EGG IT UP: Hard boil eggs in advance. Mash onto whole grain toast with some mayonnaise and top with sliced tomato and fresh herbs.

Eat fiber-rich foods: Eating enough fiber is key for digestive health and preventing chronic disease, but did you know it's also key for weight management? Fiber-rich foods like vegetables, fruits, whole grains, and beans are more filling because they slowly make their way through your digestive tract, keeping you feeling fuller for longer. Include high-fiber foods at each meal and snack. Read more about fiber on pages 27 to 29.

WE GOT YOU!

Try to eat something before drinking that first cup of coffee (we know . . . this might be hard when you're sleep deprived). Coffee can be an appetite suppressant and blunt your natural hunger cues, making you think you're not hungry (or just increasing the likelihood that you'll forget to eat!).

SARAH SAYS: *Because time was so precious when I had wee ones, I remember buying ready-to-eat, precut vegetables like baby carrots, snap peas, mini cucumbers, and baby tomatoes. I would aim for at least 4 servings per day and at least 3 different colors. Convenience was key, and this is where I cut corners and gave myself a break.*

Physical Activity

Wear your baby everywhere: We agree on this one: the best postpartum purchase we ever made was definitely a good-quality baby carrier. Instead of putting our little ones in a swing or bouncy chair, we both wore carriers for much of the time. Yup. Cleaning, cooking, playing with other children, going out for a walk, shopping in the grocery store—baby was attached! Aside from the closeness and extra bonding that comes from wearing a baby carrier, you also burn extra calories throughout the day. Win-win!

Find other ways to be active: If you can fit in exercise classes, a bike ride, or a run while someone watches baby, count yourself lucky! For many of us, exercise will likely involve both mom and baby, so you'll have to find a way! Do not give up hope—you have lots of options:

- Look for mom and baby stroller fitness, barre, aerobics, or yoga classes in your area. Baby is by your side (or in the stroller) the whole time.
- Find fellow moms and walk together with strollers or baby carriers.

- Exercise at home during naptime. Find online fitness videos that suit your exercise style (Zumba? yoga? HIIT training?) and follow along. Listen to your body—don't overdo it.
- Look online for gently used exercise equipment at reasonable prices and make a small home gym. You can get free weights, resistance bands, and a gym mat for about $20 to $30.

CARA SAYS: *I found a local stroller fitness class through a neighborhood Facebook page, and looked forward to my weekly sessions. Not only did I get to walk, stretch, and squat, but I met fellow neighborhood moms who commiserated with me about sleepless nights, breastfeeding woes, and the joys of baby smiles. I'm usually a loner during exercise, but this like-minded group turned out to be exactly what I needed when my baby was just a few months old.*

Set yourself up for success

The "see-food syndrome": This isn't about eating lobster and shrimp. We often talk about the "see-food diet" as in, if you see food, you want to eat it! Few people are immune to the allure of the cookie jar. When you leave tempting snack foods in plain sight (likely on the kitchen counter), it activates the areas of your brain that control appetite and reward, and can actually make you feel hungry. It makes food very hard to resist when temptation is right in front of you—especially when that food is a treat. The last thing you want to do when you're overwhelmed and exhausted is ALSO test your willpower. Hint: you'll likely lose. Weight loss becomes very hard when you rely on willpower alone (ahem . . . this is a big part of the reason that weight loss diets DON'T work long term), so do yourself a favor and control your environment—keep tempting snack foods out of sight and throwing some fruits and vegetables into a basket on your counter instead.

> (REALITY CHECK)
>
> Studies show that simply viewing high-calorie food images can activate the brain regions that control appetite and reward, and significantly increase feelings of hunger and desire for sweet and savory foods.

Breastfeed! Women who breastfeed exclusively for more than 3 months tend to lose more weight than those who do not. Bonus: if you continue to breastfeed beyond 6 months, you continue to lose weight. So if you're able to breastfeed,

Don't have unrealistic post-baby weight loss goals. There is an incredible amount of pressure of moms to lose weight postpartum and "bounce back" to their prebaby bodies. You may turn to dieting as a way to shed pregnancy pounds and to feel more like "yourself," but dieting in the postpartum period has been linked to poor body image, increased mental health challenges, and eating disorders. New moms who deprive themselves of food and nutrients may be creating nutrient deficiencies that can trigger a whole host of problems. Trust us when we say that postpartum recovery and healing goes much better when you nourish your body optimally.

it helps you in the postpartum weight-loss department (everyone is different, of course—and some mommas find breastfeeding has no link to their weight). Aside from the many benefits of breastfeeding, by exclusively nursing, you can burn an extra 300 to 600 calories per day. Cool!

Be your own priority: Yes, you may have a crazy toddler and a fussy baby. But that doesn't mean that you should neglect your own health and settle into a weight that doesn't feel right. We truly believe that part of being a good mom means taking care of yourself, and slowly getting back to your healthy and comfortable weight is part of that.

CARA SAYS: *Ah, social media. On the one hand, it connects us to mom groups with timely advice and realistic portrayals of life as a new parent. On the other hand, it bombards us with images of "ideal" lifestyles—perfect bodies, well-behaved kids, clean kitchens, etc. Remember that these idealized, airbrushed people on social media only post select, staged snapshots of their lives (the best possible ones), so try not to compare yourself to what you see on the screen. You have the power to choose whom you follow on social media. If fit bodies and clean homes are inspiring, have at it. But if they make you feel bad, or not "enough," unfollow them, and fill your feed with like-minded people who have positive, realistic messages that you identify with.*

What can I do to ease postpartum constipation?

We've both been there—just when we thought the pushing was over, it wasn't. Too much information?! Probably not, because you're likely going through (or will go through) the same thing. So we'll give it to you straight: pooping after having a baby freaking sucks. Constipation affects 25% to 50% of women during the first 2 weeks postpartum. It's usually caused by a combo of dehydration, pregnancy hormones (like progesterone, which slows bowel function), and perhaps a lack of fiber-rich foods (see page 27). Oh, and the fear of pushing! It hurts, especially if you had a bad tear or a C-section.

Other than stool softeners (which totally work, and they may send you home from the hospital with some), here are some things you can do to ease constipation:

Drink lots and lots of fluids, especially water: Dehydration is common among new moms, so it's important to pay extra-close attention to drinking a lot, especially water. This will help to move food through your digestive tract effectively (and help with digestion in general), and boost your milk supply!

Eat fiber-rich foods often: Foods high in insoluble fiber, such as fruits, vegetables, and bran, can increase bowel transit time (speed things up). Foods with soluble fiber, like oats, barley, beans, and psyllium, can help form a bowel movement that is easier to pass. Both are important for easing or even preventing constipation.

Limit refined, ultra-processed foods: Foods that are highly processed and refined typically lack fiber and can "bind" your stool (make it harder and not as easy to pass), which can worsen symptoms of constipation. Try to minimize them.

Consider changing your nutrition supplements: If you've been taking an iron supplement during pregnancy, continuing to take it in the postpartum period could make constipation worse. Talk to your doctor about getting blood work done again to check your iron status, and perhaps ditch the iron supplement if you don't need it. Focus on iron-rich foods such as meat, poultry, fish, eggs, beans, lentils, and leafy greens.

Can nutrition help prevent or treat postpartum mental health issues?

It's estimated that postpartum mental health complications—things like depression and anxiety—affect about 10% to 15% of women in the months and years post-baby, whether it's a new or a re-emerging condition.

Postpartum depression and anxiety develop due to a variety of factors, including physical (factors related to the body) and environmental (experiences or external factors). There is no one single factor that causes postpartum depression or anxiety, and it's often the result of many different issues combined, many of which you cannot control or prevent, like your genetics or your birth experience. Most importantly, please know, it's not your fault.

REALITY CHECK

It's important to understand that postpartum depression is a real mental illness that often requires comprehensive and professional help and treatment for healthy recovery. Better nutrition and supplements *alone* are not cures for postpartum depression and mental illness, but rather, should be part of the treatment plan and recovery.

You might be at greater risk of postpartum mental health concerns if:

- You had a previous mental illness
- You have a family history of mental illness
- You had a challenging birth experience
- You lack family or economic support
- You struggled with physical stress from pregnancy and childbirth
- You have hormonal imbalances
- Your nutrition is inadequate, and you're lacking certain important nutrients

Postpartum depression can be treated in many different ways including therapy, medication, support groups, family support, and nutrition therapy. Many women decide to use a combination of methods.

The role of nutrition and maternal mental health isn't well understood , but luckily, more research is emerging. There are several studies that have found a connection between nutrition and perinatal depression. In fact, one review of 24 studies (and over 14,262 subjects) found that "pregnancy and lactation deplete nutrients essential to the neurotransmission system," which could be one reason for the increased risk of depression postpartum.[40] Certain key nutrients are needed in greater quantities during pregnancy and postpartum (we talk all about this on pages 74 to 78), and deficiencies in these nutrients may put mom at an increased risk of postpartum depression. Make sure you get enough of these nutrients through food and supplements (if necessary):

- Vitamin D (see more on page 30)
- Essential omega-3 fatty-acids, including EPA/DHA (see more on page 24)
- Trace minerals, including selenium, zinc, and iron (see more on page 25)
- B-vitamins

To do this, aim for balance and variety in your meals and snacks (see page 13), and make sure that you're not *forgetting* to eat (which can happen easily when you're busy with a new baby!). Nutritional supplements can be great way to fill in the nutritional gaps during pregnancy and postpartum. But it is important to work with a registered dietitian to determine what supplements might be necessary and appropriate for you. Read more about supplementing post-pregnancy on page 124).

WE GOT YOU!

We both know how tiring and overwhelming the postpartum period is. And even for us dietitians, it's hard to find the time to prep food and eat well during this time. That's why we HIGHLY recommend that you accept help from loved ones and friends who offer to make and deliver meals and snacks for you. And if you get the open-ended question "what do you need?" or "how can we help?" ask for nutritious food. Trust us! The best food gifts are things like freezable dinners, nutritious baked goods, and one-handed snacks. Ordering groceries online or using meal-kit services, even just temporarily, can help to lighten your load too.

Being a parent is stressful. Am I drinking too much alcohol?

We debated writing this section in the book because it can be a bit "touchy." But we felt that it was common enough (and likely not talked about enough) that it was worth addressing. The truth is, women are drinking alcohol more frequently than ever before. In fact, alcohol abuse among women more than doubled from 2002 to 2013, according to the National Institute on Alcohol Abuse and Alcoholism.

It's a cultural phenomenon that can be drilled down to a few simple memes bearing phrases like "mommy juice" or "it's wine o'clock." And it's quite common to open a bottle of wine while making dinner, sip some during the meal, maybe a bit more post-dinner, and suddenly the bottle of wine is gone. And you think . . . "oops–how did that happen?" There also seems to be a lot more mommy groups where alcohol is the most enticing part of the gathering–even though you meet under the guise of a book club or card game.

Listen. We understand as well as anyone how stressful raising kids can be, and that wine (or vodka, or beer, or . . .) can certainly take the edge off. And sometimes it's really nice to get together with fellow mommies and have a martini or 2. So maybe you're wondering . . . is drinking alcohol safe? Or how much is too much? Here are some general guidelines about drinking alcohol when you're NOT pregnant or breastfeeding:

> **REALITY CHECK**
>
> If you are having more than one drink a day on most days, you are at an increased risk for heart, liver, and pancreatic disease, as well as at increased risk for certain types of cancer, including breast cancer. Keep track of your intake and try to limit yourself to 1 drink per day. If you have trouble sticking to this limit, talk to your doctor about seeking help.

- **If you don't drink alcohol, we don't recommend that you start.** There are no "necessary" nutrients in beer, wine, or spirits, so you're not missing out. And yep, red wine contains antioxidants, but so do grapes–so you don't actually *need* to drink wine (but nice try).

- **If you do drink, have no more than one standard-size drink per day (see page 135).** This is a safe level that most women can metabolize before alcohol builds up and causes harm (and nope, you can't "save up" and have 7 drinks on Saturday). Men can metabolize 2 drinks a day, so their daily limit is a bit higher.

SARAH SAYS: *I love enjoying a glass of wine while making dinner, and certainly share a bottle of prosecco with some girlfriends now and then. But I do try to keep my alcohol consumption in check by sticking to one drink per night (most of the time) and either saying no to more, or swapping out an alcoholic drink for a virgin one (or just water). Despite the many risks of excessive alcohol consumption, you also don't feel great the next day, which, as a mom, can make an already busy day even more challenging.*

CARA SAYS: *I'm a non-drinker in a drinking world, which makes social situations awkward. Yep, people hound me for a reason why I don't have a wine glass in my hand. I'm often asked if I'm pregnant or if I'm observant in a religion that shuns alcohol. Nope, neither. Then people assume that I don't drink because I'm a dietitian and I follow a super-strict healthy diet (ha! they should see my chocolate cupboard!) But it's not that either. It's simple: I don't like the smell or taste of alcohol. I don't even like rum balls (and they contain chocolate)! If you're out with a non-drinker, respect their choice and make sure they respect your choice too. No judgment either way, right?*

DEEP DIVE: ALCOHOL AND BREAST CANCER

More than 100 studies have looked at the association between alcohol and breast cancer, and have consistently found an increased risk of breast cancer associated with women with higher alcohol intake. A meta-analysis of 53 studies showed that women who had approximately 3 drinks per day had 1.5 times higher risk of developing breast cancer when compared to non-drinkers. But even moderate drinking correlates with increased breast cancer risk. Studies show that for every 10 grams of alcohol consumed per day (slightly less than one drink), researchers observed a 7% increased risk of breast cancer.[41]

For information about drinking alcohol during pregnancy, see page 93. For information about alcohol intake while breastfeeding, see page 135.

Top 10 Tips
for postpartum

1 Drink lots of water.
If you're breastfeeding, you'll always be thirsty! Choose water most often.

2 Remember that you need to eat too.
Taking care of a baby is hard work, but don't forget to care for yourself.

3 Eat a bit extra.
You need an extra 350 to 400 calories per day to support breastfeeding.

4 Keep snacks handy.
You will be busy (and hungry), so plan for nutritious snack breaks.

5 Eat balanced meals.
Keep energy levels up. Make sure meals have protein, whole grains, and vegetables.

6 Be realistic about weight loss.
It took 10 months to put all the weight on; you can't lose it all in 2 weeks!

7 Know that caffeine is okay.
We suggest no more than 300 milligrams of caffeine, or about 2 cups of regular coffee per day.

8 Be safe with alcohol.
If you have a drink, have it right after breastfeeding. Avoid breastfeeding for 2 or 3 hours.

9 Be your own priority.
Make time for yourself every day.

10 Ask for help.
If this is all new to you, rely on family and friends who have been through it before.

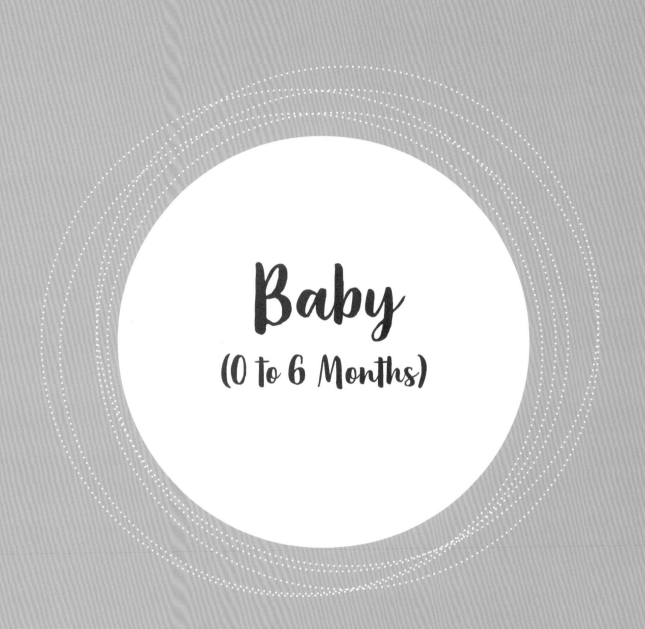

Baby

(0 to 6 Months)

Introduction

We believe strongly that "fed is best." Together, we've had 5 experiences feeding babies, each unique and different (and both rewarding and challenging in their own ways). Feeding babies is not easy for everyone, and there's a lot of pressure for moms to breastfeed their babies exclusively. And hey, if that works out for you, it's amazing and wonderful! But although it may be easy for some moms, it's not as easy for others. That's why we say fed is best—making sure your baby is nourished is priority number one, whether it's from breast or bottle, using breastmilk or formula.

We have no doubt you're going to have a ton of questions about timing of feeds, your baby's bowel movements, digestive issues (like spitting up, reflux, constipation, etc.), or maybe questions about infant formula or when to introduce solid foods. We cover it all and more in this chapter. Read on!

Nutrients

Your baby will get all of the nutrients that they need from breastmilk or formula for the first 6 months of their life. The only supplement that's always recommended for breastfed babies is vitamin D. Breastmilk does not provide very much vitamin D, so you have to give it to your baby separately using liquid drops, which are available at any pharmacy.

Commercially prepared infant formula is nutritionally complete, so unless your baby has a diagnosed vitamin or mineral deficiency, nutrition supplementation isn't usually required (even vitamin D is not needed when babies are exclusively formula-fed, and consuming at least 32 ounces per day because the vitamin D is added to the formula).

Breastfeeding and formula-feeding

When it comes down to it, deciding whether or not to breastfeed is a very personal decision. You need to make the best decision for you and your baby. Maybe that means exclusively breastfeeding, or maybe it means a combination of breastfeeding and pumping so that you can have a bit of flexibility. Or maybe formula-feeding works better for you and your family.

Even if you want to breastfeed, there can be many reasons why it's just not possible including milk supply issues, anxiety, or a medical condition. When you have tried, reached out for support, tried again, and just can't do it any longer, it can be very emotional and disheartening. But you're an amazing mom and you will still bond with your baby. Regardless of feeding method, your baby can be well nourished and you will have the opportunity to bond and reap the emotional benefits of feeding them by bottle.

> **When it comes down to it, deciding whether or not to breastfeed is a very personal decision. You need to make the best decision for you and your baby.**

Your baby's day

Many parents want a detailed feeding schedule and routine to follow, with guidance on specific amounts at each feeding too. But unfortunately, when it comes to babies, there really is no schedule. And trust us. We are both efficient, organized, type-A personalities. If there was a schedule that worked for every mom, we would have found it by now! And we would share it here. Instead, the most important thing is trusting your baby's cues (read about this on page 160).

Growth charts

When your baby is born you will likely be introduced to growth charts. Growth charts use percentiles to mark where your baby falls in relation to a reference population of the same age and gender. For example, if your baby's weight puts them on the 10th percentile, that means that 10 out of 100 babies (10%) weigh less than them, and 90 out of 100 babies (90%) weigh more. Growth charts are used to track the progress of your baby's growth over the months and years ahead. Sometimes the information they show can be alarming (why is my baby so different!?), but it shouldn't be. Kids come in all different shapes and sizes. Heck, children from the same family may fall on very different percentiles! Sarah's oldest child has been on the 75 percentile since birth, while her youngest has consistently landed on the 25.

The goal is for your baby's growth to follow a fairly regular growth pattern, regardless of where they fall on the chart. So, if your baby is born on the 15 percentile, it makes sense that they continue along that growth curve (15 percentile or thereabouts) through-out childhood. The point is to make sure that your baby is growing steadily and not jumping too much higher or lower than their natural curve, which might indicate a health or nutritional concern.

Oh, those serene images of mom shrouded in silky sleepwear, beautifully groomed, and lovingly gazing down at baby with a perfect latch. Is she floating on a cloud? Maybe. Because she sure isn't down in the real world! Hey, guess what? BREAST-FEEDING CAN BE &%$%@#$ HARD! Some moms are lucky and baby takes to it right away, mom's milk supply is plentiful, and baby has a good latch. Amazing. But sometimes it feels like a little alligator is biting at your already dry and cracked nipples. And you're raw and sore—not quite the same as floating blissfully on a cloud in breastmilk heaven. The good news is that if you stick with it, things *do* often get easier and start to feel more "natural" (but not for all, and that's okay!). Here are some words of encouragement for why breastfeeding can be worth sticking with:

Benefits for baby

Immune-supporting properties: Breastmilk provides perfect nutrition and immune-supporting properties for baby at every stage. It contains the exact right amount of protein, carbohydrates, fat, vitamins, and minerals that your baby needs. And as your baby grows, your milk changes to keep up with your baby's needs.

Brain-boosting nutrition: Breastmilk naturally contains nutrients that are important for brain development, including omega-3 fats. It also provides antibodies that are important for immune function, which protects against digestive, respiratory, and ear infections, and the development of allergies and asthma. Breastfeeding can also decrease the risk of sudden infant death syndrome (SIDS).

Possible prevention of future diseases: Some studies show that breastfed babies are less likely to develop chronic diseases such as type 2 diabetes and heart disease.

> **SARAH SAYS:** *I had 3 very different experiences with breastfeeding each child. I struggled big-time with my first, never having enough supply even with lactation consultant help, cluster-feeding, and nipple shields. I ended up pumping exclusively for 6 months and it worked wonderfully for us. With my second, I had an OVERsupply (which I was thrilled about at first, until my daughter cried and screamed constantly, likely from being overfed, gassy, and uncomfortable). Guidance from our lactation consultant really did help, and I ended up*

breastfeeding her until 1 year. With my third, everything was great—breastfed without a problem. Go figure! Even with the same boobs and same mom, breastfeeding experiences can be so completely unique.

Benefits for mom

Warm fuzzies: Some moms feel happiness and fulfillment (that nice fuzzy feeling) from the attachment that they experience while breastfeeding (some other moms don't feel this—and that's totally normal!). The feel-good feeling becomes even stronger with hormones that are released while nursing, including prolactin and oxytocin. Prolactin gives you a sense of peace and calm, which can help you to focus on your baby while nursing. Oxytocin is known as the "love hormone" because it can help to make you feel a strong sense of love and attachment while breastfeeding.

Healing: Breastfeeding can help with recovery after childbirth because the hormone oxytocin helps the uterus return to its regular size more quickly and reduces postpartum bleeding.

Lower risk of obesity and chronic disease: Research shows that women who have breastfed their babies have reduced rates of breast and ovarian cancer later in life. It also may protect moms against developing chronic diseases like type 2 diabetes, rheumatoid arthritis, and heart disease. Oh, and um, breastfeeding delays the return of your period! Need we say more?!

Some other benefits of breastfeeding:

- It's economical: breastmilk is completely free!
- It can be easy (once you get the hang of it) and can save you time and energy making up and warming bottles.
- It's always with you! Whether you're out and about running errands, at a friend's house, or out of town, your milk is always ready and available.

> **WE GOT YOU!**
>
> We encourage you to arm yourself with knowledge and support when it comes to breastfeeding, even before baby comes. We know, we know . . . you're probably only focusing on labor and delivery before baby comes— we were too! But trust us, it's good to be even a little prepared because you'll be tired and drained once baby comes home. Being prepared might include having a list of lactation consultants you can reach out to if you're experiencing challenges, and knowing how to access public health resources.

- It's better for the environment, because there's less waste and water usage with cleaning bottles.

CARA SAYS: *The biggest surprise to me was abdominal pain that I felt in the first few minutes of my baby latching on to feed. It was excruciating—like very intense period cramps. I quickly learned that it was normal—my lactation consultant explained that it was the feeling of my uterus shrinking back to its normal size. So if you get similar cramps, know that they last only a minute or 2 during each feed, and they go away within the first few days of breastfeeding.*

DEEP DIVE: COLOSTRUM

Colostrum is liquid gold. If you are breastfeeding, when you first start feeding your baby, you'll produce a type of milk called "colostrum," which is thick and yellowish. It's high in carbohydrates, protein, and antibodies, but comes out in small quantities. Newborns have small stomachs and colostrum delivers a very concentrated form of nutrients and immune protection that your baby needs in these early days. The antibodies contained in it protect your baby's mucous membranes in the throat, lungs, and intestines—which is pretty cool—and it contains leukocytes, which help to protect your baby from harmful viruses and bacteria. Colostrum also helps to establish your baby's gut microflora (healthy bacteria). It's truly liquid gold!

Colostrum also has a mild laxative effect, which helps baby to pass meconium, which is the first type of bowel movement that baby has (it's really thick, dark, and sticky—kind of like molasses). After 3 to 4 days of producing colostrum, you will start to produce regular breastmilk.

What about formula-feeding?

Infant formula is a breastmilk substitute that is safe and nutritious. It's usually made from cow's milk protein, and vitamins and minerals are added to help mimic breastmilk. Infant formulas are also often fortified with extra nutrients like omega-3 fat and probiotics (or prebiotics). There are several varieties and brands to choose from, but what's important is that it's an approved, regulated formula. You do NOT want to make your own baby formula at home—it brings on many concerns, nutrition- and safety-wise (see page 170).

Benefits to formula-feeding

Safe and nutritious: When breastfeeding isn't a viable option, formula gives parents a safe and nutritious alternative to feeding their babies.

Flexibility: Moms who formula-feed are able to have a bit of space and leave their baby with a caregiver and not have to worry about needing to be there for all feeds.

Bonding/feeding for other parent: Bottle-feeding allows both parents as well as older siblings or grandparents to experience the joys of feeding their baby, which can help with bonding and attachment.

Often fortified with nutrients that breastfed infants don't get through breastmilk alone: Commercial infant formula contains important nutrients such as iron, vitamin D, and sometimes even omega-3 and probiotics, and this may cut down on the need for giving your baby nutritional supplements.

Drawbacks to formula-feeding

Digestibility: Some babies have a harder time digesting formula versus breastmilk.

Lack of immune-boosting properties: It lacks the immune-boosting properties (antibodies) that breastmilk has.

> **WE GOT YOU!**
> Every situation is unique, and we both believe that there needs to be less judgment when it comes to how parents choose to feed their babies. Fed is best.

Not as protective for mom: It doesn't offer the same health benefits to mom (decreased risk of certain cancers and chronic diseases) as breastfeeding does.

Doesn't release the same hormones: Bottle-feeding doesn't provide the same "happy hormone" release for mom as breastfeeding. That's not to say that bottle-feeding doesn't allow for bonding, because it does!

Expensive: Formula costs money (about $100 per month).

A little more work: Bottle-feeding requires preparing formula, sanitizing bottles, warming bottles up, etc., so it may add some time to your day.

SARAH SAYS: *A good friend of mine had a deep desire to breastfeed, but she experienced so much anxiety when attempting to breastfeed in the early days that she decided to formula-feed right from the beginning. Her anxiety melted away as soon as she decided not to breastfeed, and she was able to focus on bonding and loving her babies instead of being anxious and wound up. She was a better, more relaxed mom because she chose to formula-feed. Everyone's experience is different!*

How often should I feed my baby?

We believe strongly in baby-led feeding, even with bottle-fed babies. If you're able to pay attention to baby's cues, feed responsively, and resist the urge to stick to a rigid schedule when it comes to feeding, you can rest easy knowing that your baby is getting the perfect amount for proper growth and development.

Breastfed babies

For moms who breastfeed, it's all about supply and demand. To establish a good milk supply and flow, we suggest babies are fed on demand. This is called baby-led feeding, and it helps you to recognize and respond to your baby's appetite, hunger, and fullness cues, and nurtures your baby's natural ability to eat intuitively (see page 44). Because your baby can't tell you when they're hungry, it's important to be responsive to their hunger cues, such as "rooting" (moving their mouth and turning their head toward your chest), sucking on their hand or arm, smacking their lips together, or becoming restless.

If you're able to respond to these initial signs of hunger (and not wait until your baby is so hungry that they're crying or really upset), your baby will happily start sucking and drink what they need, and they'll stop when they're comfortably full. If you wait too long, they might be too upset to feed. This can create stress and anxiety for both mom and baby and disrupt what could have otherwise been a happy and successful feed.

WE GOT YOU!

Feeding responsively and following baby's cues will encourage self-regulation and discourage the tendency to overfeed or underfeed. Although we know this can be a little easier with breastfeeding, we also truly believe that bottle-feeding can be baby-led too (see 159) as long as parents pay really close attention to baby's cues. The feeding pattern becomes more consistent and "scheduled" once you introduce solids and start to have a routine of meal and snack times.

Your breastfed baby will let you know when they've had enough or they want more. In most cases, your baby will consume most of what's available during the first 10 minutes of feeding on each breast, then might move away or doze off. When your baby is done, they may turn their head or give other signs of being done.

Bottle/formula-fed babies

Formula-fed babies, in the first weeks of life, will tend to eat a little less frequently than breastfed babies—about every 3 to 4 hours (simply because formula is digested more slowly than breastmilk). Of course, this can vary from day to day, and from baby to baby. Watch for baby's hunger cues, as mentioned above, and try not to use the clock as a guide or stick to a strict schedule.

On average, by the end of the first month, your baby should be drinking at least 4 ounces of formula per feed. By 6 months, they'll likely be consuming about 6 to 8 ounces per feed. But again, this can vary a lot.

> **REALITY CHECK**
>
> How long does it take to breastfeed a baby? Most feeds will be 10 to 15 minutes, but it's normal for babies to feed for as little as 1 minute or as much as 45 to 50 minutes. Let their hunger dictate. And how many times a day will they feed? It's whenever they are hungry, but for newborns it's usually around 8 to 12 times in a 24-hour period, or roughly every 2 to 3 hours. More or less.

Cluster-feeding

"Cluster-feeding" is when babies feed very frequently for a period of hours or even days, without warning or clear reason (usually it's because they're going through a heavy growth stage). This is when you really need to trust your baby and follow their cues—they know how much they need! Oh, and stock up on patience, humor, and any help you can get!

How do I know if my baby has had enough?

Here's the thing: babies are very intuitive and will let you know when they're full or when they want more. Watch and respond to their hunger and fullness cues.

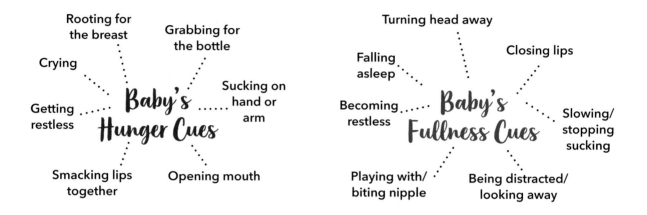

Baby's Hunger Cues
- Rooting for the breast
- Grabbing for the bottle
- Crying
- Sucking on hand or arm
- Getting restless
- Smacking lips together
- Opening mouth

Baby's Fullness Cues
- Turning head away
- Closing lips
- Falling asleep
- Becoming restless
- Slowing/ stopping sucking
- Playing with/ biting nipple
- Being distracted/ looking away

Instead of shoving the bottle or breast into your baby's mouth, wait for their cue to feed more. And if there's no cue, don't bring the bottle or breast to their mouth again. If you're not convinced that your baby is getting enough, you can use their wet diapers as a guide. Your baby will likely have about 6 wet diapers per day in the first month and about 3 to 4 bowel movements per day. Your baby will also seem satisfied and not show signs of hunger for about 2 to 3 hours after each feed if they are getting enough unless they're cluster feeding (see page 159).

> **REALITY CHECK**
>
> Your baby may lose a bit of weight in the first couple of weeks of life, as your milk supply establishes (if you are breastfeeding). Totally normal. Once they've regained their birth-weight, a great indicator that they're getting enough is if there's fairly steady weight gain from there on. Whether breast- or formula-fed, babies usually gain about 1½ to 3 pounds per month for the first 3 months of life, and then the rate of weight gain slows from 3 to 6 months—about ½ to 1½ pounds per month. Read about growth charts on page 153. If you're concerned about your baby's growth (or lack thereof), or they're failing to thrive or showing signs of being malnourished, chat with your baby's pediatrician or doctor.

Is it okay to feed my baby to soothe?

Sometimes it can be hard to decipher whether your baby is hungry or just needs soothing (right?!) because babies suck when they need soothing (and it is normal!), and this can be confused with hunger. As you get to know your baby more, you'll be able to distinguish between their hunger cues and their need for soothing. It's hard for parents to know whether to let baby suck on the breast or bottle versus a pacifier or finger. Babies suck for comfort regardless, and sometimes for sleep too, so this creates a bit of a dilemma. We wish we had a more clear-cut answer here. It's really a personal choice!

> **(SHADES OF GRAY: COMFORT FEEDING)**
>
> There are many differing opinions when it comes to comfort feeding. Some experts believe that nursing babies to sleep and for comfort is perfectly normal and beneficial, while others believe that nursing or bottle-feeding should be reserved only for nourishment.
>
> **Breastfeeding:** There's some research that shows breastfeeding can help a baby sleep, may calm them, and can help them handle stress better. Sucking releases the hormone cholecystokinin in both mom and baby, which results in sleepiness. Breastmilk also contains sleep-inducing hormones (such as melatonin), amino acids, and nucleotides, which have higher concentrations during the night and may actually help babies establish their own circadian rhythms (and help them sleep!).
>
> **Bottle-feeding:** Bottle-feeding is a little different, in that the milk is coming out at a steady stream (and often faster) than with breastfeeding. If formula is being used, it won't contain all of the additional benefits mentioned above. And if it's pumped breastmilk, it may not contain the same beneficial factors if it was pumped during the day rather than at night. So we don't recommend letting baby fall asleep sipping on a bottle for these reasons.

CARA SAYS: *I nursed my babies to sleep when they were little, and I found that their hunger level would dictate how long that would take. When they were not very hungry, a 2-minute breastfeed could lull them to sleep. When their appetite was more robust, the feed could last 15 minutes or more! Remember, babies have an innate sense of fullness (and sleepiness) that you can trust.*

What do I do if I encounter breastfeeding challenges?

If you find breastfeeding challenging (and, trust us, so many moms do!) or it's not going as you had planned, here's what we recommend:

Seek help from a lactation consultant: Lactation consultants are trained specifically to help breastfeeding moms deal with common challenges associated with breastfeeding. Often, one suggestion or little tweak will make a world of difference. They know things about nipple shields, proper positions, good latches, and the right supplements or medications to boost milk production.

If that lactation consultant isn't as helpful as you had hoped, connect with another one . . . and then another one. Not every lactation consultant will be a great fit, so if one isn't helpful, try another one. If you feel like you are being bullied or shamed (sadly, this happens), move on to someone else ASAP!

Be patient: It took both of us weeks, if not months, to establish a good milk supply and feel confident breastfeeding. Try to have patience and know that with time and a bit of perseverance, it does get easier.

Try pumping: Using a breast pump or manually expressing breastmilk instead of breastfeeding (or *as well as* breastfeeding) is a great option for moms who are experiencing challenges with breastfeeding but are producing milk. This is an option that can be discussed with a lactation consultant and can either be done exclusively (as an alternative to breastfeeding), or to supplement breastfeeding to give you a break and some flexibility.

Give yourself permission to explore other options. You're a good mom no matter what. And what's important is that your baby is fed and loved. If you're anxious, stressed, overwhelmed, in pain, and out of options to make breastfeeding work, know that there are other great options (i.e., formula). And again, you're an amazing mom no matter what.

CARA SAYS: *The fact that breastfeeding HURTS at the beginning seems to be a well-kept secret. Who knew? Certainly not me. Something that's so natural should be easy, right? Well, it's not always easy for everyone. I struggled for the first few weeks, but was well supported by lactation consultants at the hospital where I gave birth. They kept repeating this phrase over and over: "Remember, it is* breastfeeding, *not* nipple feeding.*" I had absolutely no freaking idea what that meant, until they showed me how my baby was sucking just on the tip of my breast, rather than having her tiny mouth latched higher up. Ohhhhhh. Nipple feeding. Got it. So take a look at the latch. Baby's mouth needs to be open wide when they latch on so they can develop a good strong suck.*

(REALITY CHECK)

When asked why they stopped breastfeeding, mothers give "not enough breastmilk" as the most common reason. But the reality is, insufficient breastmilk production is very rare. In most cases, this lack of milk is perceived rather than real.[42] Trust that your baby is getting what they need and consult with your doctor, lactation consultant, midwife, or public health nurse if you're curious or concerned. And turn to page 131 for our advice on foods and supplements that may be recommended to increase milk supply.

How do I pump and safely store breastmilk?

There are many reasons why women pump breastmilk. Whether you're a nursing mom returning to work, are seeking a bit of freedom to go out without baby in tow, or just want the option of feeding your baby a bottle instead of nursing, you might be wondering how to safely store your breastmilk to maximize its nutrition and minimize waste. (And if you've ever pumped and then accidentally SPILLED the gold, you know the pain of that waste!) Here is what you need to know:

COLLECTING BREASTMILK

- Always wash your hands prior to expressing or handling breastmilk.
- Collect the milk in freezer-safe milk storage bags or clean, sanitized bottles with tight screw caps. Avoid using formula bottle bags or regular sandwich-type storage bags, as they tend to leak easily and don't always seal properly.
- Label your bottles/bags with the date that your breastmilk was collected so that you can use the oldest milk first. If the milk is being used in a daycare or by a caregiver, add your child's name to the bottle or bag.
- Avoid adding freshly expressed milk to previously frozen milk, and discard milk from a bottle that was fed but not finished. This reduces the risk of bacterial growth.
- Clean your pump supplies thoroughly after each use.

THAWING BREASTMILK

- Transfer from the freezer to the refrigerator, or run the bottle or bag under warm water (or place it in a bowl of warm water).
- Do not use the microwave. Microwaves don't heat evenly, which could lead to milk with hot spots that can scald the baby. Microwaves can also damage the breastmilk and its nutrients.
- Do not refreeze breastmilk once it's thawed.

STORING BREASTMILK

Room temperature: Keep covered and as cool as possible.
- Temperature: up to 77°F
- Time: up to 6 to 8 hours

Insulated cooler bag: Make sure that ice packs are in direct contact with milk the entire time it is in the bag, and minimize opening the bag.
- Temperature: 5°F to 39°F
- Time: up to 24 hours

Refrigerator: Store at the back of the fridge, where the temperature is the most constant.
- Temperature: 39°F
- Time: up to 5 days

Freezer: Store at the back of the freezer, where the temperature is more constant.
- Freezer compartment in fridge (older models):
  - Temperature: 5°F
  - Time: up to 2 weeks

- Freezer compartment of fridge (with separate door):
  - Temperature: 0°F
  - Time: 3 to 6 months
- Chest or upright deepfreeze:
  - Temperature: −4°F
  - Time: 6 to 12 months

How do I choose the right formula for my baby?

If you've chosen to use formula, you're probably wondering which one is best. It's easy to feel overwhelmed walking down the formula aisle, pondering which one to choose: milk or soy-based? Liquid or powder? Omega-3-enriched or probiotic-enriched? You probably want us to give you 1 answer and a brand name for the formula we recommend. But the truth is, we can't. It's not that simple!

All commercial infant formula is regulated, which means it meets certain standards of safety and nutrient value, and it provides the similar nutrients found in breastmilk. Infant formulas have come a long way in the last decade or so—manufacturers are trying their best to mimic breastmilk, adding extra nutrients like omega-3 fat (which is important for brain and eye development), prebiotics, and probiotics (which can benefit baby's digestive system and immunity), and lutein for eye and brain health. There are also new formula varieties aimed to reduce spit-up and ease diarrhea, fussiness, gas, and colic, and some made especially for preterm and low-birthweight babies, older babies, and toddlers. Overwhelmed yet?! Don't worry, we'll help you figure out which one is best.

Types of infant formula

There are 3 main varieties of infant formula that are differentiated by the type of protein that they contain.

Cow's milk protein: This is the most popular and common formula, and tends to be the most economical as well. It's the most studied and tends to be the closest, nutritionally speaking, to breastmilk. Cow's milk formulas are appropriate for most formula-fed infants. Goat's milk formulas are also an option, but are less widely available.

Soy protein: Soy-based formulas are used for babies with a cow's milk protein allergy or intolerance, babies with galactosemia (a milk sugar intolerance), or babies who are being raised vegan. Experts have some conflicting opinions when it comes to soy-based formulas, and whether or not they're appropriate for preterm or low-birthweight babies. Some have questions about the effects of soy phytoestrogens, but research is not definitive.

Hydrolyzed/amino acid-based formulas: For those 2% to 3% of babies who have a true milk protein allergy, or who have multiple allergies or intolerances, there are hypoallergenic formulas (such as Nutramigen or Alimentum) that are specially formulated with predigested (already broken down) proteins and are much easier to digest. They are typically safe for those babies with cow's milk allergies.

There are also amino acid-based formulas, such as Neocate or EleCare, that are extremely costly (around $40 to $50 per can) but can be tolerated by babies who have trouble with all other formulas (including hydrolyzed formulas). It's important to talk to your pediatrician or dietitian prior to going this route.

> **REALITY CHECK**
>
> Babies who were born prematurely or at a low birthweight, or who have a compromised immune system, should be fed commercially produced liquid infant formula and not powdered formula, because of the higher risk of bacterial contamination with powders. If a parent absolutely has to feed powdered formula over liquid, it's important to sterilize the water by bringing it to a rolling boil for 2 minutes, then cooling it prior to mixing.

Trial and error

All babies are different, and the way they react to or tolerate formula is different too. You may try several varieties of formula within the first couple of months before you settle on the right one. There's no magic solution that will prevent or fix things like fussiness, gassiness, eczema, spitting up, etc. It's important to remember that fussiness, spitting up, and gassiness are all normal baby things. Babies' digestive systems are developing—some more quickly than others—and this can result in digestive woes (which might mean some long nights and tired mornings).

Give one variety a fighting chance before switching to another. Issues might even be exacerbated by trialing too many varieties in a short period. Any problems could also be the result of the feeding technique or type of bottle versus the formula ingredients. If you're really concerned and there's excess gassiness, spitting up, vomiting, or eczema, make sure to bring it up with your baby's doctor.

> **WE GOT YOU!**
>
> Make sure to get some guidance from a pediatrician, family doctor, or dietitian before starting a specialized formula, such as a soy or hydrolyzed formula. Advertising can drive decisions more than it should, so seek help from experts before making those decisions.

If your baby doesn't react well to the first formula you pick, it often simply comes down to trial and error and testing out a few different brands. If your baby has any reaction to an infant formula, see your pediatrician or dietitian to figure out what may be causing it.

CHOOSING YOUR BABY'S FORMULA

	Cow's milk protein	Soy protein	Hydrolyzed
What is it made from?	Cow's milk	Soybeans	Cow's milk protein broken down into smaller amino acids
Who should use it?	Babies with no special feeding needs	Babies who are vegan or have a milk allergy, lactose intolerance, or galactosemia	Babies who have trouble with digestion, lactose intolerance, milk protein allergy, or other multiple allergies
What's the cost?	$	$	$$$

Powdered or liquid concentrate formulas require you to add water, while liquid ready-to-use formulas don't. It's important to know that adding *too much* water to formula can put your baby at risk for "water intoxication," which may result in low blood sodium levels (not enough sodium in the blood) and can lead to low weight, irritability, and, in worst-case scenarios, coma or permanent brain damage.

Contrary to that, adding *too little* water can lead to diarrhea and dehydration, which can result in kidney issues and other serious medical concerns. Make sure to read the instructions carefully and dilute the formula exactly as directed on the can or bottle.

Also, do not keep prepared formula for more than 24 hours, and avoid keeping a bottle that's been partially consumed by your baby. Saving leftovers can introduce harmful bacteria that may cause diarrhea and dehydration.

Lactose is the sugar or carbohydrate source in milk and is present in most milk-based formulas (because lactose is naturally found in breastmilk, which formula tries to mimic). For babies who are lactose intolerant, there are a few varieties of cow's milk–based formulas that are lactose-free. Soy protein formulas or hydrolyzed formulas are available and lactose-free are as well. These are made with an alternative carbohydrate source to lactose, such as corn syrup solids, sucrose, tapioca starch, modified cornstarch, and glucose.

Should I choose an organic formula?

Certified organic infant formulas appeal to many parents who perceive them as more "natural" than conventional formulas, or who themselves are following an organic diet. Certified organic formulas have received organic certification from a certification body that has been accredited by a national food inspection agency. Organic infant formulas tend to be more expensive and trickier to source. While organic infant formulas are safe and acceptable choices, they are *not* more nutritious or safer than regular conventional infant formulas. Organic infant formulas don't have trace levels of synthetic pesticides, which makes some parents feel safer, but the levels for pesticide residues in conventional formulas are already far below the amount that would cause health concern. In a nutshell, they're both safe and nutritious so it's a personal choice! To read more about organic versus conventional *food*, turn to page 18.

What about organic European formulas?

People have been going crazy for European-made baby formulas. We've heard parents talking about Holle, Lebenswert, and HiPP Organic, so we had to investigate to see what all of the hype was about! Here's what we found out. European formulas are:

- Organic, and some are Demeter biodynamic (which is like being organic-plus). This means that the farms that raise the cows (from whose milk protein the formulas are made) use no synthetic pesticides or fertilizers. This is better for soil quality, ecosystem preservation, and animal care, and assures no genetic modification (non-GMO).
- Available in 2 stages: birth to 6 months, then 6 to 12 months. At 6 months, babies start to need more iron, and the 6-to-12-month formula is higher in iron than the 0-to-6-month version.
- Available in both cow's milk and goat's milk options
- Free of added sucrose sugar; the sugar comes from lactose or maltodextrin instead
- Free of added thickeners and gums

Some North American formulas have *some* of these features, but you have to check packages to know for sure.

> **REALITY CHECK**
>
> If you decide to give European formula a try, make sure you buy it from a reputable supplier, not a discount website (this is your baby's food we're talking about!). Also, please note that HiPP formula is made in factories in the UK, Germany, and the Netherlands, and formulations are different in each country. If your baby is used to one of them, you should consistently order the same one!

Why do some parents believe they are better?

Ingredients lists: Some parents feel safer with the European organic formulas as they have a "cleaner" ingredients list than most US or Canadian brands, perceived as such because they are made up of more recognizable words—for example, biodynamic skimmed milk, organic whey powder, organic vegetable oil, calcium carbonate, vitamin A, vitamin C, vitamin E, etc. By contrast, ingredients lists on North American formulas are longer and have scary-sounding words. But here's the thing: some of those scary-sounding words don't mean the ingredients are scary; they are just the chemical names of vitamins, minerals, and probiotics. For example, where on European formulas you'll see "iron, vitamin E, and vitamin C," on North American formulas you'll see the same ingredients listed as "ferrous sulfate, DL-alpha-tocopherol-acetate, and ascorbyl palmitate." Sounds ominous, but these aren't anything to fear.

Farming practices: Some parents believe that European farming practices are better, so the formula is naturally going to be safer. North American formulas are regulated and safe as well, of course, but European formulas do seem to have a certain "extra" that parents are looking for because they can't have *any* detectable level of pesticide residues. The same high standard is not in place for North American formulas.

As of the time of writing this, European organic formulas are hard to find and tricky to purchase in North America because they are not available at local drug stores or supermarkets. You have to buy them online. It's doable, but it requires planning as some have shipping times of up to 4 weeks.

They are also more expensive than basic North American formulas (around the same price as organic or speciality formulas), and that high cost is out of reach for many. Rest assured that whichever you choose, all commercial formula (European or North American) will sufficiently nourish your baby.

Is it safe to make homemade formula?

In short: heck NO. Homemade infant formulas are usually made based on recipes found online that contain animal milk (which may or may not be pasteurized), plant-based beverages such as soy milk or almond milk, plus coconut oil or broth. Homemade formulas are nutritionally incomplete. They are often low in iron, omega-3 fat, and other important nutrients. Formula that lacks these nutrients can lead to nutrient deficiencies in babies and growth and development concerns.

What's just as scary is that these homemade formulas could potentially include *too many* nutrients, creating an issue of vitamin or mineral toxicity, which is equally dangerous. Also, if your food sanitation habits aren't 100% perfect, you can easily introduce bacteria into the formula, and your baby could get a foodborne illness like salmonella.

Moral of the story? Don't do it. Just don't. It's not worth the risks.

Should I give my baby nutritional supplements?

Typically, you don't have to worry about nutritional supplements for your baby, with the exception of vitamin D, which is a must for breastfed babies (and formula-fed babies consuming less than 32 ounces per day). Breastmilk doesn't provide much vitamin D, which is a fat-soluble vitamin that's important for preventing rickets, a bone disease that results in deformity of your baby's bones. The primary source of vitamin D for humans is sunlight exposure (we synthesize vitamin D under our skin when it's exposed to sunlight), but as you likely know, infants under 1 year shouldn't really be sitting out in the sun, so a supplement is required.

Breastfed babies: Vitamin D supplementation for breastfed infants has been recommended for decades, and has been proven to be an effective and preventative measure against rickets. You don't want to give more than about 400 IU per day, though—anything over 1,000 IU per day, for an infant 6 months and younger, can put baby at risk of vitamin D toxicity.

Formula-fed babies: Commercially prepared infant formula is nutritionally complete, so unless there's a diagnosed vitamin or mineral deficiency, nutrition supplementation isn't required. That being said, in the very beginning, if you're feeding your baby less than 32 ounces (4 cups) of fortified infant formula a day, you should be giving your baby 400 IU of liquid vitamin D a day—starting in the first few days after birth. Continue giving your baby vitamin D until they reach 32 ounces (4 cups) of formula a day. Once your formula-fed baby has started solids and is consuming less formula, you can introduce the 400 IU vitamin D supplement again and continue throughout childhood.

Giving to baby: Liquid vitamin D supplements are recommended. And they are easy to use: you just apply 1 droplet to your nipple before baby latches on, and they ingest it while they breastfeed. Or you can also put it on your clean finger, or side of your clean hand, for baby to suck off.

CARA SAYS: *I can't tell you how many times I spied that little bottle of vitamin D drops on the counter and couldn't remember whether I had given a drop to my baby that day or not (baby brain is a real thing). So I changed my tactic and starting treating it like a meal. Every day, my baby got their vitamin D drop at "breakfast"— also known as the first feed of the day. Consistency is key to combat forgetfulness!*

Should I give my baby probiotics?

Probiotics are healthy bacteria or "microbes" naturally found in your gut. A mother's placenta does not provide baby with bacteria or "microbiome"—this doesn't start until the birthing process begins.

How do probiotics help?

Probiotics are live bacteria that can help to repopulate the "good" bacteria in the gut. When things are out of balance—let's say when a baby has to take antibiotics for an ear infection—you may want to consider adding a probiotic supplement to help replace that good bacteria that is wiped out by the antibiotics. If this isn't done, an imbalance of bacteria in the gut can occur (see the explanation of dysbiosis opposite).

Probiotics for fussiness: Look for a probiotic supplement that contains about 5 to 10 billion live cells, including the specific strains that have been researched and proven to benefit baby's digestion and prevent excess gas, colic, or fussiness; *Lactobacillus reuteri* is a strain that may help. Make sure it's specifically safe to use with babies. Ask your pharmacist, doctor, or dietitian if you aren't sure.

Probiotics to take with antibiotics: We know that antibiotics can affect a baby's gut health, essentially wiping out both the good with the bad bacteria, leading to an antibiotic-associated diarrhea. Some physicians will recommend that babies who need antibiotics also take probiotics to help prevent diarrhea. If so, the recommendation is that probiotics containing specific strains (usually *Lactobacillus rhamnosus* and *Saccharomyces boulardii*) be given within 24 to 48 hours of starting the antibiotic (and continue for the next 2 weeks at least). The probiotic should not be taken at the same time as the antibiotic—try to leave a 2-hour window between when you give probiotics and antibiotics.

Different strains of probiotics help different issues. For example, *Lactobacillus rhamnosus* and *Saccharomyces boulardii* have been shown to help protect babies and toddlers from developing antibiotic-associated diarrhea, while *Lactobacillus reuteri* (such as BioGaia) may help with colic in babies. There's just so much more research that needs to be done in this area, so we're a little ways off from making concrete recommendations.

Are there risks?

There's always the risk of giving your baby probiotics that their little digestive system doesn't need, which could upset the natural balance of microflora. Truth: no one knows for sure yet. The hope is that one day scientists will have a test that will allow us to know exactly which strains of bacteria your digestive system needs. That test isn't available yet, so until then, it's a bit of guesswork. Bottom line: speak with your doctor, dietitian, or pharmacist before randomly giving your baby probiotics.

SHADES OF GRAY: DYBIOSIS

The probiotic area of nutritional science is still pretty new, and there are discoveries all the time. Researchers are pretty sure that probiotics and gut microbiota play an important role in how food is digested, how strong our immune system is, and how we can protect ourselves against harmful bacteria, but they are still learning about the diverse roles of probiotics in health and prevention of disease.

We do know that an imbalance of bacteria in the gut—or "dysbiosis" (where harmful bacteria outweigh beneficial or "good" bacteria)—has been linked to various digestive issues, chronic and inflammatory diseases, obesity, and allergies. And although we don't know for sure, an imbalance in gut bacteria could potentially contribute to excess gas, colic, and fussiness in babies.

Some signs that your baby's gut bacteria may be imbalanced are irregular or abnormal stools, diarrhea, fussiness, excess gas, colic, reflux, and more. But there's still so much research to be done in this area. It's still unclear if bacteria are out of balance when these symptoms happen, what type of bacteria is out of balance, and how to fix it. There are trillions of microbes living inside the gut, and scientists have only scratched the surface when it comes to researching this important topic.

What can I do if my baby is gassy and fussy?

We both have many memories of fussy babies. Long, tiring nights of trial and error trying to figure out what the heck was making our babies scream. When you've tried feeding, changing, soothing, swaddling, and rocking (and repeat) for hours on end, it can become overwhelming—to the point where you feel like screaming! Know that all of us go through it, and you're not alone.

Unfortunately, babies can't tell us why they're fussy, so it often comes down to a process of elimination. Know this, though: every baby is a gassy baby. Because they eat around the clock, their digestive systems are processing nutrients all day and all night, and digestion produces gas (especially for immature digestive tracts in the case of newborns). Frequent passing of gas is not a cause for concern and is fairly normal, but your baby may become fussy when trying to get it out. What's not so normal is when gas causes ongoing discomfort and distress, but here are a few things you can do to relieve it:

Consider breastfeeding issues: Sometimes gassiness can be due to baby's latch, and trying a different feeding position can make all the difference. We suggest seeking help from a lactation consultant who can look at your latch, assess your letdown and flow of milk, and offer some really helpful tips to stop the excess air from getting into your baby's tummy and causing excess gas.

Look at bottle-feeding techniques: Perhaps it's the type of formula that you're using, the shape of the nipple on the bottle, or the angle at which you're feeding. Check to see if the nipple is full of milk while feeding—it should be. If you're using powdered formula, let the milk settle after shaking it, because that shaking motion creates extra bubbles that can translate into excess air in baby's tummy. Switching to ready-made formula can sometimes help too. When you're feeding your baby, it's important to make sure that their head is higher than their stomach so that it makes it easier to burp and not have the bubbles enter further into baby's digestive tract.

Try anti-gas drops: Over-the-counter anti-gas drops containing simethicone (such as Ovol, Mylicon, and Phazyme) can help break up bigger trapped gas bubbles into smaller ones that are easier to pass.

Try probiotics: See page 172.

What should I do if my baby is spitting up/throwing up excessively?

There's a reason why memes exist that show new parents rejoicing when they find a shirt that doesn't have spit-up on it. It's because babies spit up. On every shirt you own. And every pair of pants. And every pillow and blanket. Oh, the laundry you will do!

Spitting up soon after a feed is completely normal for young babies. Their digestive tract is immature, and the muscle connecting the esophagus and the stomach (the lower esophageal sphincter) may need a little more time to develop and strengthen. This will happen with time! If your baby is happy and growing well, and doesn't seem uncomfortable, occasional spit-up is no cause for concern (other than loads and loads of laundry). This usually resolves by 6 to 12 months of age.

However, if you notice that your baby is spitting up or vomiting often, shortly after breastmilk or formula-feeds (or even a couple of hours afterward), it may mean:

Your baby is being overfed or fed too fast: If you're breastfeeding and have a forceful letdown, an oversupply of milk, or overfull breasts, your baby may be feeding too fast and perhaps drinking too much in a short period, which could be causing them to spit up or vomit soon after. The amount of spit-up usually seems much more than it actually is. Parents might worry that their babies aren't actually keeping enough milk down. This generally isn't the case at all. If you think this is the case for you, it might be a good idea to meet with a lactation consultant who can give you some tips on how to slow the flow of milk and manage your supply.

> ♥ (WE GOT YOU!)
>
> It's important to closely watch baby's cues when they are feeding. If baby shows any signs of being done (slows down their sucking significantly, turns their head away, or starts playing with the nipple), then they're likely done. Forcing the bottle or breast back into baby's mouth so that they finish the feed is not a good idea and will likely result in baby overfeeding and spitting up or vomiting afterward. Watch your baby's cues closely. They will actively suck on their own if they are still hungry.

I often had an overabundance of milk, especially with my second child. For me, feeding from one breast over the period of a few hours, manually expressing some of the foremilk that forcefully comes out at the beginning of each feed prior to latching my baby, and limiting the time that I fed all helped to regulate my supply and therefore prevent my baby from constantly spitting up after feeds.

Your baby has gastroesophageal reflux (GER): This simply means that the breastmilk or formula that has made its way down to your baby's stomach is returning up the esophagus and into (and out of) the mouth. GER affects about 40% to 65% of babies aged 1 to 4 months and typically resolves around 1 year.

In most cases, reflux is harmless and normal, especially if you have a happy baby who is growing well. GER is a result of an immature digestive system. It takes some babies a little longer than others to develop a strong and fully functional digestive system. The muscle connecting the stomach and the esophagus (esophageal sphincter) seems to mature fully by about 6 to 12 months (this ranges from baby to baby), allowing most babies to grow out of the spit-up phase by their first birthdays. Even though GER isn't harmful, it can be worrisome, and let's be honest—messy! And kinda gross. Below are our tips for preventing, managing, and minimizing GER symptoms in your baby.

Your baby has gastroesophageal reflux disease (GERD) or another serious condition: While most cases of GER are no cause for concern, occasionally babies suffer from what's known as gastroesophageal reflux disease (GERD), which is a more severe version of GER or, even more worrisome, a gastrointestinal obstruction. These possibilities are very rare, but nonetheless good to be aware of.

If your baby is failing to thrive (not gaining weight or losing weight), refusing to eat, frequently vomiting forcefully (projectile), or frequently spitting up large amounts (and/or unusual colors such as green or yellow), these might be signs that there is a more serious problem that needs immediate attention from a doctor. Severe reflux that continues for more than 2 to 3 months can cause damage to a baby's stomach, esophagus, and throat.

Top 6 tips to prevent reflux and spitting up

1. **Feed on demand in smaller, more frequent meals.** Whether breast- or bottle-fed, your baby may experience fewer reflux and spit-up episodes if offered smaller, more frequent "meals" (versus fewer and larger feeds). If your baby's stomach becomes too full, this puts pressure on their lower esophageal sphincter (mentioned above), which can cause it to stop doing what it's supposed to do (keep stomach contents down) and allows stomach contents to creep back up. If you're breastfeeding, try cutting back on the amount of time you spend feeding if you find that your baby is getting too full and spitting up after feeds. Feeding on demand, following your baby's cues closely, is the best bet.

2. **Burp your baby more frequently.** Burping your infant during and after each feed is important to relieve some of the pressure in the stomach, helping to prevent reflux. Continue to burp every hour or so after a feed if you find that your baby is gassy. Burp bottle-fed infants often during feeds—about every 1 to 2 ounces. If you're breastfeeding, burp your baby every time they pull off of the nipple.

3. **Experiment with different nipple sizes.** If your baby is bottle-fed, they may be drinking too fast or too slow—both of which can cause excess gas to form, often triggering reflux and spitting up. The cause of too-fast or too-slow drinking is often the size of the nipple. If the opening is too large, your baby might be guzzling milk too fast, causing the stomach to overfill with milk and air, and if the opening is too small, they will likely swallow excess air, which we now know can spur on reflux. Experiment with nipples with various shapes and opening sizes.

   > **WE GOT YOU!**
   >
   > It may surprise you to find what a difference a nipple can make! Using a nipple shield if you're breastfeeding can also slow your milk flow, preventing your baby from swallowing air or gulping milk too fast. Talk to a lactation consultant if you're considering a nipple shield to make sure it's the best choice for you and your baby.

4. **Keep your baby upright for at least 30 minutes after feeding.** Babies are more susceptible to reflux because they spend a lot of their time lying down. Let's face it—their diet is mostly liquids and the muscle tone of their esophageal sphincter isn't fully developed yet. Perfect recipe for spit-up. It's a good idea to keep baby upright for about 30 minutes after a feed. This will allow gravity to do its thing—help the milk make its way down the digestive tract (and stay down). You can also elevate

the end of your baby's crib where their head is by rolling a towel or using a wedge pillow (to about 30 degrees) under the mattress to slightly elevate your baby while sleeping.

5. **Continue to breastfeed.** At this point, there is no research to show that a mother's diet causes reflux in her breastfed baby . . . although many believe that it does. See a dietitian, who can help you with an elimination diet if you feel strongly that your diet is affecting your baby's digestive health.

6. **Consider switching formulas.** If you're bottle-feeding, your pediatrician may recommend a thickened formula or perhaps a hypoallergenic formula if they suspect that your baby isn't tolerating the proteins in the present formula. But don't switch formulas on your own without talking to your baby's doctor, as it's usually not warranted.

What should I do if I think that my baby might be constipated?

One of the most common concerns among parents with infants is constipation (and their bowel habits in general). Here's the truth: your new baby's poop habits are going to be all over the place when it comes to frequency, consistency, color, and smell. There's no "normal," really. In the first couple of days after birth, newborns pass meconium, which is a really dark green-black, thick, and sticky bowel movement. Soon after, their stools become lighter in color, looser (even liquidy sometimes), and seedy, with not much of an odor (if breastfed).

The frequency of bowel movements for both breastfed and formula-fed babies can vary (although there's more variation in breastfed infants), but tend to decrease with age. Some infants might poop after every feed, and after about 4 to 6 weeks, some babies may go 3 or 4 days (or longer—even weeks!) between bowel movements. This can be normal for babies who are tolerating milk well and gaining weight appropriately.

Your baby's bowel movements can change with time and with any change in feeding, such as if you transition from exclusively breastfeeding to supplementing with formula, or even switch the formula type or brand.

CARA SAYS: *My daughter would go for long stretches without a poop and it totally freaked me out. I asked her pediatrician, and after assuring me that it was normal, he explained that breastmilk is filled with nutrients that babies use for growth and development—sometimes they use every last drop, so there is little waste to come through via poop. And I like the way it was summed up to me by a public health nurse: "7 poops in one day or one poop in 7 days—those are both totally normal scenarios for babies."*

WHEN TO CONSULT YOUR DOCTOR

In breastfed babies, constipation is very, very rare. In fact, normal bowel function can occur even when a baby has gone days without pooping, especially if they seem happy and aren't showing discomfort or straining. Often (and unfortunately), this wide range of "normal" can be misinterpreted as constipation and be treated unnecessarily, which can lead to future bowel issues. So if your baby is growing well and eating well and there are no signs of bowel obstruction, you can assume that they're not constipated. If you're concerned, consult with your baby's doctor to be sure.

If there's no bowel movement for 2 weeks, and/or there are other red flags (see list below), it could indicate that there's something wrong and that there's another underlying medical condition. This is when you want to contact your baby's doctor:

- Fever
- Hard, dry stools
- Bloated tummy
- Weight loss, poor weight gain, or failure to thrive
- Nausea and/or vomiting
- Blood in stool
- Foul-smelling diarrhea (usually accompanied by abdominal cramping and urgency)

> **REALITY CHECK**
>
> Home constipation remedies such as prune juice, brown sugar water, and corn syrup are not recommended for exclusively breastfed babies 6 months and younger.

When should I introduce solid foods? 4 months or 6 months?

Here's an all-too-common scenario that we hear all the time: You see your doctor for your baby's 4-month checkup, and they say, "Okay, it's time to introduce solids!" You look perplexed, because your Facebook parenting forums all say to wait until 6 months. What gives?

SHADES OF GRAY: INTRODUCING SOLID FOOD

Nutrition is a science, and science changes based on new research, which is why there are slightly differing opinions on this subject.

- The World Health Organization, which makes health recommendations for the entire world, recommends that infants start receiving complementary foods at 6 months.
- The American College of Allergy, Asthma, and Immunology recommends starting solids between 4 and 6 months, and some doctors prefer to use this.

There's no doubt that almost all experts think it's best to wait until *at least* 4 months to start solid foods. Introducing foods earlier (before 4 months) may increase the risk of eczema, celiac disease, type 1 diabetes, wheezing in childhood, and unhealthy pediatric weight gain.

Baby's gag reflex hasn't fully developed at 4 months, which puts them at an increased risk of choking, especially if you're feeding anything other than thin purees. Their digestive tract has also not developed to the point of being able to digest the nutrients in solid food either. That's why we like the *6-month* time frame better.

Breastmilk (and/or formula) provides 100% of baby's nutrition up to the 6-month mark. Then they enter late infancy, which is a time of rapid growth and development, and breastmilk or formula alone don't cut it anymore. Breastmilk and/or formula will still continue to provide *the bulk* of your baby's nutritional needs until they are one year old, though. The World Health Organization estimates that solid foods provide about one-fifth of a baby's needs from 6 to 8 months, and then just under half of their needs from 9 to 11 months. If you do choose to introduce solids at 4 months, stick with a thin pureed consistency because of the above reasons.

Top 10 Tips

for babies (0 to 6 months)

1   **Know that fed is best.**
Your baby can grow and thrive whether you breast- or formula-feed.

2   **Be flexible with breastfeeding.**
When it comes to babies, there is no schedule.

3   **Let baby dictate feeds.**
Feed responsively, and baby will get the right amount for proper growth.

4   **Boost your supply.**
If you breastfeed, the more you feed or pump, the more milk you will produce.

5   **Store breastmilk correctly.**
Refrigerate for 5 days; freeze for 3 to 6 months in regular freezer or up to 12 months in chest.

6   **Choose the formula brand that works best for your baby.**
Work with your doctor or dietitian to choose the right formula to meet baby's needs.

7   **Do not make your own infant formula.**
Buy a commercial one that best suits your baby's needs.

8   **Give breastfed babies vitamin D.**
Breastfed babies need 400 IU of vitamin D daily.

9   **Rest assured that constipation in babies is rare.**
If they don't poop for a few days, that's okay!

10   **Know when baby is ready for solids.**
Introduce foods at 6 months (read more in the next chapter).

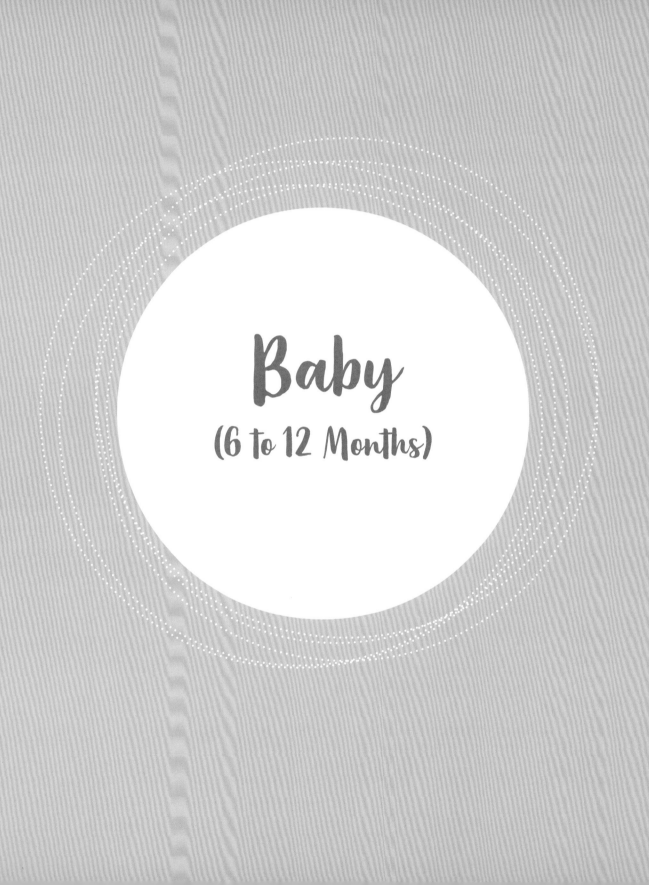

Baby

(6 to 12 Months)

Introduction

You've been waiting for this momentous occasion for months. You have the high chair set up, the bibs folded neatly in the drawer, the camera ready—it's going to be so adorable and you want to capture every moment. Welcome to the world of solid food! But wait a minute, what about the questions that you have swirling around in your brain about when, how, and what to feed solid foods your baby?

- Should I introduce iron-fortified rice cereal first like my mom did with me, or red meat like my friend did?
- Are purees best, or should I do "baby-led weaning" instead?
- What about nuts and eggs? Don't I have to wait a year to introduce those because they're allergenic?

> Starting solid foods is an exciting milestone in your baby's life, but it can also be confusing.

Starting solid foods is an exciting milestone in your baby's life, but it can also be confusing, especially when you're overloaded with conflicting information on how and when to do it.

Luckily, we know the latest infant-feeding guidelines very, very well, and we've scoured the research on introducing solid foods. And while there are some outliers, the majority of studies say that a baby's ability to manage and safely swallow solid foods develops about 6 months, so that's the age we recommend. What's more important than the *exact* age is making sure your baby is ready for food. It may be a week or two earlier or later than 6 months—and that's totally okay. All babies develop at different rates. Watch *your* baby's cues and introduce solids when they are ready (see page 192).

In this chapter, we'll answer your questions on the timing of food and bottle-feeds, how much to feed at any given time, how to wean your child off of a bottle, what the most important nutrients and foods are, how to deal with a baby who refuses to eat, and how to know whether your baby is constipated. So, fear not—we've got it all covered when it comes to introducing solid food!

Feeding styles

Spoon-feeding or baby-led weaning? The most popular question next to "breastfeed or bottle-feed?" The good news? You don't need to pick! We're all about the combination. You can spoon-feed some foods, like yogurt, oatmeal, and pureed fruit (because why not—we adults use a spoon too!), and let your baby self-feed other foods, like toast strips, soft and safe fruits and veggies, and grated cheese. Find out more on page 193—and yes, we also answer your questions about the fear of choking.

Foods to choose

You may be wondering about the best food to start with. There isn't really a perfect choice. We asked parents which food they introduced first, and you will see that the answers (on page 200) have a huge range, from vegetables to fruit to meat to grains! Any of these can be the right answer—it's really up to you. Traditionally, iron-fortified single-grain cereal thinned out with breastmilk or formula was the gold-standard first food for baby. Although it's still an option, it is no longer the only starter-food choice (and nor is it our number one pick). Turn to page 188 to see what foods we recommend.

Nutrients

IRON

Iron-rich foods should be introduced right from the get-go (as soon as you start solid foods, around 6 months), as your baby's iron needs increase around this time. The reason for this is that baby's iron stores are depleted by 6 months of age (they were built up in the womb and lasted until 6 months). Babies between 6 and 12 months of age should be offered iron-rich foods at least twice a day. Things like tender pieces of meat or finely minced, ground, or mashed cooked meat, deboned fish, poultry, well-cooked whole egg, beans, and lentils are great first foods and iron-rich choices.

PROTEIN

Babies are in big-time growth mode at this point, and protein is the building block for tissues such as muscles, organs, skin, and nails. It's important that baby is getting enough every day. They'll still be receiving a lot of it from breastmilk or formula, but it's still important to offer protein-rich foods at most meals and snacks, such as meats, poultry, fish, beans, lentils, nut butters, seeds, tofu, full-fat Greek yogurt, and cheese.

Starting Solid Food

How do I start?

Make sure that there are minimal distractions

Sit directly across from baby while feeding

Watch for baby's hunger and fullness cues (see below)

Don't put too much food on the spoon, or on their tray or plate, as this can be overwhelming

Do not feed too quickly, or chase baby's mouth with the spoon (that means no airplane trick, folks!)

How do I know my baby is hungry?

Reaches for or points to food

Shows excitement when food is offered

Opens mouth and/or follows spoon indicating that they want a bite

Uses sounds, or signs to indicate hunger

How do I know my baby is full?

Slows pace of eating

Dodges or bats away the spoon

Turns head away

Clenches mouth shut

Starts playing with food or throws it

Shakes head to say no

Simply says "no" or "all done"

DIETARY FAT, INCLUDING OMEGA-3
Omega-3 fatty acids are important for many reasons, but when it comes to babies, the most important are brain, nerve, and eye health. Offer about 2 servings of oily, low-mercury fish per week once solids have been established. (If your family doesn't include fish, read more on page 25 for alternate ways to meet omega-3 needs).

(REALITY CHECK)

It's up to you whether you breast- or bottle-feed *before* serving solid food or *after*; experiment with both and see what works. The World Health Organization says that "whether breastfeeds or complementary foods are given first at any meal has not been shown to matter. A mother can decide according to her convenience and the child's [cues]" which will change with the baby's age and feeding regime.

Your baby's day

Now that baby is starting solid food, your schedule is going to become more consistent. Remember those days of nursing around the clock and napping whenever? Those are a thing of the past. But that's good! This consistency will help put some freedom into your routine because you'll be able to predict when baby is going to be hungry. Consistency and routine is also good for baby. It helps them to learn how to self-regulate their appetite. Kind of like how you eat breakfast, lunch, dinner, and snacks. So will they—eventually!

The timing of breast- or bottle-feeds in relation to solid foods is up to you. Some parents choose to have a set breast- and bottle-feed schedule; for example, a feed in the morning, another at night, and another just before or after mealtimes. Others prefer to fly by the seat of their pants!

(WE GOT YOU!)

Time your baby's meals so they eat with you (and your family) at the table. When you eat breakfast, they eat breakfast. This will eliminate the need to transition to family meals later on (and save you time!).

Meal planning

Following a strict meal plan for exactly when, how and how much your baby eats isn't necessary, and it can set unrealistic expectations about how much your baby should eat at any given time (because in reality, this could be all over the place!). We went back and forth about whether to even include a *sample* meal plan for you—heck, we even drafted one up! But, ultimately, we decided against it. It just wasn't feeling right! Being a new parent is tough enough without that added pressure of worrying about a meal plan.

TIMING

To start, solid foods should be introduced once per day, and gradually increased to 3 meals per day by the time baby is about 9 months. Start by serving breakfast. Then, after a few weeks, try adding lunch too, and then eventually add dinner. Make sure it's a slow transition. You don't go from exclusively breast-or bottle-feeding to 3 square meals a day! It's a gradual climb to get there.

Once baby is enjoying breakfast, lunch, and dinner, this is when you can start adding solid food "snacks" in between meals. The introduction to snacks can be gradual too. Eventually, you will be feeding your little one soild food 4 to 6 times a day. Solid food snacks won't replace breastfeeds or formula feeds right away; the idea is for the amount of breastmilk or formula that you feed your baby to decrease slowly as you add more and more solid food. At 12 months, a formula-fed baby can be fully weaned from formula and receive their nutrition exclusively from solid food, unless your doctor has indicated otherwise. If you're breastfeeding, you can continue to breastfeed for as long as you and your baby would like—just be sure they are also enjoying a wide variety of nutritious solid foods.

SERVE A RANGE OF FOODS

The newest feeding guidelines state (and nutrition experts around the world agree) that a variety of solid foods should be introduced right from 6 months of age. Any nutritious whole food can be offered, with the exception of choking hazards (see pages 204), foods that might cause food poisoning (see page 205), honey (see page 206), and cow's milk (see page 196). No prescriptive meal plan, specific amounts, or a strict starting-solids schedule are required!

What foods should you serve in a typical baby meal? We recommend including at least one iron-rich food that also contains protein (meat, fish, poultry, egg, beans, lentils, nut butter, etc. are all good options). Plus at least 2 vegetables and/or fruits, plus a whole grain food. A little portion of each is fine. If your baby cues for more, serve more; let *your* baby's appetite be the guide.

Textures, Shapes, and Sizes to Choose at Every Stage

It's important to consider *how* you will prepare and serve foods to your baby, to make sure they are age-appropriate for every stage. Through the ages of 6 to 12 months, the textures and sizes of foods that are suitable to offer to your baby expands. As baby grows, they slowly develop more mature chewing and swallowing skills, as well as better finger dexterity and fine motor skills. This helps them handle firmer, smaller pieces of food.

As you watch your baby eat, you will notice changes in the size of pieces that they can pick up. Every baby develops at a slightly different rate, and that's okay! While one baby might be ready to pick up small peas and blueberries by 9 months, another might not until 11 months. The suggestions below are just a loose guideline of which textures and sizes of food to offer at each age and stage. Of course, pay close attention to your own baby to know what's right for them. The photos on page 191 show the shape and size of baby foods at different ages. As your baby becomes a more confident feeder, move to the next stage. By the time they turn one, they will be self-feeding like a pro—you got this!

6 TO 7 MONTHS

Protein/iron-rich: Start with cooked meat and poultry being pureed and spoon-fed; or minced and shaped into meatballs or patties (7); or slow-cooked then shredded. Low-mercury fish should be deboned and cooked until soft, then pureed or shaped into patties. Eggs should be hard-boiled then mashed; or cooked as an omelet and cut into strips; or scrambled (1). Beans, lentils, or chickpeas should be cooked and then mashed or pureed. Cheese should be grated (5) or thinly sliced. Plain or Greek yogurt can be spoon-fed.

Fruits and vegetables: Soft fruits (like avocado, ripe pear, or banana) should be peeled and cut into large pieces (about the size of a quarter avocado). For bananas, leave half the peel on to help baby's grip (3). Harder fruits and veggies (like green beans, carrots, zucchini, or apples) should be peeled and steamed until soft, then either mashed or pureed and spoon-fed (4), or cut in large pieces and served as finger food (8).

Grains: Whole grains like quinoa or oats should be cooked and spoon-fed, or baked into meatballs or patties. Whole grain bread should be toasted and cut into strips, then thinly spread with nut or seed butter (6). Iron-fortified infant cereals (2) and Baby's First Oatmeal can be spoon-fed (page 199).

Continue to serve any of the foods from 6 to 7 months, and progress to these textures when your baby seems ready.

Protein/iron-rich: Add medium-size, soft-cooked pieces of meat (11), poultry and fish. Try beans and lentils made into patties (15) like our Toddler-friendly Lentil Bites (page 257).

Fruits and vegetables: Add grated raw options like peeled apple, or carrot (10), and medium-size pieces of soft or steamed-soft options, like raspberries (13), or kiwi (14), or peach (16).

Grains: Try large-flake or steel-cut oats, mixed with peanut butter and mashed banana (9). Add bite-size pieces of cooked pasta, such as penne, or macaroni (12). Add firmer grain options, like farro and barley.

10 TO 12 MONTHS

Continue to serve the foods listed above, and progress to these textures when your baby seems ready. Now that baby has better dexterity, pieces can be smaller.

Protein/iron-rich: Try smaller pieces of meat, poultry (21), and fish (check out our Yummy Salmon Bites (19) on page 317). Add cooked whole beans or chickpeas (17), and cheese cubes.

Fruits and vegetables: Add smaller pieces of cooked vegetables like steamed sliced carrots (20) and small slices of tender, peeled options like cucumber (18). Try sliced grapes and small whole blueberries (24), and pieces of dried fruit, such as apricots (23) or raisins.

Grains: Include these in mixed meals (without added salt) such as ravioli with tomato sauce (22), spaghetti bolognaise, and soup.

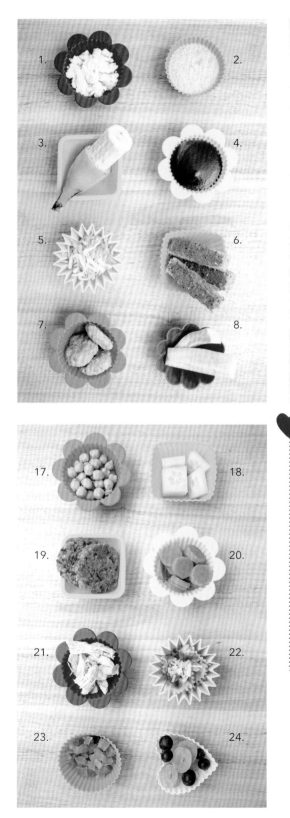

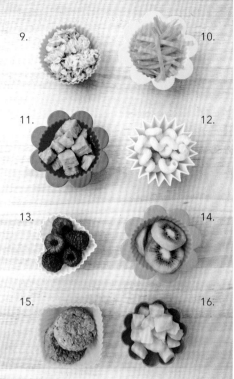

♥ (WE GOT YOU!)

It's always nice to see a visual isn't it?! Here are some of our favorite age-appropriate finger foods for babies. The photos shows foods we recommend for 6 to 7 months (top left), 8 to 9 months (top right) and 10 to 12 months (bottom left). Don't feel beholden to these ideas though—just think of them as nutritious inspiration for what to try with your own little eater!

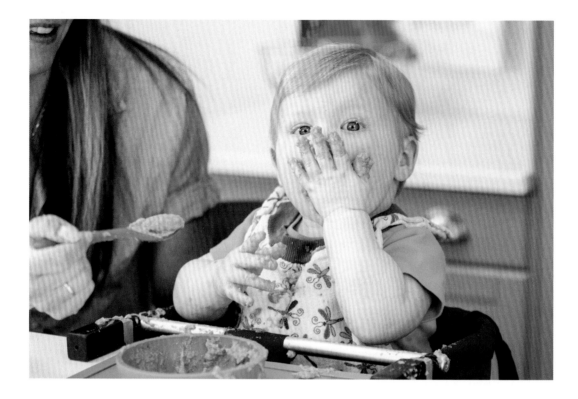

More important than the *exact age* your baby starts solid foods (read more about this on page 180) is making sure your baby is *ready* for solid food. All babies develop at different rates. Watch *your* baby's cues and introduce solids when they are ready. Signs of readiness include:

- **Baby can sit, supported.** Baby should be able to sit in a high chair, feeding seat, or infant seat, supported, with good head and neck control.
- **Baby opens their mouth when food comes their way.** Baby may be ready if they watch you eat, reach for your food, and seem eager to eat.
- **Baby can maneuver food from a spoon to the back of their throat.** If you offer a spoonful of food to baby and they push it out with their tongue and it dribbles onto their chin (the tongue thrust reflex), they may not be ready yet. You could try diluting it the first few times, then gradually thicken the texture, or you may also want to wait a week or two and try again.

- **Baby is big enough.** If your baby has at least doubled their birthweight and weighs at least 13 pounds, they may be ready to start solids.

CARA SAYS: *I was SUCH a rule follower with my first baby. I knew that the guidelines recommended feeding at 6 months, so I literally had the day marked in the calendar and was all set to give my daughter her first taste of food. Both sets of grandparents were present for the momentous occasion! My husband and I took turns trying to get the spoon into her mouth, and of course we recorded the whole session.*

With my second baby, I was a bit more relaxed (okay—a lot more relaxed). I was more confident in my mom abilities, and instead of sticking to a calendar date, I watched for cues that he was ready to feed. About 2 weeks before his 6-month birthday, he was showing all of the classic signs—sitting up in a high chair, trying to reach for food on my plate, etc. So at 5½ months, food was introduced. All good.

SARAH SAYS: *When my third baby was a week shy of his 6-month birthday, he tried his first solid food. Want to know what it was? Salmon! Not pureed, not mashed, and not mixed with breastmilk. Just barbecued salmon brushed with a bit of olive oil, in pieces that were big enough for him to pick up and soft enough to easily break apart in his mouth. The reason it was salmon? That was what we happened to be serving the night that our baby reached out and grabbed a piece off of my plate. I thought, "This is the perfect first food for you—let's start solids!" He was ready.*

> (REALITY CHECK)
>
> Starting solids *later* than 6 months (unless advised by baby's pediatrician) might make the transition to solid food more challenging and create picky eating issues. It also puts a breastfed infant at risk for iron deficiency anemia.

Should I spoon-feed my baby or do "baby-led weaning"?

When it comes to starting solids, the buzz phrase these days is "baby-led weaning," whereas spoon-feeding and purees have sort of become old-school methods. But you can safely feed your baby using either method; there is no right or wrong. As long as you're feeding "responsively" (see more about this on page 44), and offering a variety of tastes and textures in the first couple of months, spoon feeding and self-feeding are both great. A combination of both is best in our minds!

Baby-led weaning

Baby-led weaning means that you skip purees and spoon-feeding altogether. Instead, you offer your baby soft finger foods for them to feed themselves. The benefits of this method are:

- Baby learns to feed independently from an earlier age and develops fine motor skills
- Baby is 100% in charge of what and how much they eat
- It can potentially reduce picky eating later on
- It cuts down on time spent making homemade pureed baby food
- It cuts down cost of store-bought baby food

UM . . . WON'T MY BABY CHOKE?

A common concern is that baby will choke on solid foods. Now, choking is serious business (see page 208), and we would never recommend a practice that was dangerous in any way. Often, though, choking gets confused with gagging—which is extremely common when babies are starting solids (see page 217). The gag reflex keeps larger food pieces out of the windpipe and near the front of the mouth, only allowing very well-chewed foods to the back to be swallowed. It's a safety mechanism to prevent choking!

A study compared a group of babies who were fed by baby-led weaning (whose parents were trained in this method) to a control group using the spoon-fed method. While the baby-led weaners did gag more at 6 months than spoon-fed babies, they gagged less by 8 months. By this time, the baby-led weaners were used to eating solids, and the spoon-feeders were just starting! And there was no difference in the number of actual choking episodes reported between the 2 groups.[43]

Spoon-feeding

Some parents feel they are missing out on the bonding experience of spoon-feeding if they choose baby-led weaning. Plus, it's not practical to get a 6-month-old to spoon-feed themselves a bowl of oatmeal or yogurt! (That being said, between 9 and 12 months, you can start letting your baby practice self-feeding with a spoon.) So what to do? Try a combination! There is no rule to say that you have to pick one method or the other. We say do both!

SARAH SAYS: *As much as I love the baby-led weaning philosophy and approach (and truly believe in it!), I also loved the experience of spoon-feeding my babies. It allowed me to be fully engaged in the feeding experience and exchange smiles and sweet little interactions with my babies during mealtimes.*

One of the benefits of baby-led weaning is that it helps baby learn to regulate how much and how fast they eat. What many parents don't realize, though, is that spoon-feeding can also be baby-led, as long as it's done with awareness! Your baby should set the eating pace, so it's important to really pay attention to their physical cues when it comes to bringing food to their mouth and pausing between bites.

⚖️ **SHADES OF GRAY: IRON INTAKE**

Nutrition experts (and parents) worry about adequate iron intake if you choose baby-led weaning. Iron-rich foods such as red meat, fish, legumes, and eggs are important for babies over 6 months of age, as their iron stores have been depleted (read more on page 197). Babies who are fed using baby-led weaning may fall short of iron, which puts them at risk for iron deficiency anemia. It's a bit more challenging to ensure baby receives enough of this nutrient when they're exclusively self-feeding. Quite simply, they may not pick up and eat those strips of meat or pieces of scrambled egg. And you certainly don't want to force it!

The most important thing? Letting your baby lead

This means either allowing baby to self-feed and eat how much they want (without coaxing them to eat more or taking food away when they're not done), or paying close attention to their cues while spoon-feeding (see page 186 for those cues). Kids will eat when they're hungry and stop when they're full. Honoring those instincts may help them avoid overeating now and down the road.

How much food (and breastmilk/formula) should my baby eat per day?

There's no set amount of food that your baby should be eating every day—every baby is different, and every day is different. Your baby may eat a lot one day and hardly any the next—this is normal! The key? To trust your baby's cues and let them lead in terms of amounts. If you do this, 9 times out of 10 you'll see that by the end of the week, baby is getting what they need.

WE GOT YOU!

The main thing to remember is that you're in charge of WHAT, WHERE, and WHEN food is served, and the rest is up to your baby (IF and HOW MUCH they eat). Didn't we tell you that Division of Responsibility (sDOR) (page 41) would come in handy!? Start with 1 or 2 teaspoons of pureed food and/or a few bites of soft finger food, and if baby seems interested in more, offer more. If baby seems uninterested or full, stop offering—it's as simple as that!

CARA SAYS: *I often talk with parents who are SO stressed about all of the perceived "food rules"—it's complicated to ensure baby always has enough iron, omega-3, protein—ahhhhhh! Please don't stress. The guidelines are gentle and you are doing a great job! If your little one doesn't get iron at a meal or pushes that omega-3-rich fish off their tray, they will be just fine! It's the big picture that matters most, and your goal is to introduce various nourishing foods to your children over time. You've got this!*

What is the best first food for my baby?

We guarantee that if you've looked into this question, you've heard some of the following answers: Start with rice cereal! Start with pureed vegetables! Start with avocado! Start with meat! Start with banana! So which is the correct answer? They are all correct, and the first food you offer your baby is *your choice*. There's no one perfect answer for everyone. But that's more fun for you, because you get to plan your baby's menu!

At 6 months, it's safe to introduce all whole foods and some nutritionally processed foods—vegetables, fruits, grains, meat, poultry, fish, eggs, natural nut and seed butters, and pasteurized dairy products—with the exception of bottles filled with fluid cow's milk (see page 206), honey (see page 206), those that might cause food poisoning (see page 205) and choking hazards (see page 205) in any order you'd like. For more on appropriate textures and shapes at each stage, turn back to page 189.

The most important thing to remember is to make iron-rich foods the priority when starting solids. This is because baby's iron stores are becoming depleted at 6 months and they require this nutrient from food for proper growth and development. Iron-rich foods include meats, poultry, fish, beans, lentils, and iron-fortified infant cereals. They don't need to be the first foods your baby ever tastes, but you should offer iron-rich foods from the get-go.

Solid foods can be introduced in the same way for vegetarian or vegan babies who eat mostly plant-based foods. Simply replace iron-rich meat with soft or mashed tofu, beans, lentils, and chickpeas. You can also offer eggs, full-fat yogurt, and cheese (if vegetarian). Read more about raising vegan or a vegetarian baby on page 207.

Once your baby has been exposed to a variety of new foods, you can start feeding them their meals with the rest of the family. Try for each meal to include at least 3 different foods and textures, whether these are finger foods, spoon-feeding foods, or a combination of both. For example, spoon-feed yogurt and let your baby self-feed pieces of grated carrot or soft, whole grain muffin.

Iron-rich First Foods

- Soft and tender pieces of meat or poultry
- Finely minced, ground, or mashed cooked meat
- Deboned fish
- Well-cooked whole eggs , halved, quartered, or mashed
- Beans and lentils, mashed
- Iron-fortified whole grain infant cereals

DEEP DIVE: FIRST FOODS & ALLERGIES

Historically, the guidelines for starting solids were a little more structured. It was recommended that parents introduce one food at a time, waiting a few days in between to be able to recognize a potential food allergy. New guidelines aren't as strict—it's okay to introduce more than one food at a time, and there's no need to follow a certain order. Of course, this is all up to you as the parent and based on your comfort level. If you or your partner have allergies, you may want to introduce common allergens (egg, peanut, nut, soy, fish, wheat, milk, sesame) one at a time to watch for reactions (turn to page 64). This may also be the suggestion from your doctor, especially if baby also has shown signs of eczema, which goes hand-in-hand with some allergies.

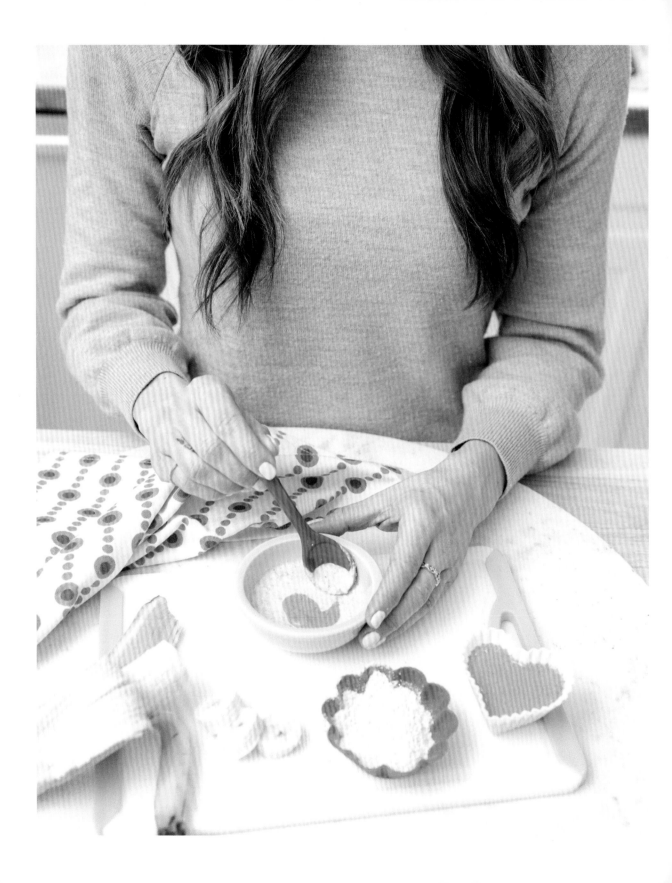

BABY'S FIRST OATMEAL

This recipe is a great way to introduce peanuts!

Makes 1 to 2 servings (depending on baby's appetite!)

½ cup rolled oats
½ cup water
Pinch cinnamon
1 tsp natural peanut butter
1 tbsp mashed banana
Breastmilk or formula, as needed

1. Pulse the rolled oats in a food processor or blender until finely ground. Store in the fridge or freezer for up to 3 months.
2. Bring the water to a boil in a small pot. Stir in 2 tbsp of the oat powder and cinnamon. Whisk for about 1 minute to ensure the oat powder doesn't clump.
3. Let simmer for 3 to 5 minutes, stirring occasionally.
4. Remove from the heat. Stir in the peanut butter and banana. If the mixture is too thick, add breastmilk or formula to thin it to the desired texture. Allow to cool.

IRON-RICH TEETHING BISCUITS

Homemade teething biscuits are oh-so-fun for babies because they can be made into fun shapes using cookie cutters. We like to make stars, animal shapes, or firetrucks. Enlist the help of your older kids for a fun activity. (Photo on page iii.)

Makes 12 biscuits

1 banana
½ cup iron-fortified oat, barley, or multigrain cereal
½ cup whole wheat flour
1 tbsp coconut oil
1 tbsp cinnamon
2 tbsp or more of water (to get sticky consistency)

1. Preheat the oven to 400°F. Line a baking sheet with parchment paper.
2. In a large bowl, combine the banana, cereal, flour, oil, cinnamon, and water. If too dry, add more water to reach a dough-like consistency.
3. Roll out the dough on a floured surface until ¼ to ½ inch thick. Use cookie cutters to cut out shapes.
4. Transfer to the prepared baking sheet. Bake for 15 minutes. Cool and serve, or store in the freezer for up to 3 months.

WHAT WAS YOUR BABY'S FIRST FOOD?

Fortified baby oat cereal. —Amanda

Banana and avocado. —Nadine

Believe it or not, I was so concerned about iron that I started with pureed meat. It did not go well. Then bananas. —Mackenzie

I started with baby oat cereal thinned with breastmilk. —Belle

Mashed avocado. —Lucille

Cooked meat, for the iron. —Ahmed

My baby's first food was iron-fortified baby oatmeal cereal. I mixed it with breastmilk. —Ezra

We started with mashed banana. It was a big hit! —LeeAnn

Mashed cooked red lentils. Cooled to room temperature. We are vegetarian so I didn't want to introduce meat. Lentils have iron too! —Daniella

Avocado and banana mashed together—for fat and sweet. —Liz

Rice cereal with water. Just a spoonful or two. —Nafeeza

Steamed apples and pears, cooled and slightly mashed. —Erica

Baby barley cereal. Then I added banana after a few days. She loved it. —Kathy-Anne

I made beef in my slow cooker. It was nice and soft, and easy to mash and feed to my little guy. —Wanda

Sweet potato baby food. It was a beautiful and hilarious mess. —Joanna

What about infant rice cereal? Should I worry about arsenic?!

There are many questions and some confusion (and worry) about the safety of rice-based infant foods, especially with the word "arsenic" being thrown around. And we don't blame parents for being confused and worried. Luckily, we're here to share the facts about arsenic in rice and to help you make the most informed decision for feeding your baby.

FIRST OF ALL, WHAT IS ARSENIC?

Arsenic is a naturally occurring element that is found in the earth's crust. It can be found just about everywhere, as it leaches into groundwater through rocks and soil. Arsenic can find its way into our food supply through the soil and water that feed and grow our food. Plants and grains tend to absorb arsenic more readily than other crops, with rice being the biggest absorber. This is because rice is grown under irrigated conditions, meaning it is exposed to an abundance of water that has potentially been contaminated. Basically, rice has more exposure to arsenic in the growing process—therefore, it has more potential for contamination than most other grains.

DEEP DIVE: ARSENIC

Arsenic is a known carcinogen (that means it has the potential to cause cancer). It can also cause cardio-vascular, respiratory, metabolic, and immune-related health issues. Although the evidence is limited, it is thought that children may metabolize arsenic differently than adults. High exposure to arsenic in childhood may affect health and development and is thought to be associated with an increased susceptibility to cancer in adulthood.

REALITY CHECK

Should you be concerned about feeding your baby rice and rice products? The short answer is yes. But that doesn't mean you need to completely avoid them. The thing is, babies are small and therefore smaller doses have a bigger impact. The amount of arsenic found in infant rice cereal, rice-containing toddler food, and organic brown rice would likely not impact your child if offered occasionally, in moderation. Some parents think that brown rice (especially the organic variety) is a healthier choice than white rice. It's true that it has more fiber and is more nutritious, but it also contains more arsenic than white rice! Brown rice is a whole grain including the outer husk, which holds arsenic. Brown rice should only be offered occasionally—not daily.

Now it's almost impossible to tell you an exact amount of rice cereal that would be safe, because there are so many factors, including age, weight, and height of baby, type of rice cereal, and how much arsenic it contains, but offering rice cereal a few times a week should be completely safe and fine, just like any other single food. But if you were offering your baby rice cereal 2 to 3 times a day, we'd say cut back. After all, variety is key when it comes to all foods, including whole grains.

Our recommendation has always been to steer more toward nutrient-rich high-fiber grains like oats, barley, and ancient grains like quinoa, amaranth, and buckwheat.

Should I make my own baby food?

Should you cook for your baby? Sure! Do you need to make gallons of pureed squash and strained green beans? No! If you are doing baby-led weaning, your child can eat many of the foods you naturally prepare for the family. If you are using salt or spicy seasonings, separate the baby portion from the adult portion; babies don't need salt added to their food, and they aren't quite ready for fiery cayenne or chili peppers (but other spices—like cumin, coriander, and cinnamon—are fine!).

If you are spoon-feeding and want to make vegetable, fruit, bean, and meat purees, they are quite easy to do—you can even just cook or steam and then mash with a fork!

Keep it simple

There's no need to spend hours cooking and blending homemade baby food. Honestly, a lot of it will probably go to waste. Spoon-feed foods that naturally require a spoon—things like yogurt, cottage cheese, porridge, soups, applesauce—and offer other nutritious foods as finger foods. Naturally soft foods such as cooked fish, bananas, berries, soft fruit slices like pear or peach, and scrambled eggs make perfect finger foods. Cut or grated hard cheese, cooked beans, whole grain toast strips, cooked bite-size pasta, and o-shaped whole grain cereals also work really well too.

Make baby part of the family

We encourage you to make small modifications to your meal to suit the baby instead of making baby a special meal. Simple things like not salting part of the salmon fillet that you're cooking, rinsing excess sauce off cooked meat, or removing some of the ground meat that you've cooked for tacos prior to adding the taco seasoning will help to cut down on meal prep time and ensure that your baby eats nutritious foods along with the rest of the family.

CARA SAYS: *If you make your own pureed baby food, don't go crazy with the quantities. I've heard from many parents that they have purchased fancy "baby food blenders" and a mass of equipment to puree, cool, and freeze baby food safely, only to find that it was a waste of money and time. Here's the thing: babies don't eat purees for very long, and some babies won't take to them at all!*

What about fruit and veggie pouches? Are they healthy?

C'mon—what parent doesn't love these things?! Delicious blends like apple-mango-banana in a convenient little pouch? So easy. Plus, they are tasty, portable, non-perishable, and don't even require a utensil. Savory pouches especially—like chicken noodle soup or beef stew—provide pureed foods in a convenient format, and are a good choice when you are spoon-feeding your baby and don't want to make your own meals from scratch. But the trouble starts when fruit and vegetable pouches are served too often, and are used to replace other, more nutritious foods in your baby's diet.

Remember, these pouches are not equivalent to real whole fruits and veggies. The look, taste, texture, and mouth-feel of pureed fruit and vegetables is very different from whole fruits and vegetables, and the true flavor of vegetables is almost always masked by the sweetness of the fruit. The nutritional values are not the same, either. Pureed fruit pouches are super high in sugar (yep, it's natural sugar from fruit, but learn why that's still not so healthy on page 35). In fact, up to 90% of the calories in fruit pouches come from sugar. Each 3 to 4 ounce pouch (containing both fruits and vegetables) typically has between 12 and 20 grams of sugar (which is the equivalent of 3 to 5 teaspoons) and only 1 gram of fiber. Compare this to a whole apple, which contains about 10 grams of sugar and 2.5 grams of fiber. Too much sugar is bad for overall health and puts your child at risk for tooth decay. Fruit pouches also often contain lemon juice concentrate as a preservative, which contains citric acid that can dissolve tooth enamel and lead to cavities. Be sure to offer baby some water afterwards to wash the acid off their teeth and gums.

So the short answer? Pouches can add a bit of variety, nutrition, hydration, and fun to your baby's food rotation. However, babies need to be exposed to real whole foods every day, so fruit and veggie pouches should not replace them in your baby's diet. Offer them only occasionally.

SARAH SAYS: *Over the years, I've become really creative with these pouches, and any leftover pureed baby food. Yes, my kids have all consumed them straight out of the pouch, but there are lots of other delicious ways to consume fruit and veggie pouches. Here are some:*

- *Add to foods like oatmeal, infant cereal, and plain Greek yogurt.*
- *Use to slow-cook meats like pork, chicken, or beef.*
- *Add to homemade smoothies and popsicles.*
- *Use as a dip or topping for French toast or pancakes.*
- *Use in baby-friendly baked foods like muffins, loaves, and cookies.*

What are the foods my baby SHOULDN'T eat?

The good news is that the "rules" for baby feeding have changed so much in the past 15 years, and are way more lenient, flexible, and easy these days. When Cara had her first baby in 2007, there were rules about not introducing egg whites until age one and no peanuts until a kid could talk! Not anymore. Research changes, and guidelines change as a result.

While almost every food is fine to feed your baby, there are a few red flags (just a few, we promise!):

Red flag 1. Foods that are "choking hazards": Before anything else, this is priority number 1: make sure you take a baby first aid and CPR training course. Find one through your local hospital, public health center, or community center. It's so important to be confident and knowledgeable about how to react in an emergency like choking (see page 213). Note that most foods that are choking hazards are round or oval, hard, smooth, and small. Use your judgment. Skip back to page 189 for a list of safe food textures, month to month.

Potential Choking Hazards

Foods	What to Do
Hard raw vegetables and fruit (e.g. baby carrots, raw beets, or apples)	Peel and steam, and/or grate
Fruits with pits or seeds (e.g. whole plum or peach)	Remove pits, seed and peel, and then thinly slice, dice or steam
Whole grapes	Slice lengthwise into halves or quarters
Fibrous or stringy foods (e.g. celery, pineapple, or asparagus)	Finely dice and/or steam
Chunks of firm cheese	Grate
Whole hotdogs or sausages	Avoid, or finely dice if necessary
Fish with bones	Debone thoroughly
Popcorn	Avoid until around age 4
Whole nuts	Avoid; thinly spread nut or seed butter on toast instead

Red flag 2. Foods that can cause food poisoning: Babies and young children are at a higher risk of foodborne illness than adults. That's why it's very important to practice safe food handling, preparation, and storage when it comes to your baby's food (see page 82) to protect against harmful bacteria such as *E. coli*, salmonella, or listeria. These bacteria can be destroyed when foods are heated to safe internal cooking temperature (see page 71). Foods that shouldn't be offered to babies or young children:

- Raw or undercooked meat, poultry, or fish
- Raw or undercooked eggs or foods containing raw eggs such as cookie dough, homemade mayonnaise, sauces and dressings, or homemade ice cream
- Unpasteurized dairy products
- Unpasteurized juices

Red flag 3. Foods that contain honey: One final food to avoid is honey. While it's totally rare, there is a small chance honey can contain spores of a bacterium called *Clostridium botulinum*, which can cause infant botulism. Symptoms include constipation, general weakness, a weak cry, a poor sucking reflex, irritability, lack of facial expression, and loss of head control.

Fewer than 5% of most honey samples contain *Clostridium botulinum* spores, and usually the number of spores is low. But there is that tiny risk. And really, there's no reason to give your baby honey (it's pure sugar, after all).

Pasteurizing honey does not use temperatures high enough to kill the spores. Neither does baking or cooking with honey. So there is also technically a risk with products that contain honey, such as baked goods. Wait until at least 12 months before you introduce honey.

When should I start giving my baby dairy foods, like cow's milk?

You can introduce full-fat yogurt, Greek yogurt, cheese, cottage cheese, and small amounts of milk (in baking, for example) right from 6 months of age. It is fine to include milk in recipes such as muffins, homemade macaroni and cheese, or an omelet, but fluid-filled bottles or baby cups of cow's milk should not be given until around 12 months. We recommend waiting until 9 to 12 months so that your baby can reap the many nutritional benefits from breastmilk and formula for as long as possible. Transitioning from breastmilk or formula to cow's milk too soon may put your baby at a higher risk for iron deficiency or anemia.

> (REALITY CHECK)
>
> Why wait until 12 months to introduce cow's milk? Milk is high in protein, sodium, and potassium—providing more than a little baby needs—but it lacks important vitamins and minerals such as iron, vitamin E, and zinc. For more information on when and how to make the transition to cow's milk, read page 231 in the next chapter!

Your child learns to eat what you eat, right? And if you follow a vegetarian or vegan diet, you may want your child to do the same. That's a personal decision and one that can be very nutritious and healthy. But because your child's nutritional needs are so high at this age, to support growth and development, you have to make sure your baby is getting all of the nutrients they need—which, of course, we can help you with!

Breastmilk, formula and plant-based milk

Since breastmilk is such a rich source of nutrients, we recommend that vegetarian (and especially vegan) moms breastfeed for more than 12 months (we encourage *all* moms to do this anyway, if they wish). If a vegan baby is weaned from breastmilk *before* 12 months, they should receive fortified vegan infant formula instead until they are 1 year old. Some examples are Neocate infant formula with DHA and ARA (by Nutricia), Baby's Only Organic Soy Formula, Enfamil ProSobee Soy Infant Formula, and Similac® Soy Isomil®.

After 12 months, vegan infants who are not being breastfed can either continue on with a vegan follow-up formula until age 2, or consume full-fat soy beverages fortified with calcium and vitamins B_{12} and D. Don't use a fat-free or unsweetened version of soy beverages—choose one that's marked "original" flavor. Do you have concerns about soy? Read more about it on page 233.

Avoid introducing other plant-based milks such as rice, almond, hemp, cashew, or coconut at this point, as they don't have the right amounts of nutrients for proper growth and development. Plant-based milks are lower in calories, fat, and protein compared to cow's milk (see chart on page 235). Soy is the only plant-based milk with protein levels comparable to cow's milk. Serve soy milk beverages in an open cup with meals—no need to let your little one sip on it all day (this might displace other foods and nutrients!). See more on appropriate amounts of milk to serve after 12 months on page 231.

WE GOT YOU!

We recommend that all breastfed infants get 400 IU per day of supplemental vitamin D starting shortly after birth, and this should continue for all babies into the toddler and childhood years. Vegetarian and vegan babies are no different! Learn more about vitamin D requirements and food sources on page 30.

Planning for nutrients

Protein: The first question you may have about a vegan or vegetarian diet for baby is "what should I serve as a source of protein if we don't eat meat?" Until 6 months of age, baby's protein requirements can be met with breastmilk or formula. After that, when you introduce solids, it's important to include lots of plant-based proteins that both you and your family enjoy. See the lists opposite and remember there's also some protein in vegetables, fruits, and whole grain products, so it's really not difficult to meet your child's protein needs!

Iron: Anyone (this includes babies, children, and adults) following a vegetarian or vegan diet may fall short of iron, a mineral that's required for red blood cell formation. Preventing iron deficiency among babies and children is crucial, and can easily be done by ensuring that your child eats enough plant-based iron-rich foods (see pages 25, 197 and 368).

Omega-3 fat (DHA and EPA): You probably know that omega-3 fat is abundant in fatty fish like salmon, but that's not the only place where it is found. Smaller amounts are also found in omega-3-enriched eggs, for vegetarians. For vegans, omega-3 DHA and EPA can be found in foods or supplements made with algal oil. (Algae from oceans is high in omega-3 fat—fish eat algae, and that's why they contain omega-3 fat!) There's also a type of omega-3 fat called ALA, which is found in plant-based foods like nuts, seeds, and oils like flax, hemp, chia, and walnuts. Learn more on page 24.

(REALITY CHECK)

You can plan a vegan diet without cow's milk, but it's not as simple as just replacing cow's milk with almond milk (read more on page 233). If you are hoping to go vegan with your toddler, make an appointment with a dietitian. They can help you plan the optimal diet that will meet all of your toddler's needs.

Calcium: If your vegetarian diet includes dairy products, calcium needs can be easily met. Interestingly, vegetarians actually have a relatively high intake of calcium, often exceeding recommendations—probably because vegetarians who include dairy rely on dairy foods (milk, cheese, and yogurt) as protein sources and get the calcium as an added bonus! Vegan diets are different because they don't include dairy and are often lower in calcium, falling short of the recommendations. For those we recommend adding calcium-rich beans, soy, leafy greens, broccoli, almonds, calcium-fortified plant-based beverages, and calcium-set tofu. See the chart on page 369 for daily requirements of calcium.

Vitamin B$_{12}$: This unique vitamin in the B family is mostly found in animal-based products like meat and dairy. Vitamin B$_{12}$ levels are usually lowest in vegan diets rather than in vegetarian diets, which may include dairy and eggs. Vegans need alternative sources of vitamin B$_{12}$, such as fortified soy or other plant-based beverages, fortified soy products (like soy burgers), fortified breakfast cereals, nutritional yeast (some people call it "nooch"), or a vitamin B$_{12}$ supplement (talk to your child's doctor prior to giving).

Vegan Protein Options

BEANS: kidney beans, red beans, cannellini beans

PEAS: chickpeas, split peas, black-eyed peas

LENTILS: red, black, brown, or green

SOY PRODUCTS: tofu, tempeh, edamame, soy beverages

NUTS AND NUT BUTTERS: almonds, cashew, peanuts, pecans, pistachios, walnuts etc.

SEEDS AND SEED BUTTERS: pumpkin, sunflower, sesame, hemp, chia

Vegetarian Additions

DAIRY & EGGS: cheese, cottage cheese, kefir, milk, yogurt (especially Greek and Icelandic Skyr), eggs

When should I introduce common allergens (peanuts, milk, eggs)?

Up until recently, the recommendation for introducing peanuts was to wait until after age 3. We now know that delaying the introduction of all allergens (including peanuts) isn't necessary and that it's safe to introduce them as early as 4 to 6 months, even for babies at a high risk of developing a food allergy.[44] In fact, early exposure to common allergens may even prevent allergies from developing! While we think this is great news, we also know this can be confusing for new parents.

According to Food Allergy Research and Education (FARE), only about 8% of US children have a food allergy.[45] To look at it another way, that means 92% of kids *do not* have a food allergy. So please know that there's only a very small chance of your child being allergic to peanuts or eggs or milk. Babies are at a higher risk of developing a food allergy if one or both parents have allergies, or if siblings have allergies (or allergic conditions such as eczema and asthma). Turn to page 64 to read more about food allergies. If you are concerned that a food is causing your baby to have an allergic reaction, stop giving that food to your baby and talk to your doctor.

Turn to page 64 to read more about food allergies.

(REALITY CHECK)

The most common food allergens (in descending order) are peanuts, cow's milk, eggs, fish, seafood, wheat, soy, sesame, and tree nuts. You may have read that the incidence of peanut allergies has gone up by 10% to 20% in the past 10 years.[46] That sounds so scary, right? Let's put it into perspective: only 2.5% of all US children are diagnosed with peanut allergy. So yes, while the number has gone up, it's still relatively low.

DEEP DIVE: WHEN TO INTRODUCE PEANUTS

If you want the clinical rules on introducing peanuts, we've got you covered. Below we've summed up the advice from the National Institute of Allergy and Infectious Diseases:

If your baby has severe eczema, an egg allergy, or both, they are at higher risk for a peanut allergy. In this case, introduce peanut-containing foods as early as 4 to 6 months to reduce the risk. (We recommend 6 months.) Worried about doing this on your own? You may want to introduce peanuts at the doctor's office in case of a reaction. In some cases, your doctor may suggest an allergy test BEFORE introducing peanuts (testing may indicate that peanuts should not be introduced at all because your child may already have an allergy).

If your baby has mild to moderate eczema, introduce peanut-containing foods around 6 months of age to reduce the risk of developing a peanut allergy. Your doctor provider can tell you whether your child's eczema is mild to moderate. You may then choose to introduce peanut-containing foods at home or in a doctor's office if you prefer.

If your baby does not have eczema or other food allergies, freely introduce peanut-containing foods. This can be done at home together with other solid foods.

Lilianna's son Jeremy was 6 months old when she met with a dietitian. She was wondering when and how to introduce peanuts to her baby. Her older sister told her she had to wait until the baby was at least 2 years, because that's the advice her sister was given. But the public health nurse in her "mom and baby" class said she could introduce peanuts right from 6 months. Her sister couldn't believe that advice!

The dietitian said researchers worked with 2 groups of babies in a study: the first group was fed peanut products daily, while the second group avoided peanuts until age 5. They found that introducing peanut foods early (especially to those babies at high risk for developing peanut allergies—for example, if they have eczema or other food allergies) reduced the risk of developing peanut allergies by over 80%.

So, was Lilianna supposed to pop a peanut in her baby's mouth? Definitely not! Peanuts are a choking hazard because of their size and shape. She was told to try any of the following:

- Mix thin natural peanut butter with some breastmilk and feed very small amounts on a spoon (about the size of a pea).
- Swirl a bit of natural peanut butter into yogurt or oatmeal (see recipe on page 199).
- Sprinkle powdered peanut butter on infant cereal, yogurt, or fruit puree.
- Thinly spread natural peanut butter on whole grain toast and cut into strips.
- Try a peanut puff (it will dissolve easily), such as Bamba or Puffworks Baby.
- Serve crushed peanuts sprinkled on yogurt, mashed banana, or oatmeal.
- Try specially formulated baby food. Some baby food pouches include 1 of 8 common allergens (including eggs, peanuts, tree nuts, fish, and shellfish). The pouches contain a small amount of allergen protein blended with an organic fruit puree.

Finally, Lilianna learned that introducing peanuts just once was not enough—rather, peanuts and products made with peanuts should be part of a varied diet (served regularly). She now regularly swirls peanuts into yogurt and has learned that her son is particularly fond of peanut butter and banana oatmeal!

My baby gags A LOT. What should I do?

Your baby will likely gag during meal and snack times. Babies have a great natural gag reflex—and that's a good thing! Gagging is a safety mechanism to prevent choking. It helps them move food that has traveled too far to the back of their mouth so that they don't choke. They may make a funny face and a gagging sound, but if you wait for a few seconds, you'll see that your baby is an expert at this and will not choke.

Babies are developmentally ready to handle solid finger foods at 6 months of age (assuming baby wasn't born premature), so it is very unlikely that your baby will actually choke on food. If you freak out when your baby gags, your baby will freak out too. To swallow effectively, a baby needs to learn how to gather food into a "bolus" or small ball in their mouth and propel it to the back of their throat to swallow, bypassing the windpipe. If they don't swallow strongly enough (a learned skill), which often happens when babies first start solids, they will gag and the food will move forward into their mouth again. Totally normal. Gradually, gagging will lessen and your nerves will quiet down.

WE GOT YOU!

Your baby will gag. A lot! Especially in those first few weeks of solid foods and if you're letting your baby self-feed with finger foods. The best thing to do is to remain calm and cool and encourage your baby to work it out by staying positive, smiling, and NOT PANICKING. This is hard, but really important. If your baby sees you freak out, they might too, and it may possibly turn a normal experience into a scary one.

SARAH SAYS: *I introduced solids to my second and third babies using the baby-led weaning method (I let them self-feed right from 6 months). Not everyone in our family was comfortable with this, thinking that it was unsafe and that the babies would choke. In fact, many times, their dad and/or their grandparents would freak out and jump up in a panic when they gagged, unintentionally scaring them! After I explained the mechanics of swallowing and the benefits of baby-led weaning (and the fact that freaking out was counterproductive), they calmed down and could enjoy the experience a little more. If you choose to practice baby-led weaning or let baby self-feed, explain to family members why you've decided to do this, and warn them that there will be gagging (and that this is normal and okay!).*

In contrast to gagging, choking occurs when the airway is blocked. That's why it's vital to avoid the foods with potential choking risk listed on page 204. Here are some other strategies to prevent choking.

Top 7 strategies to prevent choking

1. **Let your baby self-feed.** If you put food into baby's mouth, it may quickly fall to the back of their throat without them having a chance to control it with their tongue and chew it.

2. **Watch your baby while they eat.** You can hear your baby gagging, but you can't hear them choking, which can be silent. Ideally, include baby in family meals.

3. **Use a proper high chair.** Make sure baby is sitting upright and not in a reclining position. Any other position, whether it's on an incline, lying down, in a car seat, in your arms, or standing up, isn't safe and poses a choking risk.

4. **Don't offer foods that are potential choking hazards and don't offer food in choking-hazard size.** Your baby's air pipe is about the width of one of their fingernails, so it's important to serve thinly sliced foods. Again, see page 204 for the list of choking hazards and alternative ways of serving them.

5. **Offer soft foods.** Peel and steam fruits and vegetables and test the foods to make sure you can squish them with your tongue on the roof of your mouth. It's much easier to cough up (or swallow) a piece of soft food than hard food. See pages 188 and 191 for a list of age-appropriate foods to offer.

6. **Take away distractions.** Don't let your baby play with toys or watch TV during meals. They need to focus on the task at hand—eating! And a distracted baby is more likely to choke.

7. **Be prepared.** Take an infant CPR course so you know what to do in the event of choking.

> **REALITY CHECK**
>
> The most common food that baby-led weaners choke on is full apples. Instead, serve apples lightly steamed, peeled, grated, or thinly sliced.

CARA SAYS: *It's crazy how many parents have a choking story about their child. But choking can happen, and the best thing you can do is take a CPR class to learn what to do in case of an emergency. You can't just call an ambulance—there is no time. You need to react FAST. And I know this firsthand, because we have a choking story about my son. He was about 18 months old and was finished eating. We took him out of his high chair and he was wandering in the dining room when my husband noticed a strange look on his little face. My husband's CPR training kicked in and he dislodged a blockage by doing a back blow like he learned in the training class. Out came a chunk of waffle. My little guy must have had it balled into his fist when he got up from the table, and put it in his mouth when he was walking about. We didn't know. When you get baby out of the high chair, check their hands! Crisis averted, thankfully. But it left an indelible mark on my husband, who still cringes every time we have waffles.*

What do I do if I think my baby is constipated?

First, let's establish what constipation is and what it's not:

- **Constipation:** Baby's stools are hard, dry, and painful to pass, and this lasts for more than 2 weeks.
- **Constipation is *not*:** Baby doesn't poop once a day. It's normal for babies to poop daily, or to skip a few days.

If your baby *is* constipated, they may not feel like eating due to a tummy ache. It's pretty common for babies to get constipated, especially when solids are first introduced. It's a huge change to their system. So what can you do? First, don't panic. Constipation is common when kids either don't get enough fluids or don't get enough fiber (or both). Sometimes a simple fix is to offer some water (via sippy, straw, or open cup) and amp up servings of fiber-rich foods like beans, lentils, nuts, seeds, vegetables, fruits, and whole grains (see page 29). If upping the fiber and fluid isn't working, try these strategies:

- **Baby exercise!** When baby is lying on their back, gently move their legs like they're riding a bike.
- **Introduce stewed prunes.** They can work wonders on backed-up babies. Start

with a small amount, like a couple of teaspoons—they don't need a lot!

- **Cut back on refined infant cereal or other refined grains like white bread.** Use whole grain cereals like oat, barley, or multigrain (and other whole grains like oatmeal, whole grain bread, or whole grain pasta) instead, because they contain more fiber.
- **Try a very soft tummy massage.** This often stimulates the bowels. Try it a few times a day.

If nothing seems to work and baby is going weeks without a bowel movement and appears to be in pain, talk to your doctor.

What should I do if my baby doesn't want solid food?

Many babies make the transition to solids fairly smoothly. But of course, all babies are different, and some really love breast- or bottle-feedings and have little interest in solid food. Some babies progress really quickly through different textures and food groups, while others take longer to adjust to solids.

Keep in mind that breastmilk and/or formula still provide the majority of baby's nutrition up until the age of 9 months, which means that although it's important to introduce a wide variety of foods early on, these first few months are for learning more than for pure nourishment.

And before you panic that your baby isn't eating well, it's important to troubleshoot. Here are some common reasons why your baby is rejecting solid foods:

Baby comes to the table full: There is no rule that you must breast- or formula-feed your baby prior to offering solid foods, but many parents feel more comfortable doing this. The issue with this strategy is that your baby may come to the table feeling full and will not be as open to eating solid foods. Make sure that you give your baby a bit of time before offering solids after a full breast- or formula-feed—an hour or so to develop a bit of an appetite.

Baby is too hungry: On the other hand, you want to make sure that your baby isn't too hungry when they come to the table—fussiness may deter your baby from trying new foods. Ideally, your baby should be alert and slightly hungry when they come to the table.

The environment is too distracting: If your baby is distracted by toys, music, screens, or siblings, they may become too distracted to focus on their food. Try to create a healthy and distraction-free environment (preferably at a family table) for your baby to test and enjoy solid foods.

Baby is too tired: If you bring your baby to the table and offer solids right before a nap or bedtime, you may find that they are fussy and disinterested. Make sure that you're offering solids when your baby is alert and happy.

Baby is uncomfortable: If your baby comes to the table with clothes that are too tight, has a full diaper, is gassy or constipated, or is in pain due to teething, you may have little luck getting them to eat. Babies may take a solid food hiatus or prefer softer textures when they are teething.

Baby prefers a different texture: Some babies prefer purees over soft finger foods, or vice versa. Before spending hours pureeing many months' worth of homemade baby foods, experiment to see what your baby prefers. Try to have an open mind and be creative with how you present foods to your baby—they may want to transition to a lumpier texture (or self-feed with finger foods) sooner than you think! For example, your baby may not like mashed banana, but may enjoy picking up a half banana.

Baby can't grasp foods: If you choose to feed your baby finger foods early on, you may be tempted to cut the food into teeny tiny, eensy weensy pieces so that baby doesn't choke. Unfortunately, babies don't have the fine motor skills to pick up these tiny pieces of food and bring them to their mouths until they are around 8 or 9 months old (or older). This may be why baby isn't eating much at mealtime, when really, they want to! It's so important that you make baby's food pieces large enough that baby can grasp them on their own. Or, for slippery soft foods, try coating larger pieces (e.g. banana or avocado) in infant rice cereal to add grip!

But you're worried about choking, right? Cut foods in long, thin strips rather than chunks, and choose soft foods that melt in the mouth easily. Try cooked sweet potato, boneless, skinless chicken thigh cut lengthwise, or a long slice of ripe peeled pear.

A piece of whole grain toast with some butter on it cut into thick strips would be appropriate too. Your baby should be able to pick up their food, bring it to their mouth, and "gum" away at it. It is normal for baby to "miss" their mouth or drop their food, but as long as they can bring it to their mouth, it is likely appropriate in size.

SARAH SAYS: *It's important to understand that every baby is different, even when it comes to siblings. My eldest child, Ben, preferred to be spoon-fed as a baby, whereas my daughter, Lylah, spat purees out and swatted the spoon that I offered, yet happily gobbled up soft finger foods right from 6 months of age. Had I assumed that Lylah was rejecting her food and was a "picky eater," I may have created problems that were never there to begin with. Instead, I was able to keep an open mind and one day allowed her to grab the banana out of my hand and devour it whole. We never looked back at purees again. There's no right or wrong way; what's important is having an open mind, experimenting with different textures and flavors, and, above all, having lots of patience (and fun!).*

What to avoid

It's important to have the proper tools (remember the Division of Responsibility (sDOR), page 41) to help your baby overcome any early feeding difficulties in a way that doesn't make matters worse or perpetuate the problem further.

Try not to become forceful or domineering when feeding, or feed in a way that doesn't respond to your baby's natural cues (e.g., putting a spoonful of food into baby's mouth when they aren't ready or willing to take it). Any form of pressured feeding can lead to mistrust and anxiety when it comes to eating and can create picky eating issues later on.

Be patient and allow your baby to control what and how much they eat right from day one. That's called "baby-led feeding"—and it allows a baby to feel confident that their own cues are enough and can be trusted. Ultimately, this contributes to a healthy relationship with food for life. Read more about our approaches to feeding on page 41.

> REALITY CHECK
>
> Common old-school feeding techniques such as the airplane trick (distracting a baby by pretending the spoon is an airplane and then landing it into baby's mouth) aren't beneficial long-term and can actually create more issues. While these techniques get the job done NOW, it's important to put your long-term lens on. What you teach your baby about feeding will affect their long-term relationship with food.

Reasons to seek help

If your baby rejects or doesn't swallow any of the food that is offered at first (even for the first couple of weeks), know that this is normal and to keep trying, in a non-pressured way. If your baby continues to reject foods into the seventh month, whether offered by spoon or as soft finger foods put on baby's tray, it may be time to seek professional help from a dietitian or feeding expert to see if there's something more complex going on.

If none of the reasons above seem to make sense in your case, contact your doctor who can refer you to the proper specialist. This is the case if baby has trouble chewing or swallowing; vomits frequently during or after meals; is not eating family foods by their first birthday; is rejecting solid foods altogether; or is consistently fussy/crying at mealtimes.

I'm worried my baby doesn't eat enough. How do I know?

Remember the Division of Responsibility (sDOR) from the introduction (page 41)? It explains that babies and children are responsible for *how much* they eat. We are all born intuitive eaters. Some parents may assume that their baby doesn't know how much food they need, when in fact it is the opposite—babies know better than anyone how much they need. They are extremely intuitive and will eat when hungry and stop when comfortably full if given the chance (see page 44)!

Infants naturally stop eating or give cues that they are done once they feel full. When a baby's feeding cues are ignored or bypassed, mistrust develops between the baby and parent and may serve as the root for feeding issues down the road. Have faith that they are getting enough by trusting their appetite and following their cues. For a list of hunger cues and fullness cues from baby, refer back to page 160.

SARAH SAYS: *Many parents tell me that they feel as though their baby hardly ingests any of the food that is served, because after the meal, the high chair is covered with bits of food. Know that this is normal and that your baby is likely eating what they need—if you are paying close attention to baby's cues.*

> (REALITY CHECK)
>
> Do your job of feeding so that your baby can do their job of eating. Parents have the important job of providing babies with a variety of nutrient-dense foods in a safe and healthy eating environment. Babies are in charge of deciding whether and how much food is eaten. This is the backbone of the sDOR.

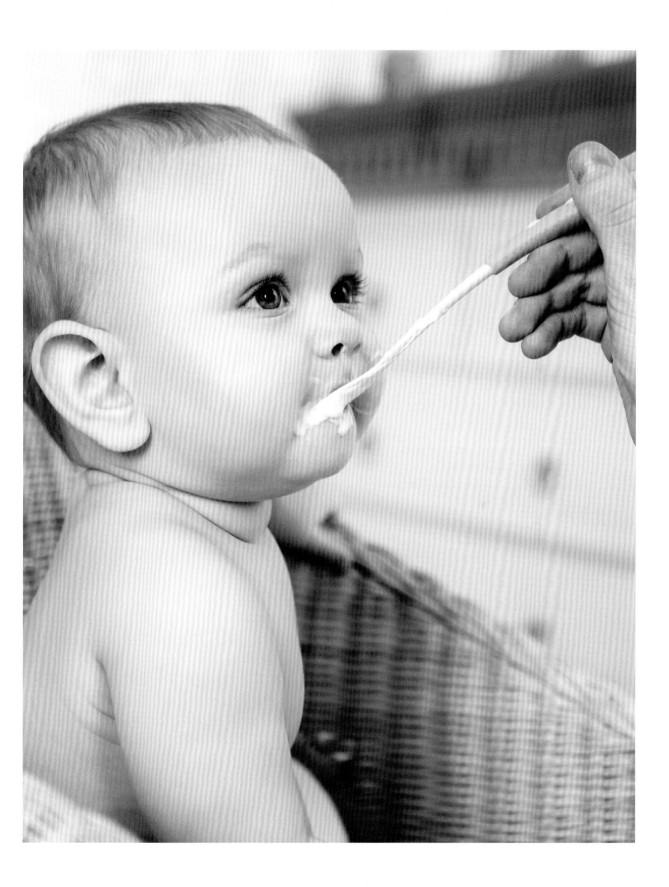

Sandra and her husband went to a dietitian for nutrition counseling when their baby, Aria, was 10 months old. They had introduced solids by doing baby-led weaning and had just fed Aria the same foods that they were making for the rest of the family (with the exception of choking hazards and salty or sugary foods).

They were concerned that their daughter wasn't eating enough solid food. In recent weeks, Aria's appetite seemed smaller and she didn't seem interested in finger foods anymore. She was fussier than normal and having some trouble sleeping, which was unusual for her.

The dietitian asked Aria's parents to take some videos of her while she was eating. Upon viewing the videos at the next appointment, the dietitian saw that Aria wanted to eat—she was still interested in food—but every time she put a piece of food in her mouth, she winced in pain. Turns out she was teething! When Sandra and the dietitian looked inside of Aria's little mouth, they noticed that she had 3 teeth that were about to surface—she was REALLY teething!

When babies teethe, their gums are so sensitive that it's hard for them to gum or chew food. It's just a phase. The dietitian suggested that they offer some smoother-textured foods, such as oatmeal, yogurt, smoothies, unsweetened fruit and vegetable sauces, and softer meats and fish, rather than finger foods that needed chewing—just temporarily until Aria's teeth surfaced. It worked like a charm—Aria devoured her softer foods, it all made sense to her parents, and soon enough, they were back to baby-led weaning and offering family foods.

My baby rejects lots of foods that I offer. What should I do?

When presented with a new food, some babies may make funny faces or spit it out right away. Some parents take this as rejection and assume that their baby isn't a fan and likely won't be for a long time. Not the case. It's just new, and your baby is learning. In most cases, the reaction that babies give to a new and unfamiliar food is a normal reaction to something unknown.

Okay, imagine you are at a cocktail party and a waiter offers you a weird pink mushy-looking ball

♥ (WE GOT YOU!)
Keep trying! It can take many exposures until baby likes the food. Of course, there may be some foods that baby NEVER likes, and that's fine too. Even adults have a short list of foods they don't like!

with some green and black dots on it. You're talking to the party host, who encourages you to try it. So you pick it up, maybe sniff it, and slowly take a bite because you're unsure what to expect. Will it be salty? Sweet? Sour? Do you like it? Will you spit it out? THAT'S how a baby feels too—a little apprehensive, a little curious, somewhat unsure . . . Although baby may reject a new food after the first several offers, with repeated non-pressured exposure (where baby is in charge), they may eventually warm up to it and accept it. If you limit your baby's menu to only what they love now, they won't have the opportunity to widen their palate. If you're worried about picky eating, read more on page 49.

What type of cup should my baby be drinking water out of?

You can start giving your baby water at around the time they start solid foods—about 6 months. When it's time to do this, it seems like the go-to cup of choice for parents of babies and toddlers is the sippy cup. Sippy cups are easy and convenient and prevent a mess, but they're not our first choice for everyday use for a few reasons (outlined in detail on page 241). Instead, babies can be introduced to regular, open cups at 6 months of age, when they start solid foods. The most recent infant-feeding guidelines say that open cups are the best choice right from the get-go.

Seriously? What about the spill factor? When your baby is first learning, you'll likely need to reserve open cups for family mealtimes at the table, when you can help and be on spill watch. And of course, you don't want to fill the cup with too much fluid (it's just more to clean up).

When on the go, a better option is a straw cup. Straw drinking is harder work than sipping from a sippy cup. It develops the same oral muscles needed to successfully and safely manipulate food in a baby's mouth, and the same muscles needed to make sounds and talk! Babies are typically ready to learn

REALITY CHECK

By choosing a straw or open cup, you're helping to build a stronger foundation for developing these important skills. And if your toddler is struggling with solids or speech, moving away from a bottle or sippy cup might just help! Even if you continue using a sippy cup once in a while (which is okay!), try to use an open cup when you can. Even better, slowly wean your little one from the sippy and start using a combination of open cups and straw cups. Your little one will surprise you at how quickly they learn!

how to drink from a straw cup at 9 months of age, but you can start right from 6 months (or sooner). They might cough or liquid may go "down the wrong pipe" at first—this is normal. If it happens often, though, try putting a thicker liquid into the cup (something like a smoothie) until they get the hang of it.

SARAH SAYS: *I found that introducing an open cup at 6 months helped both my daughter and my son "get it" sooner. By the time they were both a year old, they were using regular cups fairly independently without too many spills.*

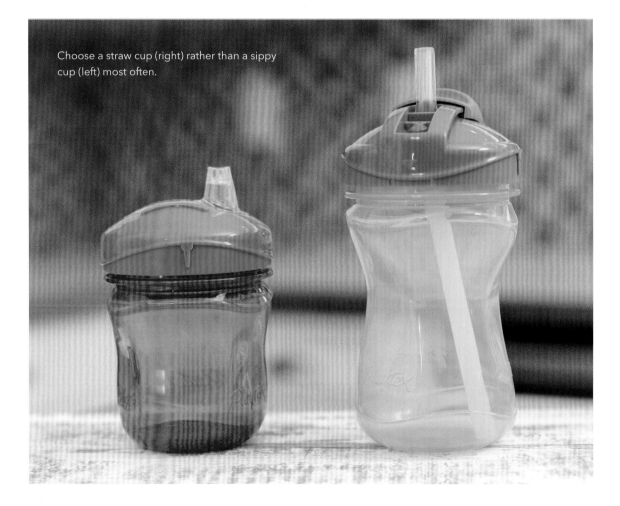

Choose a straw cup (right) rather than a sippy cup (left) most often.

Top 10 Tips

for babies (6 to 12 months)

1 Introduce solids.
Baby is ready to eat solid foods by 6 months (and this is the right time to start!).

2 Choose the first food.
Baby cereal, fruit, vegetables, meat, beans–anything goes for the first taste of food!

3 Choose iron-rich foods.
Baby needs iron-rich foods at least twice a day.

4 Limit rice cereal.
Try iron-enriched infant whole grain, barley, or oatmeal cereal instead.

5 Be aware that some foods are choking hazards.
Take an infant CPR course!

6 Feed with the combo method.
Try both spoon-feeding and letting baby self-feed soft finger foods, even at the same meal!

7 Know that gagging is normal.
It's a natural reflex that prevents choking. Stay calm, and baby will be calm too.

8 Don't delay allergenic foods.
Peanuts, tree nuts, milk, eggs, soy, and other possible allergens should be introduced at 6 months.

9 Know your role.
Let baby be responsible for how much they eat. Don't force-feed!

10 Introduce a cup.
At 6 months, try water in a cup. It will be messy at first, but baby will learn quickly!

Toddler

(12 to 24 months)

Introduction

Welcome to the toddler years! Having a toddler is fun, fascinating, and frustrating all at the same time, especially when it comes to eating! As your child transitions from babyhood to toddlerhood, you'll notice developmental and social changes, which can impact their eating habits too. With better balance and coordination, and the desire to master fine motor skills, self-feeding becomes easier. Plus, their newly developed sense of self will help them actually want to control more of their own food intake. It's a good thing! This chapter will explain how to help your toddler wean off bottles, learn to drink from a cup, and successfully feed themselves with a spoon (if they are not doing that already).

You'll probably notice that your toddler's eating habits become a bit more unpredictable too. At this stage, kids' appetites and food intake may start to slow down along with their growth, which is totally normal. But it typically means they become more selective about their food choices as they yearn for independence and control—enter: picky eating (see all about it on page 49)! Your toddler may love a food one day but refuse it the next, toss an entire bowl of freshly cooked oatmeal on the floor, or throw a tantrum at the sight of a previously loved food. Your once stellar eater may not be as adventurous anymore (or maybe they will be—all kids are different!). Please know that these things are NORMAL and your toddler is learning and experimenting. It's all part of the process of learning to eat, and it does pass.

> As your child transitions from babyhood to toddlerhood, you'll notice developmental and social changes, which can impact their eating habits too.

Although your child has (hopefully) participated in family meals since they started solids, toddlerhood marks the time when they're able to communicate and engage with family members at the table in a more meaningful way. Family meals become increasingly important at this stage. They present many great opportunities for bonding, sharing, and learning—not just about food, but about tradition, rituals, language, and life! Toddlers will start to really feel like a part of the action and will begin to model after their parents and older siblings. It's really fun to watch. Welcome to the adventure-filled world of toddler feeding!

Nutrients

IRON

Iron continues to be important during this stage as toddlers are at higher risk of developing iron deficiency anemia until about 18 months. At least 2 servings of iron-rich foods, such as meat, poultry, fish, eggs, beans, or lentils, should be offered daily for this reason.

VITAMIN D

Your toddler's vitamin D requirements jump from 400 IU (10 micrograms) per day to 600 IU (15 micrograms) per day. Even with the addition of cow's milk (if you choose to serve milk), vitamin D supplementation needs to continue. It's very difficult to meet requirements through food alone, since few foods contain vitamin D. Continue with a 400 IU supplement daily. We find the drops work well.

DIETARY FAT

Babies and toddlers need enough fat in their diet for healthy brain and nervous system development. Studies have shown that omega-3 fat (specifically DHA and EPA) has beneficial effects on brain, nerve, and eye development in babies, toddlers, and kids. Babies and toddlers 6 to 24 months should be getting about 10 to 12 milligrams of DHA per kilogram per day. So if your toddler is 20 pounds (9.1 kilograms), they should be getting about 91 to 109 milligrams of DHA per day. At least 2 servings of oily fish per week will cover this, and more. If you go the supplement route, most supplements will contain both DHA and EPA, but what you should look for is the correct daily amount of DHA. See the lists of foods rich in DHA and EPA on page 367.

> Family meals become increasingly important at this stage.

PROTEIN

Young toddlers need at least 13 grams of protein per day to meet their requirements. (But that's just a minimum—of course they can get more than 13 grams!) If they are not big eaters, don't worry: 13 grams of protein equals just 1 egg and 1 serving of Greek yogurt. Or it could be a couple of tablespoons of meat, some milk, and a small piece of cheese. Not much!

Your toddler's day

Because of their slowed growth, young toddlers don't need to eat as much or as often as they did as babies, and they may be more selective. It's important that nutritious meals and snacks are offered at regular and predictable intervals (about every 2 to 3 hours). Try to stay relatively consistent with your schedule so that your child learns that eating isn't a free-for-all, but something that happens at roughly the same intervals every day. This will help them develop a healthy meal pattern so they don't graze all day or say "hungry!" and ask for food. Consistency is key.

At this stage, establishing mealtime boundaries around WHAT, WHEN, and WHERE they eat is important so that your toddler can learn how to manage their hunger and fullness (self-regulate) and eat intuitively. The more regular and predictable your meal and snack timing can be (with a bit of flexibility, of course—let's be real), the easier it is for young toddlers to learn how to manage their appetite and food intake. Although you established feeding roles when you introduced solids, these roles are strengthened *big-time* in early toddlerhood, which can help to set them up for a healthy relationship with food. That's right—these boundaries may be a bit of a struggle, but they are worth it because they lead to less picky eating, better weight management, and healthy thoughts and behaviors regarding food as they grow. Refresh your memory on the Division of Responsibility (sDOR) again (page 41).

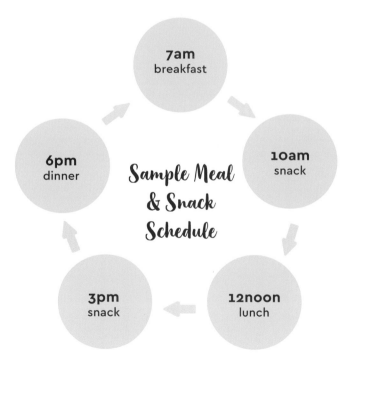

STRUCTURED MEALS AND SNACKS

To the left you'll see a suggested meal and snack schedule for your toddler. These times aren't meant to be exact, so don't worry if they don't match your routine. What they show is a nice pattern of meals and snacks that you can recreate on your own time.

Foods to choose

Your toddler may still be breastfeeding or drinking expressed breastmilk, which is encouraged for as long as it feels right for you and your toddler. Breastmilk offers so many nutritional and immunological benefits! At this stage, however, food *can* provide 100% of a toddler's nutritional needs if breastfeeding has ended. And cow's milk can be safely introduced to replace breastmilk at around 12 months of age.

Formula-fed, healthy-weight babies can be weaned from formula at 12 months (and should be fully weaned by about 14 to 18 months), unless your toddler's doctor has advised otherwise (for example, if your child is not growing well, the doctor may recommend formula for a longer period). Read more about why on page 238.

On average, toddlers need about 1,300 calories per day for proper growth and development, and these calories need to come from a variety of foods so they get all of the vitamins and minerals they need. But that word "calories?" We say it really cautiously, because we certainly *do not* want you to be counting your toddler's calories—this isn't necessary, nor is it healthy! As long as you're following the Division of Responsibility (sDOR) (see page 41), your toddler should get what they need for proper growth and development on their own.

> Because of their slowed growth, young toddlers don't need to eat as much or as often as they did as babies, and they may be more selective.

We hesitate to give you guidelines on exactly how much 12-to-24-month-olds should eat each day because it can be SO varied! We don't want to you stress or worry if your child eats more or less than what a silly chart says (you have enough stress already!). So instead of focusing on how much your child should eat, we're going to suggest *what* to offer your child to eat. Leave the rest up to them—they know their appetite. If they eat it all, great. If not, that's fine too! Turn to page 230 for some sample meal and snack ideas.

Sample Meals and Snacks for 12-to-24-month-olds

Sample day 1	Sample day 2
Breakfast	
Banana	Oatmeal
Whole grain toast, strips	Almonds, slivered
Peanut butter	Blueberries
Whole milk	Whole milk
Morning snack	
Plain unsweetened full-fat (at least 3.25%) yogurt	Peaches, diced
	Whole grain toast, strips
Watermelon, cut into wedges	Nut or seed butter
Lunch	
Cooked chicken thigh, cut into strips or chunks	Cooked zucchini and squash
	Whole grain pita
Cooked quinoa	Flaked light skipjack tuna (low-sodium)
Steamed broccoli with cheese on top	with mayonnaise
Afternoon snack	
Steamed whole garden carrots	Unsweetened applesauce
Strawberries	Plain unsweetened full-fat (at least
Homemade hummus	3.25%) yogurt
Dinner	
Cooked beef, or tofu, sliced	Homemade chili
Whole grain pasta with sauce	Cheese
Cooked sweet potato, diced	Whole grain bread
Whole milk	Whole milk

Is cow's milk essential in my toddler's diet?

In short, no. Cow's milk is not essential, but some of the nutrients in cow's milk—like calcium, vitamin D and protein—ARE essential. Cow's milk is certainly an easy way for your child to get all of those nutrients in a drink (that most kids enjoy!), but it's not the only way to get those nutrients. So if you choose not to offer cow's milk, that's totally fine! If your child will not be drinking milk (perhaps your family follows a vegan diet or your toddler has a milk allergy), it's important to pick complementary foods to replace the nutrients found in milk with other food sources. See pages 364, 369 and 371 for a list of foods (beyond milk) that contain calcium, protein, and vitamin D. If you're not sure how, make sure to consult with a dietitian.

How do I introduce cow's milk to my toddler?

Whole cow's milk can be safely introduced to replace breastmilk or formula at around 12 months of age. Before this age, your baby's digestive tract isn't mature enough to handle large quantities of the nutrients in cow's milk. A bit of milk in a recipe is fine, but you do not want to fill bottles or cups with milk until 12 months.

> **WE GOT YOU!**
> If you don't want to feed your child any dairy foods, that's totally fine. Dairy foods are not "must-haves," but the nutrients in dairy foods—like calcium and vitamin D—are vital.

The transition to cow's milk

The easiest way to transition to milk is to start with 1 or 2 tablespoons a day, mixed into formula or expressed breastmilk, then slowly increase the amount of milk over a few weeks until you are serving pure milk. Some moms like to breastfeed morning and night and serve cow's milk after lunch. Then eventually they replace the morning feed with cow's milk too. There's no exact pattern you need to follow. Just take it slow to give baby a chance to adjust. Cow's milk is not as sweet-tasting as breastmilk, so your child may not like it right away. Be patient! You can start this right at 12 months or a little earlier if that fits better with your schedule.

HOW MUCH SHOULD I GIVE?

Toddlers can have up to 16 ounces (2 cups) of milk per day. If they also eat cheese and yogurt, you can reduce the amount of milk they drink.

WHOLE MILK

Be sure to stick with whole milk to start; you don't want to feed your baby reduced-fat or fat-free milk until after the age of 2 because they need dietary fat found in milk for proper growth and development. Depending on where you live, this milk may be called whole, homo, homogenized, full-fat, red cap, red lid, or 3.25% milk fat.

When it's time to introduce milk, don't rush it! You want to give your little one time to adjust to the new proteins and other nutrients in cow's milk by starting with 1 or 2 tablespoons a day. You can slowly increase this amount until fully transitioned, which typically takes time—anywhere from 2 to 6 weeks.

> **PROBLEM SOLVED: FORMULA OR COW'S MILK?**
>
> Mara was planning to return to her job after maternity leave, and was weaning her baby Sabrina off breastmilk as she transitioned her to more solid foods. Mara's first day back at work would coincide with Sabrina's 11-month "birthday," and Mara sought advice because she was confused about the optimal fluid to fill Sabrina's baby bottles. She felt stressed about the idea of pumping breastmilk every day, so that was not an option. She wondered if she should introduce formula or start Sabrina on cow's milk before the 12-month date that her doctor suggested. Ultimately, Mara opted for cow's milk for several reasons:
>
> 1. Formula has a strong flavor, and it's tough to introduce it at 11 months of age, especially after a child has been breastfed for so long.
> 2. Formula is more expensive than cow's milk.
> 3. The daycare that she was taking her child to had milk on the menu beginning at 12 months, so it was only 4 weeks away. She didn't want to transition Sabrina to formula for 4 weeks, then transition again to milk. It was easier to make only 1 transition!
> 4. Her dietitian and doctor assured her that while the transition to cow's milk was optimal at 12 months, it was safe to introduce it at 11 months, especially if it coincided with a work start date (or a vacation, or any other reason).
>
> Sabrina settled into daycare drinking cow's milk (and occasionally goat's milk), through an infant straw cup—something that she was used to sipping water out of already.

Is it okay to serve my toddler plant-based milk alternatives?

Milk alternatives such as rice, hemp, coconut, oat, cashew, or almond beverages don't contain enough calories, protein, or fat to directly replace breastmilk, formula, or cow's milk. Using these milk alternatives alone won't provide proper nutrition for growth and development, especially before 12 months of age. Of course, it's totally fine to whip up a smoothie and add a bit of almond milk, or to stir some coconut milk in baby's oatmeal. But these milk alternatives should not be used as a replacement for cow's milk, breastmilk, or formula, because they are simply not nutritious enough.

LET'S BREAK IT DOWN . . .

Beginning at 12 months, if you are no longer breast- or formula-feeding, your best options are:

- **Whole cow's milk:** This milk contains the essential protein, dietary fat, vitamins, and minerals your baby needs. And don't use skim or 2% milk—whole cow's milk contains extra fat, which is important for growth and development.
- **Goat's milk:** Goat's milk is comparable to cow's milk in its nutritional qualities. It has similar amounts of protein, calcium, and vitamin A. Choose one that's whole-fat, pasteurized, and fortified with folic acid and vitamin D.

Turn to page 235 to see the nutritional value of cow's and goat's milk versus plant-based alternatives. This will give you a good sense of the differences between milks, and also the alternative sources of nutrients you should look for more of should you choose a plant-based milk.

WHAT ABOUT SOY MILK?

Soy milk has about the same amount of protein as cow's milk, but only about half as much of dietary fat. Some dietitians recommend it as the best option for vegan children along with adding more dietary fat to their diet in other ways (with healthy oils, nuts, seeds, salmon, etc., turn to pages 27 and 366 for more on dietary fat.).

> **REALITY CHECK**
>
> No plant-based milk is 100% nutritionally equivalent to cow's milk. Be sure to read the labels of milk alternatives: almond, coconut, hemp, or rice beverages are often fortified with similar vitamins and minerals as cow's milk, but they don't contain nearly enough protein or dietary fat to be considered a safe or healthy 1:1 alternative for this age group.

Surprise, surprise—there is some controversy in the nutrition world about certain milk alternatives for toddlers, and soy milk is at the top of the list. Some nutrition experts believe that since it's lower in calories, fat, and protein than cow's milk, it's not a suitable alternative. Others believe it's okay because it's the closest plant-based option (nutritionally speaking) to cow's milk.

In cases where cow's milk is not an option (maybe your child has a milk allergy or is vegan), you can offer full-fat, fortified, "original" (not unsweetened) soy beverage instead of milk as long as there are no growth or development concerns (because in that case, your child will need to consume a high-fat/high-calorie diet, and soy milk will not suffice).

Some conventional soy products come from genetically modified soybeans and may contain traces of synthetic pesticides or fertilizers. If this is a concern to you, choose an organic soy beverage. Check your package carefully to ensure that the soy beverage is fortified with vitamins and minerals (such as calcium and vitamin D), which are added to mimic the nutrients found in cow's milk.

Beyond the nutrient content, there's another soy controversy you should know about. Soy contains antioxidants known as isoflavones, which may protect against certain diseases. That's good news. Isoflavones have a mild estrogen-like effect, and that's where some people kinda freak out a little. Estrogen is a sex hormone that plays an important role in reproduction, so some people wonder if soy will make their daughter go through puberty too early or make their son grow man-boobs. These are legitimate questions. The answer is mostly that we don't know. Very few studies have been conducted that involve children and soy intake, and the few that do exist are very small or are funded by the soy industry (and are obviously supportive of soy).

At the end of the day, it's your choice as a parent whether you want to offer soy milk as an alternative to cow's milk, because there isn't enough science to make a truly non-biased, evidence-based decision.

NUTRITIONAL VALUE OF MILKS (PER CUP)

	Calories (kcal)	Protein (grams)	Fat (grams)	Sugar (grams)
Whole cow's milk	157	8	8	12 (from lactose)*
Whole goat's milk	178	9	10	11 (from lactose)*
Unsweetened soy milk	80	7	4	1
Original soy milk	110	8	4.5	6
Unsweetened hemp milk	60	3	4	0
Original hemp milk	140	3	5	14
Unsweetened coconut milk	45	0	4	0
Original coconut milk	60	0	4	3
Unsweetened almond milk	35	1	2.5	0
Original almond milk	60	1	3	7
Unsweetened rice milk	70	0	2.5	1
Original rice milk	130	1	2	14
Unsweetened cashew milk	40	1	3	0
Original cashew milk	50	0	2.5	5

*There is no added sugar in cow's or goat's milk. The sugar comes from naturally occurring lactose.

Could my baby be lactose intolerant?

There is no routinely used lactose intolerance test for babies, but check with your doctor. If they suggest your baby may have lactose intolerance, you can try lactose-free milk in place of regular cow's milk, offered in the same quantity. If your baby has been diagnosed with a milk allergy, you may want to consider continuing breastmilk or formula (or follow-up formula) until the age of 2 to ensure proper nutritional needs are met. There are soy or hydrolyzed protein/hypoallergenic formula varieties for babies with milk allergies (see page 165).

My toddler wants milk all the time. How much is too much?

Sometimes parents (and toddlers) rely too heavily on milk for nourishment, and this can lead to undernutrition and picky eating. If milk is served in a bottle or sippy cup, it can be used for nourishment AND comfort making it a hard habit to break. It also puts your toddler's little teeth at risk of cavities. Drinking too much milk can become a problem for a couple of reasons:

It can displace other nutrients: Milk is nutritious. It contains calcium, vitamin D, magnesium, phosphorus, and about 12 other essential nutrients. But it also has a strong satiating effect—that's the fancy way of saying that it makes you feel full. Milk contains both fat and protein—nutrients that make toddlers with small tummies feel really full. Of course, if they drink too much milk throughout the day (especially between meals), they won't be hungry at mealtime! Too much milk can displace other nutritious foods in their diet.

> **WE GOT YOU!**
>
> Don't freak out about tooth decay, because it can easily be prevented. You can use a toddler toothbrush with non-fluoride toothpaste to scrub away any bacteria that builds up on their little teeth. You can also rinse their mouth with water. The American Academy of Pediatric Dentistry recommends that a child's first trip to the dentist happen at one year. At the appointment, the dentist will check for any decay.

Those teeth! Milk also contains lactose, a naturally occurring sugar. When toddlers are drinking milk all day (especially out of a sippy cup), the sugar can wreak havoc on their teeth. Known as baby-bottle tooth decay, it can happen when any sweet liquids (yes, even milk!) cling to teeth. Bacteria in the mouth will thrive on sugar and create acid that harms teeth and leads to decay.

HOW MUCH IS TOO MUCH?

Toddlers need only about 2 cups of milk per day. And the best time to offer this milk? With or just after a meal. Offer about ½ cup at mealtimes (or right after), which leaves room for another ½ cup before bedtime, if that is part of your routine. Water should be the only fluid offered between meals for hydration. And if your toddler doesn't like milk, or you'd prefer not to serve it, that's okay, as long as they are getting those essential nutrients from other sources.

When should I wean my child from breastfeeding?

Deciding when to wean your child is a very personal decision, and it can depend on a few different factors. Some moms decide on a specific age to start the weaning process; others go with child-led weaning (i.e., letting their child decide when they are done nursing). Regardless of what you *think* you want, you may find yourself nursing your 18-month-old toddler, even when you didn't expect to! There's no one size fits all. What's important, is to wean gradually to let both your body and baby to adjust.

Setting boundaries is okay: Beginning at 12 months, we suggest setting a breastfeeding schedule that works for you (unless your little one gets sick, in which case they may breastfeed more for comfort). Just like the Division of Responsibility (sDOR) for meals, it is the same for breastfeeding: you decide when to offer a breastfeeding session (not the other way around), and then your toddler decides how much and for how long they breastfeed during that session. There can be some give and take when it comes to breastfeeding your toddler—it's a relationship that goes both ways. Perhaps breastfeeding sessions are limited to first thing in the morning and before bedtime (if that's what's most convenient for you), or maybe they happen between mealtimes. Set the schedule that works for you both, and stick with it.

Weaning doesn't always happen linearly: Know that your toddler may want to nurse more at certain times—during growth spurts, when they're sick, or when they're teething—and that's okay, and normal as long as you feel comfortable with it. We encourage you to continue offering regular and balanced meals during these times, and leave some time between nursing sessions and solid food feeds for them to build up an appetite. During mealtimes, let your toddler self-feed solid food and eat as much as they want, without pressure (see Division of Responsibility (sDOR) on page 41).

CARA SAYS: *I nursed both of my children until around 15 months, and as they became more mobile and busier, they were less interested in breastfeeding. The key to weaning is to take it slowly so your breasts can adjust. (Because, ouch! Weaning too quickly = sore, engorged breasts, rapid hormonal changes, and a very unhappy mommy.) I dropped a feed every few weeks until we were just left with the morning cuddle feed and the goodnight feed. Then I gradually dropped the morning feed and kept that night feed for another month, then replaced it with milk before bed, in the same cuddle chair with the same story book. Worked like a charm.*

My toddler prefers breastfeeding over solid food. Should I worry?

Your toddler should be eating a variety of nutritious foods and participating in family meals, regardless of whether they are still breastfeeding or not. It may seem like your toddler isn't eating as much as other children the same age, and this is probably because of the additional calories and nutrition they receive from breastmilk. But if they're eating a variety of foods—and they're happy and growing well—don't worry! Breastmilk is still a very important part of their diet because it's where many nutrients come from!

Now, if they're not eating a well-balanced diet and you're concerned that they'd fall short without breastmilk, you can read more about how to deal with picky eating on page 49—though we also suggest seeking out personalized help from a dietitian.

I can't get my toddler off the bottle and onto a cup. Any tips?

Weaning a toddler off of their milk bottle can be challenging, especially because it often serves as a source of comfort. For many parents, it can be a long, frustrating process, and can easily be put off, because . . . life. The trouble is that the longer you wait, the harder it becomes for your little one to wean. We get it—sometimes the bottle can be just as soothing for us parents as it is for a toddler! But there are several reasons for weaning your toddler from the bottle:

Tooth decay: Little teeth that are exposed to bottled formula or milk (or worse, juice, fruit punch, or soda) throughout the day are at an increased risk of cavities.

Oral motor skills and speech: Young toddlers should be developing and strengthening their oral motor skills and speech at this stage, and ditching the bottle can help with this.

(REALITY CHECK)

By 12 months, babies should be relying on solid foods for their nutrition, so formula isn't required anymore (in most cases). So it's recommended that babies be weaned from bottles around the 12-month mark; however, it may take a few months for the process to be complete. Your toddler should be fully weaned by 18 months and drinking from open cups or straw cups instead (see page 241).

Mealtimes suffer: Parents often rely on bottles for peace of mind, using them to "top up their toddlers" if they feel that they haven't eaten enough. But too-frequent bottle-feeds (whether formula, cow's milk, or breastmilk) can fill a toddler up, making them full at mealtime and displacing other nutritious foods in their diet. Snowball effect: they eat poorly at mealtime. Parents worry. And then feed their tot a bottle afterward for peace of mind. See the cycle?

Can slow eating and drinking skills: Overreliance on bottles can be a double-edged sword. It can create picky eating habits as well as delay of mature drinking skills.

SARAH SAYS: *Make sure that you either brush your toddler's teeth after their bottle (before laying them down to sleep) or, at the very least, let them sip on water afterward. With all of my toddlers, I kept a clean toothbrush beside their rocking chair in their room to quickly brush after I breastfed them or if they had warm milk before bed—I'd also get them to have a few sips of water before laying them down. This will prevent the natural milk sugar from sitting on their teeth during their nap. Gradually do the same with the bedtime feed.*

(WE GOT YOU!)
Are you wide-eyed and panicking yet? Don't worry—it's a process and it can take some time. As moms who have weaned a total of 5 babies, we get it.

Top 5 tips to help wean your toddler off the bottle

1. **Start slow, one bottle at a time.** Start by eliminating a bottle in the middle of the day first (perhaps after a nap), and then work your way out to eliminating bottles in the morning and afternoon. It's much easier to take bottle-feeds out that don't happen directly before naptime or bedtime, because they tend not to be as comforting. Then slowly transition away from the naptime bottle by offering a bit of milk (warm or cold) in a straw or open cup right before the nap, just like you would do with a bottle. Eventually, you can transition away from offering milk completely, and replace it with water before naps and bedtime. There's no "right" way to do this, so go with what works best for you and your toddler.

2. **Use the transition away from infant formula.** This is as the perfect time to switch to cups! Formula-fed toddlers associate the taste of infant formula with the bottle, so if you can start the transition away from formula at 12 months WHILE you transition away from bottles and onto cups, it will be easier! In other words, don't just replace formula with cow's milk in a bottle. Create a new association between cow's milk and cups.

3. **Offer foods every 2 to 3 hours.** Make sure that you're offering 3 nutritious and balanced meals a day, with smaller snacks (whole foods rather than treats; for the difference between these see page 16) in between if meals are longer than 3 hours apart. This will ensure that your little one is getting the nutrition that they need, and they'll rely less on the calories from the bottle.

4. **Break the associations.** Whether it's a bottle in the stroller on the way to drop older siblings off at school, or a bottle in the car, or a bottle before naptime or bedtime, associations between bottles and times of day can be hard to break. Replace bottles with something else comforting such as a favorite stuffed animal, a blanket, or snuggles with you. This will be hard at first, and associations will likely take a couple of weeks to break—consistency is key!

5. **Relax and have faith.** It's hard to have faith that your toddler—who has been so dependent on breastmilk or formula-feeds until this point—will get the nutrition needed for proper growth and development through food and milk alone. We get it. Please know that as long as you're feeding responsively, they will get enough!

I've heard that sippy cups aren't ideal for drinking out of. Is this true?

Sippy cups are the go-to cup of choice for many parents of toddlers, simply because they're easy and convenient and they prevent a mess! They're also perfect for on-the-go sipping, which is key. But you may have heard that they aren't ideal cups for toddlers, that they don't support proper oral motor development or mature drinking skills, or even that they can delay speech development.

The truth is, we all just need to take a deep breath and relax. Sippy cups are fine to use occasionally, especially when you're first introducing water in a cup at around 6 months—sippies are easier for babies to use in the beginning because they're very similar to bottles, and, let's be honest, they're easier for parents too. We used them when on the go with our babies and toddlers too. But, as dietitians, we know that they're not the ideal cup for toddlers, for a few reasons:

Coordination: Sippy cups prevent the opportunity to practice mature oral motor and swallowing skills. Toddlers use an infant-like sucking motion when drinking from a sippy cup (similar to when drinking from a bottle), and the spout prevents the front of the tongue from elevating during a swallow. Using sippy cups multiple times a day and for an extended period can prevent a toddler from developing the independent lip, jaw, and tongue movements needed for successfully drinking from a regular open cup at an appropriate age (which is around one year).

Comfort: The spout of most sippy cups is similar to a baby's bottle and can easily become a pacifier (a source of comfort) for a toddler. The more comfort the sippy cup provides, and the longer this goes on for, the harder it is to change. If the sippy cup is full of milk or formula, an association can be formed between milk and comfort as well, which can cause issues such as dependence on milk and drinking too much (regardless of what type of cup it comes out of). This can displace other nutritious foods in your child's diet.

Cavities: Sippy cups often serve as a vehicle for sugary drinks like formula, milk, or juice. When toddlers sip frequently throughout the day (which they will if there's a sippy cup hanging around), they're exposed to excess sugar, which can lead to an increased risk of cavities. We especially caution parents not to send their child to bed with a sippy cup full of milk, juice, or formula—the sugar can sit on the teeth all night putting them at risk for cavities.

SO WHAT DO WE USE INSTEAD?
Regular open cups are the best choice for kids 6 months and up (especially after age one) when they are sipping water. Read more about how to introduce an open cup on page 238. For on-the-go drinking, we suggest using a portable straw cup by the time your child is 12 months (and suggest starting this at about 9 months). Read more about why we like straw cups in the previous chapter on page 221.

WE GOT YOU!

If you have a 2-year-old who is still slurping exclusively from sippy cups, don't beat yourself up about it. Just start introducing a regular cup at meal and snack times (your child will need your help at first), and be patient—you may be surprised at how quickly your little one catches on to a regular cup!

Are there any foods that I shouldn't feed my toddler?

By 12 months, your toddler can eat everything that the rest of the family is eating, and should be enjoying a wide range of flavors and textures of food. There are 2 exceptions to this "eat everything" rule:

Avoid choking hazards: Whole grapes, popcorn, etc., should not be served. See page 205 for a list of common choking hazards.

Avoid sweets: Young toddlers don't need candy, cookies, ice cream, and cake. No fun, right?! But until they're at least 24 months old, their tummies are too small and their nutrient needs are too high, so there's little room for cake and ice cream! It's more important to fill their tummies with nutritious foods. Of course, we are realists—it's okay for your toddler to try cake at a party or some holiday sweets, but these should not be staple foods in the diet (read more on page 16).

My toddler throws food off the tray constantly. What should I do?

The first few times your baby grabs food off their high-chair tray and throws it on the floor, you laugh, pick it up, smile, and say in your gentlest voice, "No throwing, honey." You might even snap a picture because it's so adorable. But when the cuteness wears off and food throwing becomes a game—one where you're the loser—it can become frustrating (the mess!) and worrisome (there's more food on the floor and wall than in your baby's mouth!).

Food throwing is a popular topic since most parents deal with it at some point with their little ones. This is the most important takeaway: it's normal! Most kids go through a food-throwing phase in their early years. Ours sure did! Some things to keep in mind about food throwing as your baby grows:

- **For babies aged 6 to 8 months:** It's rarely intentional. It's often a result of your baby learning how to control and coordinate food with newly minted fine motor skills.
- **For older babies, 9 months plus:** It becomes an exercise in learning cause and effect: What will happen if I throw this bowl full of oatmeal? Will it make a noise? Where will it go? Will it come back?
- **Fast-forward to toddlerhood:** Now it becomes an intentional attempt to trigger a reaction—positive or negative—and can turn into a power struggle, creating stress at mealtimes.

Playing with (mushing, squishing, stacking, organizing) foods politely is a normal and positive way of becoming familiar and comfortable with a food, and should be encouraged, especially with foods that haven't yet been accepted or eaten. Food throwing, on the other hand, especially at this stage, is not as innocent and productive.

SARAH SAYS: *There's a big difference between a toddler playing with and exploring foods, and deliberately being messy with or throwing foods. My son James was a champion food tosser—definitely intentionally trying to get a reaction. I clearly remembering lunging toward his highchair to catch a full bowl of uneaten spaghetti when he was about 2 and being unsuccessful. It took everything in me to not react negatively. I calmly cleaned it up, replaced it with fresh food, and told him that food stays on his tray.*

Fast forward to having 3 kids, and my 2 older kids often egged on my youngest when he threw food—it became their mealtime entertainment! But this attention fueled the food-throwing fire and usually intensified it. When I encouraged them to "teach" their younger brother how to keep his food on his tray instead, they felt proud and their little brother followed their lead! Toddlers crave attention and a reaction, so it's best to remain calm and neutral and focus on what you WANT them to do, versus what they should not do.

Top 7 tips to stop food throwing

1. **Don't react.** Babies and toddlers are natural attention-seekers who thrive off a reaction. To avoid encouraging the behavior, do your best to stay calm and neutral.

2. **Try returning the food to the table.** But don't engage in a game of drop-and-pick-up. Replace it just once or twice, then take the hint that your toddler is done eating and is now playing instead. That teaches your toddler that once food is thrown, it's gone. Toddlers are smart, they'll learn quickly and will change their behavior!

3. **Talk to your toddler.** To reinforce your message, say something like "food belongs on the tray". Choose a phrase that indicates what you *do want* to happen, as opposed to a phrase like "we don't throw food," which indicates what you don't want to happen.

4. **Get everyone on board.** Talk to older siblings (um, and your spouse) about why it's important not to react to food throwing. And be careful not to react yourself by laughing! Make a family plan to stay really calm and not react when the young one throws food.

5. **Ditch the tray.** When older babies are learning about gravity and can see over the edge of a tray, it makes the food-throwing game more enticing. Consider removing the tray and pushing the high chair up to the table so it's harder to see the floor. Bonus: it also offers more opportunity to model healthy eating.

6. **Keep the dog out.** When you're a toddler, what's more fun (and distracting!) than throwing food and watching the dog gobble it up and beg for more? Try letting the dog out during mealtimes—you can invite them back in for cleanup!

7. **Take a hint.** Flinging food might very well be your toddler's last-resort effort to tell you, "I'm full!" If they're giving you the sign that they're full, you need to respect that. Serve portions that aren't large or overwhelming, offer more if your child indicates they want more, and take the pressure off.

> **WE GOT YOU!**
>
> If you can weather the food-throwing storm, stay calm, and focus on teaching your toddler what you want them to do (keep food on the tray or table), it will pass, and mealtimes will become more positive and less stressful all-round.

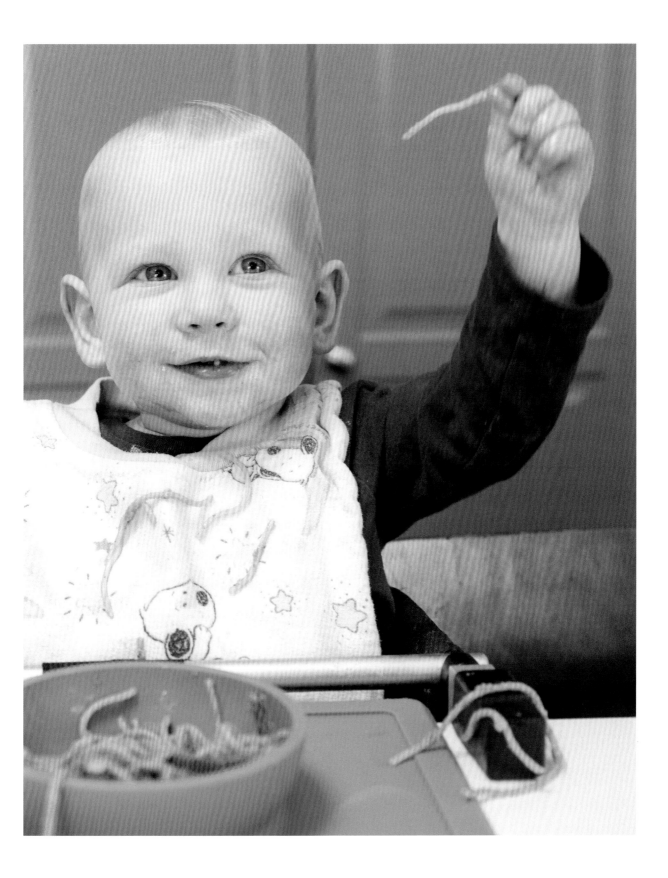

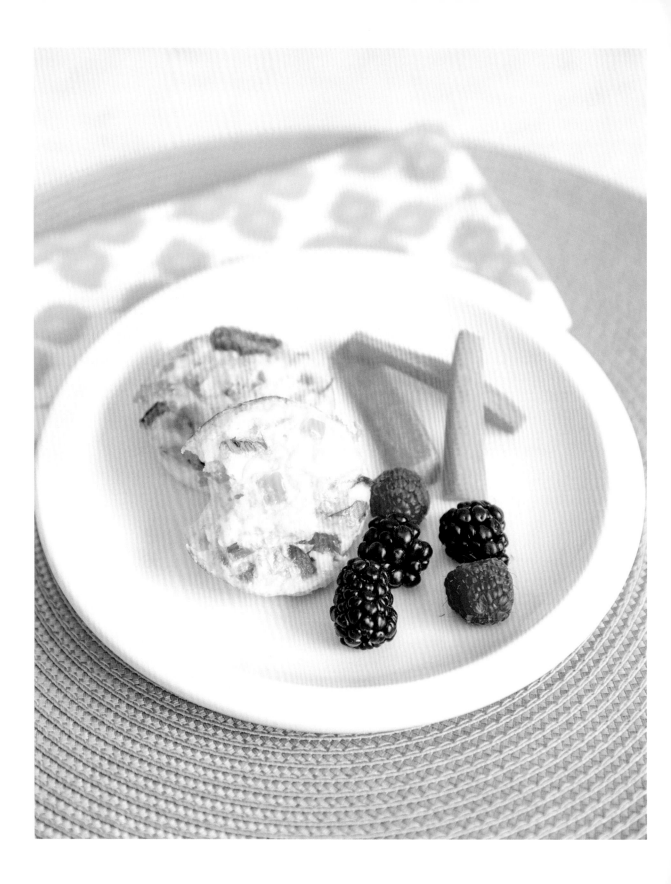

MUFFIN-TIN VEGGIE FRITTATAS

This is a great all-purpose recipe. You can freeze them for up to 3 months, reheat them, and eat them for breakfast, brunch, or dinner—and kids love them too! If you'd like, swap out the veggies: try spinach, kale, broccoli, and grated carrots.

Makes 12 mini frittatas

6 large eggs

⅓ cup milk

½ tsp salt

¼ tsp pepper

1 tomato, chopped

2 button mushrooms, chopped

½ bell pepper, seeded and chopped

2 tbsp chopped green onions

½ cup grated Cheddar cheese

1. Preheat the oven to 350°F and grease a 12-cup muffin tin.
2. In a large bowl, whisk together the eggs, milk, salt, and pepper. Add all the vegetables to the egg mixture and stir well.
3. Using a ½-cup measuring cup, scoop the egg mixture into the prepared muffin cups. Top each with 1 to 2 teaspoons grated cheese.
4. Bake until set in the middle and lightly browned, about 20 minutes.

I feel like I'm wasting so much food. How can I reduce waste?

Amidst the chaos of feeding, one big important factor can get missed: food waste. Every year in North American food waste costs the economy $278,000,000,000 USD, and is enough to feed 260,000,000 people! Wow. Little changes make big differences though (and save you time and money, too), so consider these tips:

Serve less: We tend to overserve at meals, only to throw away perfectly good half-eaten food. The solution? Serve less. A small serving of each food will suffice (and bonus: is less overwhelming for kids). If your child asks for more, serve a little more! And keep unserved leftovers for future meals.

Give foods a chance: Don't be so quick to toss food that can be repurposed. Bananas over-ripe? Freeze them for muffins. Bread almost stale? Make it French toast.

Keep your fridge and freezer uncluttered: Forgotten food creates *huge* waste. Try a "first in, first out" strategy: when you buy groceries, move the existing products in your fridge to the front first so they don't spoil at the back.

My "great eater" has suddenly become picky. Why?

Don't panic: picky eating behaviors are completely normal, and we talk about the reasons and some possible solutions in full on pages 49 to 63. In addition, here are some common reasons while your child might not be eating at meals (and what to do!):

Top 10 reasons for picky eating

1. **Too much pressure.** Don't hover over your little diner. Aim to create a calm, family-friendly space at mealtime, and let your child self-feed.
2. **Not enough control.** Involve your child in shopping, prepping, and cooking so that they feel part of mealtime choices (see page 56 for ideas). Serve meals "family style," where bowls are placed in the middle of the table and each diner gets to serve themselves (with help for small hands, of course).
3. **Simply not hungry.** Accept "I'm just not hungry" as an answer, and remind your child that the kitchen will be closed after mealtime. It's important to set boundaries around the timing of meals and snacks so that eating isn't a free-for-all, but it's just as important to let your child oversee how much they eat at these times.
4. **Too many distractions.** Remove screens and toys from the table and turn off screens and audio in other rooms. Seat kids at the table so that they can't touch, poke, or bother each other, and add a footstool under your child's feet (see page 289 for reasons why).
5. **Portions are too big.** Too much food can be intimidating to a little kid (and create unnecessary food waste!). Serve a small amount of everything, or let your child serve themselves. If they are still hungry, they can have seconds.

SARAH SAYS: *Portion size was definitely a problem with my daughter. I used to serve her the same amount that I served her older brother, but then after many meal rejections, I realized that I was serving her too much. We were wasting food and my daughter was overwhelmed with the portions that I was offering. When I cut her portions down (by more than half!), she started eating her meals again and sometimes even asked for more.*

6. **It's a texture thing.** Your child may simply not enjoy a certain food served a certain way. That's fine! You probably have food preferences too, so don't force your child to clean their plate or eat anything they don't like. Turn to page 283 for suggestions on different textures to try.

7. **Too many snacks.** If kids graze all day, they won't be hungry at mealtimes. Avoid letting your child eat throughout the day, and aim to have at least 2 hours between eating opportunities.

8. **Too tired.** Is sleepyhead falling asleep at the table? Try moving dinner to an earlier time and be consistent with nap schedules. But remember, the odd sleepiness at mealtime is not cause for alarm—they will make up for missed nutrients/calories at another time (let them sleep!).

9. **Not feeling well.** You know that being sick puts a damper on your appetite. Don't force it—your child's appetite will return when they feel better. Focus on fluids and hydration, and try serving blander foods such as bananas, rice, toast, and soup.

10. **Too much milk or juice.** Milk can fill little tummies. Stick with a maximum of 2 cups per day for small eaters. Avoid juice, but if it is a must-have, stick to no more than ½ cup unsweetened fruit juice per day.

CARA SAYS: *When Kasey was a baby, she loved broccoli. At age 2, she outright rejected it. One day, when we were driving, I calmly asked "Hey Kasey, you used to love broccoli but don't seem to like it anymore. Why is that?" And her two-word answer was simple but so insightful: "too crunchy." She was right, of course. When I stir-fry, I like the vegetables to retain some crunch. But for a 2-year-old's teeth, they were the wrong texture. The next day I made minestrone soup, where the broccoli simmers in the broth to a tender consistency. She ate 2 bowls!*

How can I have a successful meal at a restaurant with my toddler?

You can't. Ha ha—no, we're just kidding. It is totally possible to dine out with kids if you just remember the 5 Ps: place, plan, patience, prepare, and . . . pizza! A restaurant meal can be a nice break for you and can be a fun family night out. Speaking from experience, though, eating out with a toddler can also be stressful, frustrating, and embarrassing, especially if you're not prepared, or they are overly tired or hungry—and that's not fun for anyone. So we've come up with some tips that might help you decide (a) if it's worth it, and (b) how you can make it the best experience for everyone. Turn the page to read our 5 Ps.

The 5 Ps for Restaurant Meal Success

 PLACE: Choose wisely! There's no sense going to a restaurant if you're going to be stressed. Choose a family-friendly restaurant with high chairs and staff that tolerate noise and thrown food! Not sure if the restaurant will embrace the chaos of little ones? Call ahead to find out.

 PLAN: Before you leave, check out the restaurant's menu online and decide what you're going to order ahead of time. And when you get there, order right away!

PATIENCE: Never take a tired or overly hungry toddler out. Pick an opportune moment for a restaurant visit—one that won't test your patience—and don't feel bad canceling plans at the last minute—people understand!

 PREPARED: Be ready to move or leave if you have to! It's not reasonable to expect a young toddler to sit still in a high chair for much longer than 20 minutes (if that), so be prepared to go for walks around the restaurant (or outside) one or more times throughout your dining experience.

PIZZA: There's no shame in ordering in instead! In fact, if you ask either of us, we'd likely choose this option over going out.

SARAH SAYS: *When we go to restaurants with the kids (which is . . . almost never), we ask for vegetables and dip as soon as we get there—often the kids are hungry, and this is a great way to get 1 or 2 vegetable servings into them and keep them occupied until our food comes.*

CARA SAYS: *I always have some "just in case" snacks in my bag. If the kids really can't wait 5 to 10 minutes for the food to come, I let them have an "appetizer" that I've brought from home. Cucumber slices seem to be the big winner for my kids.*

WE GOT YOU!

So many things can go wrong when you're dining out with a toddler, but it's often worth the risk. Why? Because they will get used to the experience of being in a restaurant. The more exposure they have, the easier it will be to dine out as they grow up (it does get easier!). Soon they will learn how to sit still for longer than 20 minutes, then they will understand the rules of decorum in restaurants, and then they will learn the proper manners to use (like saying "please" and "thank you" to the servers). Those milestones will be proud moments.

How do I ensure my toddler is well nourished at daycare?

Having your little one enter childcare can be emotional and stressful, and finding the optimal childcare situation can be challenging, to say the least! No one will ever care for your child the way you do, and feeding won't look exactly the same (as much as we wish it would). Whether it's a nanny or a daycare, there will be new schedules, routines, and feeding styles.

Do your homework: It's important to keep nutrition and feeding top of mind when you're looking for a childcare provider. When interviewing daycares or nannies, ask a few key questions, such as:

- What will meals and snacks consist of?
- Where is the food sourced from?
- What kind of feeding style do the caregivers use? (For example, do they use the one-bite rule? Do they spoon-feed when a child is not eating well themselves? Do they pressure the child to eat if they don't want to?)

Top 10 Nutrition Questions to Ask a Daycare

1. How many meals and snacks are served during the day?
2. How much time is there between meals and snacks?
3. What is the meal and snack timing and is it structured the same every day?
4. What types of foods are served at meals and snacks? Do you follow a set menu plan? (If so, can I please see the menu?)
5. Is the food homemade? Catered? Store-bought?
6. What is your nutrition and feeding philosophy?
7. Do you enforce any mealtime boundaries (e.g., kids need to be seated at the table until excused)? What are they?
8. Are snacks given upon request or are those structured too? What is typically served?
9. Are treats or desserts given? How often? What types?
10. What is given as a beverage at meals (water, milk, juice, etc.) and between meals?

Answers to these questions will give you a good idea of whether the feeding strategies and philosophies align with your own.

Decide what's negotiable: You can also decide what you're willing to compromise on. Maybe you care more about the types of foods versus how and where meals are served. Or maybe you have a really selective eater and the feeding dynamics are more important than how balanced or nutritious the food is. Every situation and child are different, so it's important that you align your top values with your childcare provider.

Reasonably speaking, we don't suggest bombarding your potential childcare provider with a million nutrition questions (you might scare them away!), but choose a few to focus on, depending on what's most important to you. The point is to get a sense for what their feeding style is and if it matches with yours. Ideally, the types of foods and feeding styles your child experiences when in childcare are similar or in line with what's going on at home.

> **WE GOT YOU!**
> What matters most is what happens at the family table. Even if you don't 100% agree with the types of foods or the way they are served by your childcare provider, your child will learn the most valuable eating lessons and habits around the family table in the evenings and on the weekends when you're at home.

Julia was going back to work after her second maternity leave, and was not only nervous to leave her baby and toddler, but also very concerned about her older daughter's picky eating, considering that they had been struggling for a while and had just established new, more structured mealtimes. It was important to Julia that her daughter have the same feeding routine and boundaries in childcare as those that they had just established at home.

She decided to go with a live-in nanny for a few reasons, one of them being the issue of feeding and picky eating and wanting a consistent routine. Her nanny was open to suggestions and guidance on how to establish a healthy meal dynamic and keep things consistent for Julia's daughter (which Julia was relieved about). Julia invited their new nanny to eat a few meals with them to get a sense of what the mealtime dialogue was and how to feed in a non-pressured way. This really helped the nanny and also put Julia at ease. Julia even put up a printable plan on the fridge that reminded them of their newly established mealtime boundaries. It took a few weeks to create a flow, but after some time, the routine was set and everyone was happy with the eating pattern.

If you decide to hire a caregiver, it's not a bad idea to provide them with a list of easy meal and snack ideas that you know your child and likes and that you feel good about.

Top 10 Nutrition Questions To Ask a Nanny or Au Pair

1. How do you structure meals and snacks when looking after children?
2. Are you comfortable with food prep? Cooking?
3. What breakfasts, lunches, and snacks do you feel comfortable preparing?
4. Are you comfortable making dinner, or doing prep for it?
5. Would you prefer a detailed meal plan from me, or do you like to make your own plan?
6. What are your mealtime "rules" for children? For example, what would you say if a child didn't want to eat something?
7. What are your thoughts about snacking? Do you offer snacks all day long or structure them to be offered between meals?
8. Do you ever bring outside food in to serve to children? If so, what types and how often?
9. Will you be eating with the children or will they eat while you tend to other things? Will you be eating the same foods as the kids?
10. What types of drinks do you serve the kids you're looking after, and when are these offered?

How do I get my spoon-fed toddler to self-feed?

Sometimes babies or toddlers (and parents) become a little too dependent on spoon-fed pureed or mushy foods. They're seemingly safer, and it feels easier to control how much and what your little one eats. The older your child gets, the trickier it can be to get them to feed themselves and introduce new textures and tastes. If you find that your toddler still prefers to be spoon-fed at 12 months, it's time to ramp up and progress to soft finger foods and self-feeding.

> REALITY CHECK
>
> Babies as young as 6 months can start self-feeding, by 9 to 12 months they can start feeding themselves with utensils, and by 24 months, should be using them independently.

Reasons to encourage self-feeding

Mature feeding skills: Your toddler is ready. Physically, cognitively, and developmentally, they've got the tools! And the more you can encourage self-feeding and let them practice, the more efficient and independent they'll become.

Family meals: One of the perks of feeding your toddler (or baby) finger foods is that they can eat the same meal as the rest of the family. This lessens the work for you and helps your toddler to better participate in family meals—they will feel like part of the crew! It also gives more opportunity to model healthy eating. If your little one sees you picking up and munching on a piece of broccoli, they're more likely to mimic you and do the same!

Self-regulation: When toddlers feed themselves (versus spoon-fed), they're able to fully control how much they eat. Toddlers are *really* intuitive eaters—they'll eat just the right amount and stop when they're full. Spoon-feeding your child into toddlerhood can create a painfully hard-to-break habit that doesn't lend itself to growing independence, self-regulation, or mindfulness when it comes to eating.

How to encourage self-feeding

Wean them off spoon-feeding: Place a nice variety of foods (the same foods that the rest of the family is eating) on their tray in easy-to-pick-up pieces, and let them eat independently. Offer more if they finish what's on their tray, but respect signs of being "done," such as leaving food on the tray, throwing food, or getting frustrated.

Use leftover pureed baby food as dips: There's nothing that toddlers love more than dipping! If you have purees that you need to use up, add them to your toddler's plate as a dip! Another way to use them up is to add them to toddler-friendly muffins, loaves, cookies, or smoothies.

Teach them how to self-feed with a spoon: Patiently show your toddler how to properly hold their kid-friendly fork and spoon, and guide them on how to gather food and bring it to their mouth. Start with foods such as oatmeal, yogurt, and applesauce. This is going to take some time, patience, and consistency. It might take them longer to eat at first (and it might be messy!), but that's okay.

Give more time to eat: Aim to have at least 20 minutes for each mealtime and no more than 30 minutes. You'll need this to comfortably eat, deal with inevitable spills, and spend time with your toddler when teaching them how to self-feed. When you feel rushed or stressed, you will be more tempted to spoon-feed your toddler, you'll be less patient and attentive, and your child will feel rushed and anxious as well. Giving them more time also gives toddlers an opportunity to learn how to be more mindful and "listen to their tummies" so that they can decide when they've had enough.

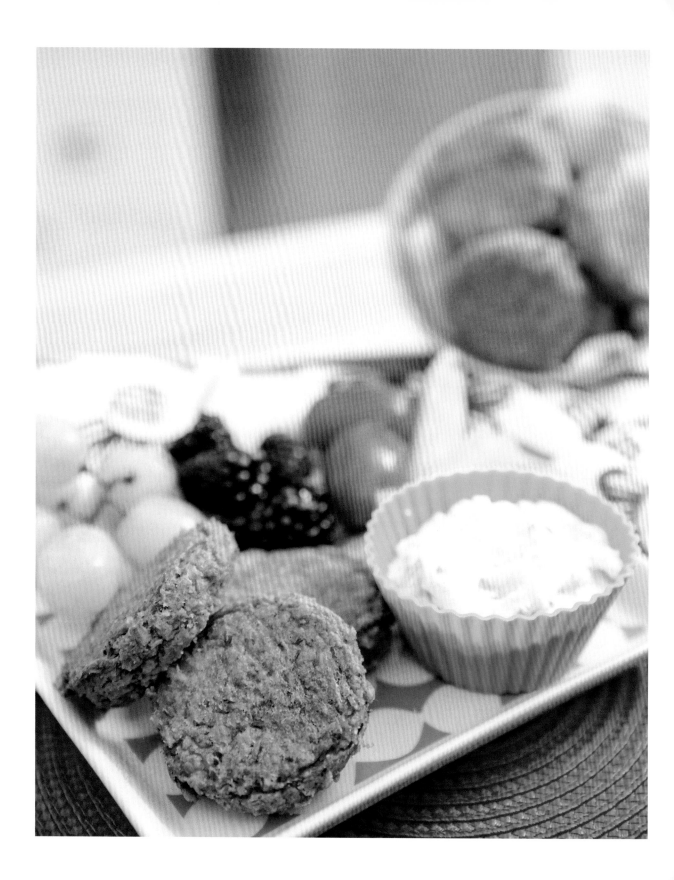

TODDLER-FRIENDLY LENTIL BITES

These bites are the perfect size for little hands, but are equally loved by older kids and the adult eaters at the table. You can double or triple the recipe and freeze leftovers for quick snacks.

Makes 12 bites

1 (19 oz) can lentils, rinsed under
  cool water and drained
¼ cup rolled oats
2 tbsp hemp, chia, or flaxseeds
2 tbsp fresh lemon juice
2 tbsp chopped fresh basil
1 tsp ground cumin
1 clove garlic, minced
2 tbsp olive oil

1. Place the lentils, oats, seeds, lemon juice, basil, cumin, and garlic in a food processor, and blend until smooth. Add a few teaspoons of water if needed.
2. Working with about 1 tablespoon at a time, roll the mixture in your hands and then mold into 12 little patties. Place patties on a plate.
3. Heat a large skillet over medium-high heat, and add 1 tablespoon of the olive oil.
4. Gently transfer 6 patties to the skillet and pan-fry for about 2 to 3 minutes per side, until golden brown on both sides. Remove from the skillet and allow to cool. Add the remaining oil and fry the remaining 6 patties.
5. Serve alongside a yogurt-cucumber dip (like tzatziki—see page 285).

My toddler still seems to gag a lot. Is this normal?

Gagging is extremely common when babies are starting solids (page 212). In fact, it's a safety mechanism to prevent choking—so thank goodness they have it! But gagging should become less frequent as babies get older and enter toddlerhood, because they gradually develop the oral motor skills necessary for eating and learn how to coordinate, chew, and swallow food efficiently. Here are some reasons your toddler may be gagging:

They need more time: If your toddler hasn't been exposed to more advanced textures until now (like soft finger foods) and is stuck on purees, they haven't had the opportunity

Kids' brains are malleable, and it's easy for them to learn new things and form new connections. The more toddlers are exposed to foods in a positive and unpressured way, the more time they have to experience them and form those new connections in their brain, which leads to more positive responses and reactions to the food.

to develop the oral motor skills necessary to coordinate food in their mouth. It may just take more practice. When these skills aren't coordinated, or their tongue muscles are weak, it's a very challenging maneuver to chew and swallow food. If your toddler gags AFTER trying to eat food, this is likely the cause.

It may be a sensory thing: If your toddler gags right after a food touches their tongue or even if they just look at it, they may have a texture aversion or sensory processing issues. In the first few years of life, kids spend their time at meals processing the sensory input they're getting from food. In toddlerhood (when picky eating typically surfaces), sometimes the touch, smell, and taste of food becomes "yucky" or displeasing. In some cases (perhaps in more extreme picky eating cases), experiencing some foods can be really uncomfortable for kids—like nails-on-a-chalkboard uncomfortable.

REALITY CHECK

Turn to page 61 to read about extreme picky eating. And if you're worried that your toddler's nutrition is suffering because of gagging, or if mealtimes are becoming really stressful, seek support from your doctor who can refer you to a dietitian, speech language pathologist, or an occupational therapist who specializes in feeding issues.

How do I avoid giving dessert to my toddler if their siblings get it?

What happens when you have older children who are offered desserts or treats? Do you make your young children a no-sugar-added version? Do you offer them a piece of fruit instead? Or just not serve them anything? This is a dilemma that both of us have faced as parents—and it's a tricky one! Here are some tips to try:

Serve something naturally sweet but nutritious: Dessert doesn't have to be ice cream. It can be fruit with a little cinnamon sprinkled on top or paired with a Greek yogurt dip. Cut the fruit into a fun new shape and it's THAT much more exciting!

Offer something similar, but different: Serving your older kids ice cream? Blend some frozen berries and/or bananas in a food processor and scoop it out like ice cream for your little one—they won't know the difference, and your older children might even prefer it!

Try a no-added-sugar alternative: If you're serving homemade cookies, offer your toddler a cookie sweetened with fruit instead. There are many no-added-sugar recipes for cookies, mini muffins, and bars that would make perfect toddler-friendly dessert options! See page 199 for our baby biscuit recipe.

SARAH SAYS: *We often make no-sugar-added smoothies (made with fruit, yogurt, chia seeds, milk, etc.) and make smoothie popsicles out of the leftovers. It gives us a delicious and nutrient-rich dessert option that the kids love.*

How do I strengthen my toddler's immune system?

If you have a toddler in your house, you also have germs—and lots of them! This is especially true if your toddler goes to daycare or if you have older kids in school who carry germs home every day. And when one kid gets sick, siblings tend to follow (and sometimes parents!).

It's normal for toddlers to get sick periodically, especially during the winter, and this can actually help their long-term immunity. But if you're finding that they're sick all the time, and that it's starting to affect their energy level, nutrition, and even their weight, it may be time to focus on some new strategies.

There are a few ways to help prevent colds, like regular hand washing, getting enough sleep, being active, decreasing stress levels (too many activities?), but one that often gets overlooked is nutrition. Fortunately, certain foods and supplements can help support a normal immune system. And what's recommended nutrition-wise to support immunity isn't far from what we already recommend for general nutrition!

Serve colorful fruits and vegetables daily: Bright and colorful fruits and vegetables— such as tomatoes, butternut squash, carrots, strawberries, spinach, broccoli, and beets— contain phytonutrients (a bioactive plant-derived compound associated with positive health effects) such as vitamin C and carotenoids. These nutrients can increase the body's production of infection-fighting white blood cells and interferon, an antibody that coats cell surfaces, blocking out viruses. Aim to offer at least 4 different colors a day for variety of vitamins, minerals, and phytonutrients, which can help to strengthen immunity.

Support the Immune System

- Serve colorful vegetables and fruits daily.
- Serve fish (like salmon) twice a week, or add fish oil supplements if kids won't eat fish.
- Serve probiotic-rich foods such as yogurt, kefir, tempeh, kimchi, and miso.
- Give 400 IU vitamin D drops, where just 1 tiny droplet is the daily dose.

SHADES OF GRAY: NUTRITION AND IMMUNE SYSTEM

There are still relatively few studies of the effects of nutrition on the immune system of humans, and even fewer studies that tie the effects of nutrition directly to the development (versus the treatment) of diseases. However there is some evidence that certain micronutrient deficiencies—for example, zinc, selenium, iron, copper, folic acid, and vitamins A, B_6, C, and E—change immune responses in animals as measured in a lab.[47] However, the impact of these immune system changes in humans isn't so clear, and the effect of similar deficiencies on the human immune response has yet to be studied.

Include oily fish: Omega-3 fatty acids play an important role in kids' brain and eye development, but many parents don't realize that the omega-3 fat found in oily fish like salmon and trout also helps immunity by increasing the activity of white blood cells that eat up harmful bacteria. Omega-3 fat also decreases inflammation, which may help to protect little lungs from infection. Serve your child oily fish (like salmon) at least twice a week, or consider giving them a children's fish oil supplement (read more about omega-3 on page 24).

Consider probiotics: You've likely heard that the beneficial microbes (probiotics) found in yogurt, kefir, and supplements can help maintain a healthy digestive tract. But did you know that about 70% of the immune system resides in the digestive tract and is also affected by these microbes? It's true!

Probiotics are "good" bacteria, and when consumed in sufficient amounts, they provide many health benefits. There has been some promising research showing that probiotics may help shorten the duration and lessen the symptoms of colds, specifically with the probiotics *Lactobacillus* and *Bifidobacterium* strains (such as *Bifidobacterium bifidum*). Look for supplements or yogurts that specifically carry that strain.

Although yogurt contains probiotics, all brands have different amounts. Some won't contain enough probiotics to help with your toddler's immune system. Some studies show that you need to take probiotics about 3 months before cold season begins in order to get the best effects. If sniffles start in November, start probiotics in August!

Continue with vitamin D: Vitamin D increases the body's production of proteins that kill viruses. A landmark meta-analysis published in the *British Medical Journal* in 2017 looked at 25 studies on vitamin D and respiratory infections (coughs and colds). Researchers found that taking vitamin D supplements can protect against respiratory infections. And while you give your child that drop of 400 IU of vitamin D, you can take your 1000 IU dose too! Try drops, where just 1 tiny droplet is the daily dose.

SARAH SAYS: *As soon as my son started preschool, all of a sudden the whole family was getting sick, seemingly very often. Even my breastfed baby caught colds and stomach bugs from my older son. Know that this is totally normal (and not fun), and it will pass.*

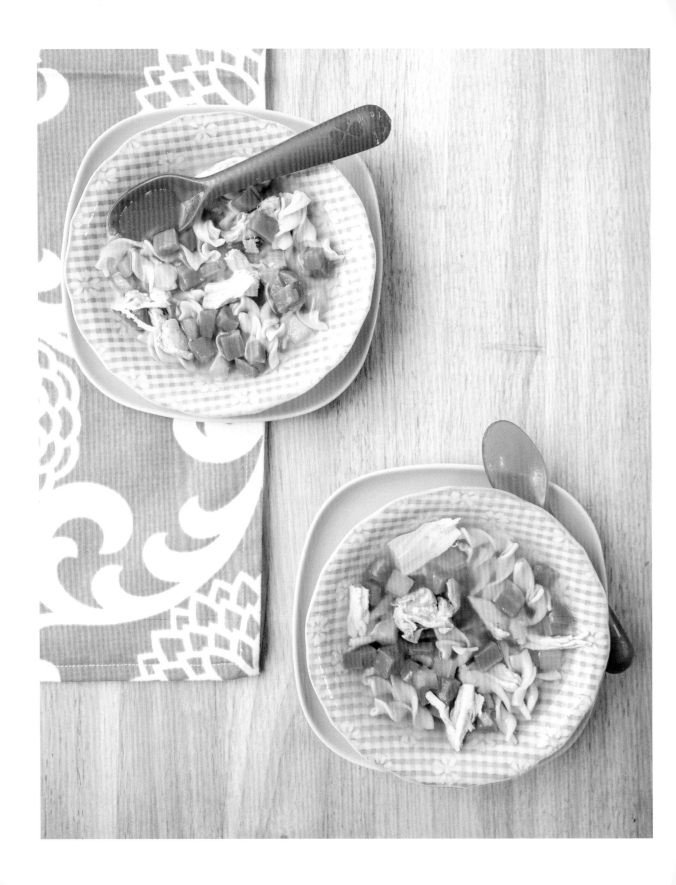

SLOW-COOKER CHICKEN NOODLE SOUP

This recipe was adapted from Sarah's friend Maija Craig's recipe for Crockpot Chicken Noodle Soup. It's an easy and delicious option when your little one needs some comfort food. Bonus: your house will smell amazing!

Makes 6 servings

2 tsp olive oil

3 medium carrots, peeled and diced

2 ribs celery, diced

1 onion, peeled and diced

2 slices fresh ginger (about ¼ inch thick each), peeled

3 sprigs fresh rosemary or thyme

2 cloves garlic, minced

10 boneless, skinless chicken thighs

4 cups low-sodium chicken broth

2 cups water

1 tsp salt

¼ tsp freshly ground pepper

2 cups egg noodles

1. Coat your slow cooker with olive oil. Add the carrots, celery, onions, ginger, rosemary or thyme, and garlic. Arrange the chicken on top of the vegetables. Add the broth, water, salt, and pepper.
2. Cook on low for 8 hours.
3. Remove the chicken, shred with 2 forks, and put back into the pot.
4. Add the noodles and cook on high for 20 to 30 minutes.
5. Ladle into bowls and enjoy.

Without a doubt, one of the most frustrating and heartbreaking parts of parenting is watching your child suffer from coughs, runny noses, fevers, and other cold and flu symptoms. You will read 1,000 different opinions on what's best (Go into cold air! No, sit in a steamy bathroom! Try garlic! Take some high-dose vitamin C!), and some of these remedies will provide momentary relief, but the truth is, kids get sick. A lot. It's not your fault, and yes, it happens in all families.

You may wonder if there are specific foods you should offer your child when sick. The best answer is to let their appetite lead. Some kids aren't hungry at all when they're sick, and that's fine. When hunger does hit, offer small portions of easy-to-digest foods, such as toast, chicken noodle soup, oatmeal, rice, pasta, bananas, or other soft fruits. Really, anything your child enjoys and that brings comfort is on the "serve" list when they are sick. Little ones may want to breastfeed more often too, and that's great. It's comforting to them and can help them feel a bit better—in fact breastmilk DOES have immune-enhancing properties (read more on page 154).

Some people swear that extra vitamin C helps when they have a cold, but the majority of studies don't justify it as a treatment (some small studies show benefit, but the larger, rigorous studies don't). Of course, if one chewable fruit-flavored vitamin C tablet or effervescent vitamin C drink makes your child feel better, it won't cause any harm either.

Overall, the diet during illness or injury mirrors the eating plan that we advocate for every other day of the year. It's mostly whole foods, lots of vegetables and fruits, and fewer ultra-processed foods that contain lots of sugar, salt, and preservatives. The most important thing? Keep your child hydrated. Offer lots of water, broth, chicken soup, smoothies, and popsicles etc.

REALITY CHECK

Yep, your grandma was right: chicken soup actually does help to relieve colds! It works in several different ways. It's a natural decongestant because it's a fluid and provides comforting steam. The typical ingredients (including garlic!) have anti-inflammatory properties that stop the action of neutrophils (cells that may cause coughing and runny-nose symptoms and make you feel lousy).[48] And it's warm and comforting to eat, which is sometimes exactly what the doctor ordered. See our recipe on page 263.

WHEN YOUR KIDS ARE SICK, WHAT ARE THEIR FAVORITE COMFORT FOODS?

Chicken noodle soup. —Nellie

Buttered toast. —Scott

Popsicles or other frozen treats. I don't serve these often, so my kids get excited when they have a sore throat because they get to eat popsicles. —Alma

Noodles with butter and salt. —Carla

Soup! Usually chicken soup with noodles. —Ken

Smoothies for sore throats. —Alana

For my kiddo it's veggies, steamed, in a soup or salad. If her tummy has been off, rooibos tea and plain toast. —Mary

Eggy soup was my favorite when I was sick, and now it's my daughter's. —Angie

Chicken noodle soup, soda crackers ("sick crackers"), and "medicine yogurt" (vanilla yogurt with probiotics). —Kristyn

Pasta with olive oil and peas. —Maria

Peeled apples or chicken soup. —Daniella

Udon or ramen noodle soup. —Shona

Decaf herbal tea with honey. —Amanda

Noodle soup—the little packets from the box. —Cheryl

My own chicken noodle soup. —Marni

Bubbie's chicken soup. —Kim

Miso soup. —Karla

Toast with honey. —Danielle

Avocado toast. —Pam

Mashed potatoes when their appetite returns. —Shawna

Poached eggs with buttered toast. —Kate

Cantonese soup, also known as bone broth. —Valerie

Toast with peanut butter and jelly. —Vanessa

Grilled cheese, frozen yogurt, and smoothies. —Andrea

Chicken noodle soup or chicken pho. —Leyah

Cream of wheat with a little butter and sugar. —Ylva

Mac and cheese. —Ericka

Popsicles! —Erin

My mom would bake chocolate chip cookies when I was home sick from school. Not sure it helped with my cold, but it sure cheered me up! —Melissa

Congee with ginger. —Alice

Top 10 Tips
for toddlers (12 to 24 months)

Introduce milk.
Your toddler can drink cow's milk at 12 months. If you are still breastfeeding, that's great too!

Use cups.
By 12 months, begin to transition from bottles to cups if you haven't already. Straw cups are better than sippy cups.

Teach self-feeding.
Teach your toddler how to use spoons and forks (and fingers!) to self-feed.

Keep it fun.
Reduce mealtime stress by keeping it calm. Don't hover, force-feed, or pressure your toddler to eat.

Set a schedule.
Your toddler should be enjoying 3 meals and 2 to 3 snacks each day to fill their small tummy.

Give vitamin D.
Continue with vitamin D supplements (400 IU per day).

Know that food throwing is normal.
It's a phase that will pass if you stay calm. Provide easy instruction like "food stays on the tray."

Don't label picky eaters.
That moniker reinforces the problem. Kids are learning about food. Being picky is a normal phase.

Avoid treats.
There's no room in a toddler's diet for candy, soft drinks, and cake—not yet anyways. They require nutrient-rich foods to fill that precious and small tummy space.

Be a role model.
Your toddler is watching and learning from you. Mirror healthy behaviors (yup, you have to eat vegetables!).

Toddler
(2 to 3 years)

Introduction

All right! You've entered the fun-filled, challenging, and *very busy* older toddler stage! We both agree that this stage is equally as cute and lovely as it is crazy and frustrating (the terrible twos can be a real thing). Deep breaths—you can do this!

Older toddlers are discovering themselves, asserting themselves, and seeking control wherever they can get it. They're developing little personalities and exploring everything around them with curiosity. This age bracket presents new feeding challenges—in particular, typical but frustrating picky eating tendencies that can easily translate into mealtime battles and power struggles, and evolve into more serious picky eating habits if not dealt with in a healthy, constructive way. But that's why we're here to help!

> Older toddlers are discovering themselves, asserting themselves, and seeking control wherever they can get it.

In this chapter, we want to ease your mind by telling you that the challenges you're facing are *normal* and by answering some of the most common feeding questions during this older toddler stage.

After the age of 2, growth starts to slow and stabilize a bit, and toddlers come out of their critical nutrition period, which means their food intake and appetite diminish. Combine this with their newly discovered independence and desire for control, and it easily translates into—you guessed it—mealtime battles. We can relax, though, because most of the time, kids get the nutrition they need over the period of a week, even though it appears they eat next to nothing on certain days. As long as you're serving a nice variety of nutritious foods throughout the week, it will all balance out (and don't worry—we'll help you figure this part out).

Here's a little nugget of information that might ease your mind too: It would be unusual if your child wasn't a "picky eater" to some extent at this stage. You're not alone in this struggle! Toddlers often turn their noses up to foods like meat, vegetables, and even (surprisingly) fruit, after they've readily accepted them as babies and young toddlers. It's normal—don't worry. Our advice is to try not to obsess or stress about your toddler's food intake (or lack thereof), because the more focus put on getting your child to eat (eat something . . . *anything*!!!), the more pressure they'll feel and the more turned off they'll become.

The key is to be patient, calm, and positive. The way you react to typical toddler feeding challenges can either create bigger, more serious eating issues down the road, or it can help your child grow their relationship with food in a healthy way. Kids learn at their own pace, and you as the parent need to respect the pace at which your child learns, and practice lots of patience in the process.

This is the stage when unhealthy feeding and eating patterns can develop and worsen, especially if there's a lot of pressure, coercion, or negative energy at the table. It's difficult to be patient and trust that your toddler is getting enough to eat (especially when it seems like they're getting nothing at mealtime), but it's imperative that the mealtime dynamic remain positive. You don't want the focus to be on "getting my kid to eat!" You want to focus on spending quality family time together, modeling healthy eating habits and making mealtimes positive. Read more about approaches to food on pages 41 to 47.

Nutrients

In the last chapter, we outlined some key nutrients for young toddlers (see pages 227; these guidelines still apply to older toddlers). Now please don't go and start counting the grams of protein your toddler is consuming every day; that would be exhausting and totally unnecessary. As long as you're offering a variety of nutrient-rich foods at meals and snacks, your toddler should meet their requirements.

At this age, it's still important to ensure your toddler is getting enough calcium and iron for proper growth and development. Omega-3 for brain development remains crucial too, as does vitamin D. See the charts on pages 364 to 372 for more information.

It's all about the HOW

You'll discover in this chapter that the trick to raising a competent eater, particularly at this stage, is all about HOW rather than WHAT. If you focus on your responsibilities as the feeder (the *what*, *where*, *and when* of feeding) and then leave the rest up to your toddler (*whether* and *how much* they eat), they will grow to accept and enjoy a variety of foods. Trust us! Read more about the Division of Responsibility (sDOR) on page 41.

SELF-FEEDING

Self-feeding should be in full swing now—older toddlers should be eating independently and shouldn't be spoon-fed. They should be participating in family meals, eating the same foods as other family members, and choosing which foods (and how much) they eat from what's offered.

BOOSTER SEATS AND HIGH CHAIRS

Children under age 3 should be sitting in a strapped booster seat or a high chair if they still fit in it appropriately. If you've already left booster seats and high chairs behind, we will tell you that it is worth every effort to bring them back into your child's life. Most toddlers don't have the attention span or interest in eating long enough to sit still, and you will be fighting a losing battle until you can start the meal in a strapped position.

Your toddler's day

If toddlers are not pressured, they will eat intuitively and consume what they need. And research shows that there's a direct relationship between how many times you offer a food (pressure-free) and subsequent food preferences. So patience really is key.

STRUCTURED MEALS AND SNACKS

Older toddlers should be served 3 balanced meals and 2 to 3 snacks between meals, depending on timing (the diagram here is suggestion only). You can offer them something to eat every 2 to 3 hours, first because their stomachs are still quite small, and second because structure is crucial. A food free-for-all (aka "grazing") may lead to mealtime battles and picky eating habits. Structure may be harder at first, but it will make eating easier in the long run.

FAMILY MEALS

Family meals continue to be key for toddlers. It's important to try to eat together at least once a day—breakfast, lunch, or dinner. Family meals give

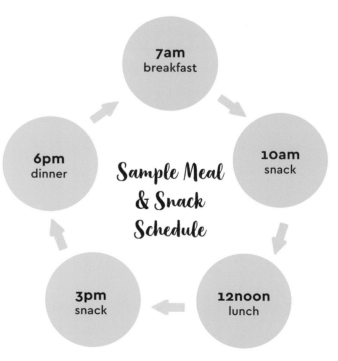

Sample Meal & Snack Schedule

7am breakfast

10am snack

12noon lunch

3pm snack

6pm dinner

you the opportunity to model healthy eating and bond as a family. And check this out: research shows that regular family meals are great for kids as they grow. They boost self-esteem and ensure kids have stronger vocabulary skills—and teens end up with a lower likelihood of developing disordered eating patterns, substance abuse, and depression. Of course, you don't associate these things with your 3-year-old, but if you make family meals a habit starting when your child is young, they will reap the benefits long term!

SARAH SAYS: *In my nutrition counseling practice, parents are often surprised when I ask them more questions about how they feed their kids and how meals are structured, versus what exactly their child is eating on any given day. Don't get me wrong—the "what" is very important too—of course it's important to ensure that your toddler is meeting their nutrition requirements for optimal growth and development. We all know this. But if the feeding relationship isn't healthy, or if proper mealtime boundaries aren't in place, or if the dialogue or energy at the table is negative and stressful, you'll be in for a world of hurt when it comes to feeding your child. And your child won't be set up for a healthy relationship with food long-term.*

Foods to choose

On the next page is a rough daily food guide for toddlers aged 2-to-3. What does this focus on? Whole food. Delicious food. Your job? To offer a selection of nutritious foods from each of the food groups listed below, every day. A word of warning: your toddler will eat less and/or ask for more than what's listed below—rarely will they actually eat exactly what's served, and that's totally normal and fine! This is only a rough guide to give you a place to start.

We don't provide guidelines on exactly how much your 2-to-3-year-old should eat, because it can be SO varied! Instead of focusing on how much your child should eat, we're going to suggest what to offer your child. Your toddler may eat more than you do one day and hardly eat the next. It's totally random—but know that it's normal, and try not to worry. Toddlers are really intuitive—they know how much their bodies need and will eat accordingly. Try not to compare your toddler's food intake to their siblings or to other toddlers (or even to themselves the day before)—they will never be exactly the same!

Sample Meals and Snacks for 2-to-3-year-olds

Sample day 1	Sample day 2
Breakfast	
Berries	Almond butter
Oatmeal	Whole grain toast
Whole milk	Whole milk
Morning snack	
Plain (at least 3.25%) yogurt with a drizzle of honey	Whole grain muffin
Seedless grapes, cut into pieces	Cheese cubes
Lunch	
Hard-boiled egg, cut into quarters	Whole grain pita
Whole grain crackers	Flaked canned salmon, mixed with mayonnaise
Apple, cut into wedges or grated	Cooked carrots and peas
Whole milk	Whole milk
Afternoon snack	
Cucumber, sliced	Melon cubes
Grape tomatoes, cut	Cottage cheese
Black beans	
Dinner	
Cooked chicken, diced	Cooked lentils
Quinoa	Steamed broccoli
Cooked sweet potato, diced	Whole grain pasta
Whole milk	Cheese
	Whole milk

"Mommy, can I have a snack?" Said with whiny intonation, and repeated over and over until you give in. Sound familiar? Chronic snacking is common in toddlerhood, and we know that it's often easier to give in than endure the impending "hangry" (hungry + angry) meltdown. Healthy snacking is important because it helps fill nutritional gaps from mealtimes and satisfy small tummies between meals. But remember we told you that as the parent, you are responsible for what food is offered and when and where your child eats (read it again on page 41)? The same is true for snacking.

The trouble with grazing

Reduces intuitive eating: All-day grazing likely won't allow your child to learn what true hunger or being comfortably full feel like—both important components for regulating their appetite and their weight. Read more about intuitive eating for kids on page 44.

Mealtimes suffer: A lack of structure means your toddler may not be hungry at mealtime (cue: meal struggles) or may be hungry when you don't have snacks handy, like in the car—we've so been there! (cue: meltdown).

Picky eating: Snack time should be fun and enjoyable, but it shouldn't take over the day. If it happens too often, it can create or exacerbate picky eating. Picky eaters have a hard time trying new foods to begin with, let alone when they come to the table full on snack foods.

Unhealthy habits: Snacks are more likely than meals to include unhealthy choices such as candy, desserts, sugary beverages, and chips (which are actually treats, not snacks; learn the difference on page 16). If all-day snacking becomes a habit, kids can easily consume excess empty calories that they don't need and that displace healthier foods, which can lead to unhealthy weight gain and poor choices that can extend beyond the childhood years.

THE SOLUTION: SET A SCHEDULE

Snacking is not something that we should give up or phase out. In fact, young kids require more frequent eating opportunities than adults do because of their smaller stomachs. It's how and when snacks are offered that cause problems for our kids.

Creating more structure around them will not only improve their overall nutrition, but make *mealtimes* much more enjoyable for everyone.

It's important that you stay relatively consistent with your schedule so that your child learns that eating isn't a free-for-all, but something that happens at roughly the same intervals every day. See page 274 for a sample meal and snack schedule.

Once your child knows that they will be given eating opportunities at regular intervals, according to when you decide, they will be less inclined to ask all day long, and more inclined to fill their tummy at meals. Creating this structure helps kids to learn self-regulation when it comes to their hunger and fullness. Of course, this pattern is just an example, and you can set your own schedule that works well in your family. The idea is to ensure that kids get on a schedule, and you decide what that schedule looks like.

Top 3 tips for handling random snack requests

1. **Acknowledge.** Times of whining, meltdowns, and chaos are not times to have a productive conversation. In a calm moment, acknowledge the request by saying something like "It sounds like you would like to eat right now" or "I understand that you want a snack."

2. **Empathize.** Empathize by saying, "I know it's hard not getting what you want right when you want it" or "I know that those muffins look really yummy and you probably want to eat one right now." Explain that even though it's not time to eat NOW, there will be another opportunity to eat soon. As soon as kids know that there is a future eating opportunity, the desperation to eat RIGHT NOW tends to dissipate. Try not to say "No" but rather, "Yes, but now is not snack time. Snack time will happen ___."

3. **Remind.** Encourage your child to fill their tummy at mealtime, because the "kitchen will be closed" afterward and snack requests will be kindly turned down. If they request a snack soon after a meal, remind them again by saying "it's not snack time now—we just ate dinner and now the kitchen is closed. Next time, remember to fill your tummy enough at mealtime."

> **WE GOT YOU!**
> Establishing new boundaries and routines with kids is not easy! Resistance is almost inevitable. A new routine will likely take at least a week to feel established. But once established, it will drastically reduce the constant snack requests because they simply won't be as hungry once they eat every few hours in a consistent pattern!

CARA SAYS: *My son would often request a snack about half an hour after eating a full lunch, so there was little possibility that he was actually hungry. It was more likely that he noticed some food, which triggered the idea that "food tastes good"—even though his tummy was full. If I knew he had just eaten and didn't need a snack, I would remind him that we had just eaten, and remind him to listen to his tummy (intuitive eating). I'd then get him busy with something—finger painting, toy cars, blocks, reading books together—and 100% of the time, this would distract him from his food request. And of course, I knew his next snack was not far off in the schedule!*

SARAH SAYS: *I have many parents tell me that they child is a "grazer." That's just how they are! They prefer snacks all day over structured meals. Well yes—if any child is given the opportunity to "graze" all day they will most certainly and most happily take on the title. Kids love snacking! But reality is, the child should not be responsible for deciding when eating happens. That's the parent's job in the Division of Responsibility (sDOR). And kids need meal and snack structure to learn how to self-regulate their appetite, and get what they require nutrition-wise.*

> (REALITY CHECK)
>
> Grazing all day can have negative nutrition and health consequences. Studies show that young kids are snacking way more now than ever before in history, and calorie intake for kids has increased significantly—just from snacks! This can set kids up for unhealthy eating patterns that continue through to adulthood.

WHAT'S YOUR TODDLER'S FAVORITE SNACK?

Celery with peanut butter and raisins. Yup, ants on a log. My mom made it for me, and I make it for my twins! –Celeste

We make homemade energy bites–we use oats, nut butter, seeds, and honey, then roll them into bite-size rounds and keep them frozen for easy snacks. –Lauren

Granola bars, and I try to buy ones without a ton of sugar. No chocolate coating. No marshmallows. –Lisa

Apples, bananas, and pears, usually cut into slices. –Yvette

Hard-boiled eggs are a big hit in my house. Sometimes we do "hard-boiled egg bowling"–we set up some cucumber sticks or apple slices and knock 'em down with a rolling egg on the plate! –Kevin

Pasta. Any shape. Any time. –Monique

My son is happiest with a bowl of berries. Really ripe strawberries, blackberries, or blueberries will make him so happy! –Sophie

My daughter likes crunchy snap peas, green beans, red pepper sticks, and other sweet-tasting vegetables. I made the mistake of steaming them once–and learned very quickly that she prefers them raw. –Andrew

Peas, corn, edamame, and any other little once-frozen vegetables or beans. –Dee

Dried cereal or some cereal with milk. –Nancy

Cheese. Sometimes crackers with cheese. Sometimes string cheese or those round wrapped ones. As long as there is cheese, she is happy. –Diane

My son loves yogurt, and I add some pureed fruit from a pouch, or some fresh berries. –Karryann

My toddler often refuses to eat at meals. What should I do?

There's nothing quite as frustrating as putting time and energy into a healthy family meal, only to have it be rejected completely. Toddlers are unpredictable when it comes to eating, and it's important for parents to stay calm and rational, and to react in a way that keeps mealtimes positive and nurtures long-term healthy eating habits rather than creating bigger issues. For all our picky eating advice turn to page 49.

How do I get my toddler to eat more veggies?

Vegetables are such an important part of a toddler's diet because of the vitamins, minerals, and fiber that they contain. And if toddlers get used to eating vegetables from an early age, they may just adopt this healthy habit! Read more about picky eating on page 51, and below are our top tips to get your child to eat more vegetables:

Take the pressure off: You now know that you're not responsible for deciding *if* and *how much* your child eats. In other words, it's not your job to make sure that your child eats their vegetables—it's theirs. Although vegetables and fruits are not 100% nutritionally equivalent, you can relax knowing that vegetables aren't *essential* for a nutritionally adequate diet. If your child has a varied fruit intake, this can largely make up for a low vegetable intake, for now. It's still important to continue exposing them to a variety of vegetables every day, even though they may reject them. This will increase their chances of accepting them later.

Rename veggies: Choose fun and kid-friendly names to make vegetables more appealing. C'mon—a "Hulk smoothie" tastes so much better than a kale smoothie! There is no trickery in renaming a vegetable something creative and fun, and it makes for a more exciting experience for your child.

Offer choice: Toddlers and preschoolers can be really finicky when it comes to how their food is served. Some kids prefer all of their food separate, and it's fine to serve foods that way. Ask your child how they would like their food served prior to serving it: "Would you like your peas inside your macaroni or on the side?" You will be amazed at the answers you'll get and, perhaps, the change in acceptability.

Change the offer: Raw vegetables with some sort of dip are much tastier than plain. Make a homemade tzatziki sauce (see page 287) and serve with peppers, cucumbers, and cherry tomatoes. Or serve carrots and celery with hummus or ranch dip. Some kids love vegetables done with a spiral tool to make fun springs. Or try steamed broccoli with melted cheese on top. Read more ideas about making veggies "yummier" on page 242.

SARAH SAYS: *My son has never known a smoothie to be without some kind of vegetable in it. He also helps me chop (with his plastic knife) vegetables to go into casseroles and sauces. If you expose your child to vegetables early, it is more likely that they will accept them as they grow older.*

Think about textures: Ask your child what they don't like about vegetables. If they're too crunchy, steam them so they are soft. Too mushy? Serve them raw instead. Figuring out what your child doesn't like can help you offer options that they DO like. The great thing about vegetables is their versatility. Check out the chart on page 283.

Give them a choice of 2: Instead of saying "We are having steamed broccoli with dinner," try giving them a choice by saying "Would you like broccoli with cheese sauce or raw vegetables and dip?" By doing this, you are handing over some of the control (which toddlers and preschoolers crave) and allowing your child to decide what they are eating, while still ultimately being in control. We call this giving kids "structured control," and we're often surprised by the answer, "Both, Mommy!" You could also offer BOTH at mealtime and let each family member decide how much of each they'd like.

Remember repetition is okay: There is nothing wrong with serving the same accepted vegetable over and over again. If your child loves peas but rejects every other vegetable, offer peas as an option, alongside 1 or 2 additional vegetables, even if you know that your child won't eat them. The more exposure your child has to a variety of vegetables, the more likely they will be to eventually try them.

CARA SAYS: *My son will eat mushrooms and sweet peppers raw but not cooked, yet prefers cauliflower cooked and not raw. The important thing is that he's trying a variety of vegetables and can recognize them by name and point them out at a grocery store. With this familiarity, maybe one day he'll expand his preferences, and I'll keep offering a wide variety of options.*

Let them pick: Take your toddler to the grocery store, farmers market, or pick-your-own farm. Let them choose a new vegetable or pick a recipe to cook with you. If children have a hand in choosing and preparing vegetables, they are more likely to try them.

Let your child help with meal prep: As messy as it gets, let your child prepare dinner with you—it has countless benefits. They may munch on vegetables that you're chopping or become adept at throwing ingredients into a blender (and every other cooking skill). It gives kids a sense of pride and accomplishment and they will also be more likely to sit down to the food that they helped prepare. Read our suggestions for getting your kids into the kitchen on page 308 and 357.

Eat vegetables yourself: If your child repeatedly sees you enjoying vegetables, they will grow up learning that eating vegetables is normal and healthy. Eat the way you want your child to eat, because you are their role model. Try to have at least 2 vegetable sides at family dinners, with lots of color.

SARAH SAYS: *My daughter has always been a selective eater, especially when it comes to green vegetables like broccoli. She would always push them to the side or remove them from her plate (which we allowed her to do), until one day when she was intently watching me happily eat vegetables (including my broccoli). I saw her look down at her broccoli, touch it, and then lick her finger. She then picked it up and took a tiny bite (I pretended not to watch her or make a big deal). She shrugged and said, "Hmm . . . not too bad." And ever since, she will always have a bite or two of broccoli when it's served.*

Make Vegetables "Yummier"

"VEGGIFY" SMOOTHIES! A big handful of "superhero spinach" won't change the taste of a fruit smoothie, but will add a lot of nutrition! Other vegetables that go well in smoothies are cucumbers, kale, carrots, and beets.

MAKE IT SAUCY! Add carrots or mushrooms (or both!) to tomato sauce, marinara sauce, or homemade salsa.

SERVE AS SOUP! Butternut squash, mushroom, tomato, or broccoli soups are a delicious way to include more vegetables.

MAKE THEM INTO RIBBONS OR SPIRALIZE! Try a "ribbon" salad with zucchini or cucumber. Or add spiralizer vegetables (like carrots) to regular pasta with sauce—yummy!

SERVE WITH CHEESE! Cheese makes everything yummier, doesn't it? Add Cheddar cheese to steamed broccoli or cauliflower, or finely grate some Parmesan cheese and dip raw or steamed vegetables into it!

DIP THEM! Serve raw vegetables with a yummy dip.

PAIR THEM WITH FRUIT! When you add some sweetness to vegetables, it takes away from their natural bitter taste and makes them more palatable. Try spinach with strawberries in a salad, or add tomatoes, peppers, and mango to a salsa. Or try sprinkling dried cranberries into a sweet broccoli salad.

ROAST THEM! Make them into "fries" or "chips": toss in some olive oil, sprinkle with a bit of salt and pepper and herbs/spices of choice, and bake! Best vegetables for this: yams, sweet potatoes, zucchini, and carrots.

Try New Vegetable Textures

To make vetables . . .	Use this technique . . .	It works best with . . .
Soft	Steam in a pot, using boiling water and a steamer basket	Broccoli, cauliflower, green beans, carrots, peas, potatoes, sweet potatoes, squash
	Roast in a baking dish in the oven at 400°F	Cauliflower, sweet potatoes, beets, fennel, asparagus, squash, turnips, rutabagas, potatoes, Brussels sprouts
	Serve raw—some vegetables are naturally soft	Avocados, tomatoes (both are technically fruits, but are used as vegetables in the culinary world), leafy greens
Semisoft	Stir-fry in a wok or frying pan with oil and garlic over medium heat	Broccoli, cauliflower, green beans, carrots, zucchini, asparagus, sweet peppers, mushrooms, snow peas
	Grill on the barbecue or an indoor grill	Eggplant, zucchini, sweet peppers, mushrooms
Crunchy but easy to chew	Serve raw, thinly sliced with a mandoline	Cucumbers, carrots, jicama, sweet peppers, mushrooms, snow peas
Hard	Serve raw, sliced into sticks	Carrots, celery, kohlrabi, celeriac, beets, fennel, cucumbers, radishes

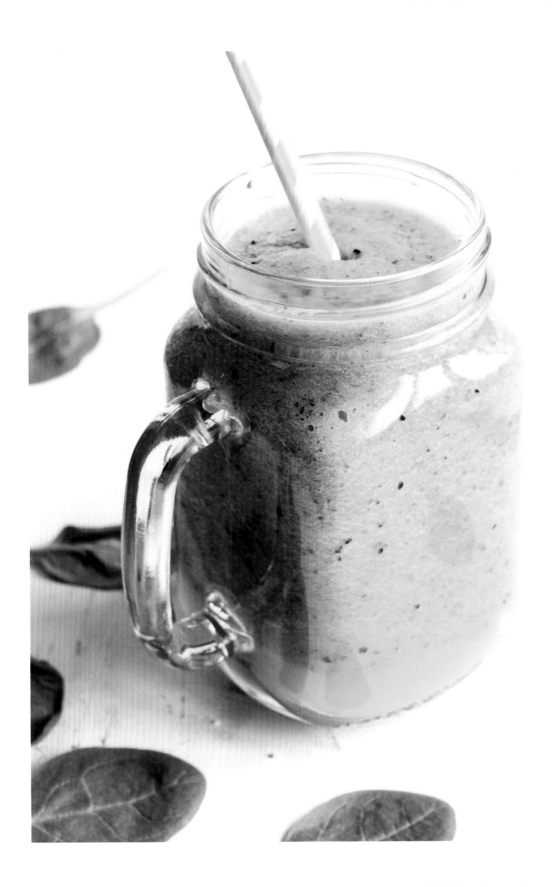

TODDLER-APPROVED TZATZIKI

The base of this dip is a protein-rich Greek yogurt (full-fat, reduced fat, or non-fat), and it's a better choice than store-bought dips, which may be loaded with salt.

Makes 3½ cups

2 cups grated cucumber
1½ cups plain Greek yogurt
Pinch garlic powder
½ tsp salt
1 tbsp fresh lemon juice
1 tbsp extra virgin olive oil

1. In a bowl, mix together the cucumber (you can peel it first if your child doesn't like "green" food), yogurt, garlic powder, salt, lemon juice, and olive oil.
2. Serve with vegetable sticks such as carrots, cucumbers, or red pepper. Store in the fridge for up to 3 days.

CARA SAYS: *My son loves to dip! Sometimes I make this tzatziki recipe, and sometimes he asks for my "ranch dressing." It's similar, but instead of cucumber, I add dried herbs—a pinch each of chives, parsley, and dill. So yummy! You can also use fresh garlic instead of powdered garlic, if your family prefers more of a "kick."*

KID-APPROVED TROPICAL GREEN SMOOTHIE

This is a fun way to introduce spinach to kids. Prepare this recipe together so they learn how to use green vegetables in delicious ways!

Makes 4 kid-size smoothies

1 banana
1 cup frozen tropical fruit, such as
  mango and pineapple
1 cup fresh spinach
¾ cup plain Greek yogurt
¾ cup milk of choice
1 tsp chia seeds

1. Place all ingredients in a blender and blend until smooth. Add more milk if needed.
2. To drink as a smoothie, pour into 4 small cups and add a straw (optional). For a smoothie bowl, pour into a bowl and add toppings of choice, such as fruit, shredded coconut, nuts, seeds, and granola. Store smoothie mixture in the fridge for up to 2 days or the freezer for up to 3 months (thaw in the fridge overnight before drinking.)

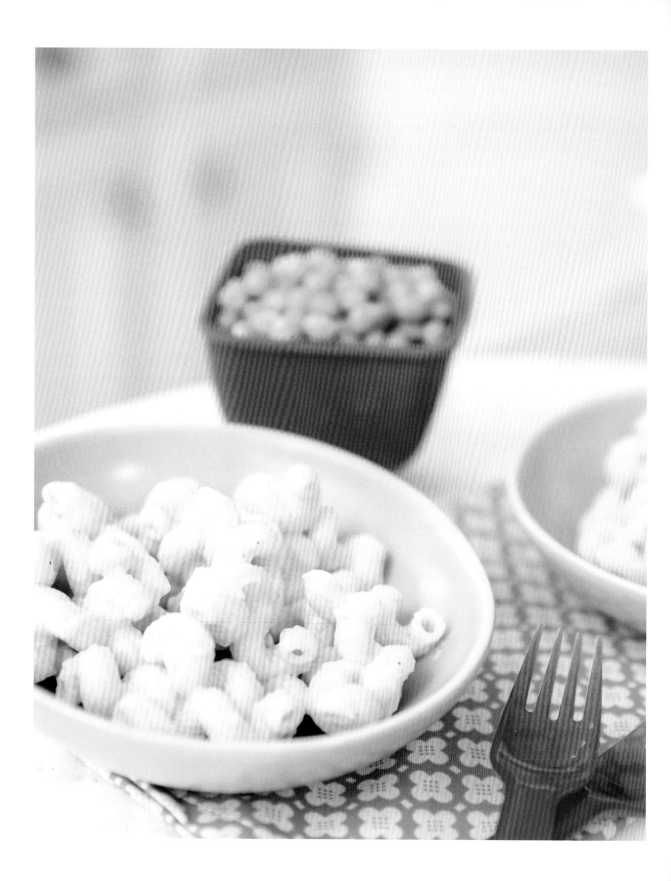

ROASTED SQUASH MACARONI AND CHEESE

Instead of serving veggies on the side, this recipe has them built right in. It's creamy comfort food that your child is sure to love.

Makes 6 servings

2 cups peeled and diced butternut squash (½-inch dice)

2 tsp olive oil

1¾ cups bite-size pasta (macaroni, fusilli, rotini, etc.)

1 cup broth

1 cup milk

2 tbsp butter

1 tsp garlic powder, or more to taste

1 tsp dry mustard

⅛ tsp freshly ground pepper

3 cups grated cheese (use a combination of Cheddar, mozzarella, and Parmesan)

Salt to taste

1. Preheat the oven to 400°F. Line a baking sheet with parchment paper.
2. Arrange the butternut squash on the baking sheet, drizzle with oil, and toss. Bake for 25 to 30 minutes, until fork-tender.
3. Meanwhile, boil water over high heat and cook pasta according to the package directions. Drain and set aside.
4. In a large stockpot set over medium heat, combine the roasted squash, broth, milk, butter, garlic powder, dry mustard, and pepper. Stir constantly while heating, about 5 to 10 minutes.
5. Remove from heat. Using an immersion blender or transferring to a blender or food processor, blend all of the ingredients.
6. Once blended, add the sauce back into the pot, then slowly add the cheese, mixing constantly until all of the cheese is melted.
7. Add the cooked pasta and gently stir until coated with the sauce. Transfer to a large serving dish and allow to cool for a few minutes before serving. Salt to taste.

Is it okay to sneak vegetables into my toddler's meals?

Years ago, hiding pureed vegetables in children's food was an emerging trend. The advice was simple: add a dollop of pureed cauliflower to pasta, a spoonful of kale to meatballs, and a scoop of beets to brownies. (Brownies? Yes. Brownies.) But we don't love this tactic. You see, kids should learn to enjoy the tastes and textures of vegetables and should not be tricked into eating them. It can backfire in so many ways.

Okay, so say your child noticed you adding pureed carrots to a tomato sauce that they LOVE, but they HATE carrots. They will be mad at you and lose trust. They may never eat that sauce again! Or when a piece of zucchini doesn't puree properly and becomes visible in your child's favorite cookie, they will become suspicious. If they catch you in the act (which they eventually will) and learn that you are not being up-front with them, those "yucky" vegetables are suddenly much "yuckier". "Now these vegetables are SO gross that my parents had to hide them in my food," they may think. If you demonize vegetables as something you have to sneak in, you create a food hierarchy and make vegetables even less desirable.

> **REALITY CHECK**
>
> Vegetables that are cooked, pureed, and then cooked again in a meal may lose their nutritional value. Vitamins degrade and fiber gets lost.

WHAT TO DO INSTEAD?

So here's the deal. It's fine to add leafy greens to fruit smoothies or pack extra vegetables into spaghetti sauce. There is nothing wrong with adding vegetables to a dish to boost the nutritional quality of it—as long as you're open and honest with your child. You'll have an even harder time long-term if you lose their trust.

If you openly (not sneakily) add pureed vegetables to foods for a nutritional boost, you should still serve whole vegetables as a side dish at meals. Children need to see that meals always include vegetables, and it helps to see BOTH parents eating their vegetables too. If your child likes a meal that includes pureed vegetables—say lasagna or burritos—have them prepare the recipe with you the next time you make it. If they already enjoy it, it shouldn't be a problem to see the vegetables being added in. For more tips about helping kids learn to enjoy vegetables, see page 279.

My toddler won't sit still at mealtimes! What should I do?

It's important that your toddler can sit still at meals, for a few reasons. A wiggly tot who is getting up and down from the table during a meal will be distracted and, like with other distractions, will end up eating less overall. Letting your child "graze" throughout a meal (which happens with getting up and down and wandering) can be a slippery slope to unstructured and chaotic family meals, power struggles, and picky eating issues. We also know, firsthand, how utterly frustrating wiggly bodies fleeing from and coming back to the table can be.

So let's talk about how to keep your kid properly seated for a meal so that they can eat safely without it turning into an epic battle:

Bring back the booster! If your child is under 3, we would highly recommend a strapped booster seat or even a high chair if they still fit in it appropriately. Most toddlers don't have the attention span or interest in eating long enough to sit still, and you will be fighting a losing battle until you can start the meal in a strapped position. If you've already left booster seats behind, it's worth every effort to bring them back, even if that means investing in a new one. You could call it a "big kid chair" or get them excited about saying "you get to wear a seatbelt!"

Make sure there is a solid surface for their feet: If your toddler's feet are dangling, they'll feel unbalanced—which means more time trying to keep their body upright and balanced, and less time focused on their food. If there isn't a ledge for their feet on the seat already, add something like a stool or a chair beneath them. This will allow them to feel more stable and go a long way toward lessening the wiggles.

Get into optimal sitting position: Chances are your child isn't sitting at an appropriate eating height at your table. In fact, it's rare that kids under 10 (or even older) sit and eat meals at an appropriate height (most kids aged 3 to 9 years need a booster seat and a stool under their feet). When this is the case, they start to wiggle and slide off their chair. Imagine what it would be like to sit at a really big table in a chair that left your feet dangling. It would feel pretty awkward! You will know that your child is seated in the best position if:

- Their feet sit flat on the ground or another surface like a stool
- Their hips, knees, and ankles are all at 90-degree angles

Help a kid out! Give them a fighting chance: if you've followed the above suggestions and are still struggling with a kid who can't stay seated for meals, ask yourself:

- **How long are you expecting them to sit at the table?** For toddlers, this should be only about 10 to 20 minutes, 4 to 6 times per day (meals and scheduled snacks).
- **Have they had enough time for active play and physical activity?** If you've just walked in the door from a long car ride or just watched an hour of television, then your child is probably going to be a little antsy. Before they come to the table, make sure they have had some time to run off some of their excess energy or "get their sillies out."
- **Are there clear boundaries and mealtime rules?** It's important to approach this subject outside of mealtime, when everyone is calm and attentive. Talk to your child about the mealtime boundaries and let them know that it's important to come to the table (even if they choose not to eat) and that food will not be offered again until the following meal or scheduled snack.
- **Are they looking for attention?** Remember that when a toddler refuses to eat or can't sit still at the table, they might be looking for attention—at least to a degree. Try giving them some extra attention in other areas of their life, and that might be the surprising solution.

SARAH SAYS: *My younger son wanted to sit in a regular chair so that he could be like his siblings, so we let him and it was a bit of a disaster—it was too soon, and he got up and down about 100 times every meal. We decided to try a new chair that was portable and was able to attach to the table so that he felt as though he was a part of the meal and still sitting in a "big boy chair." It worked like a charm and he loved it!*

Should I be worried if my toddler eats a lot of food and really fast?

If you have a toddler who is passionate about food and can't get it in fast enough, you're not alone (we both have a child like this!). Parents either celebrate their food-loving kids or worry that their toddler overeats. But it's important not to stress about it (in fact, projecting stress, pressure, or worry will make it worse). Instead, focus on your role as the "feeder" and trust that your toddler will do their job as the "eater."

Some kids just love food or need more than others. Often there's no obvious reason for this, and it can fluctuate depending on whether they're going through a growth spurt, what their activity level is, what they ate the day before, and so many other factors. Here are some reasons for and strategies for dealing with a toddler you think eats too much or too fast:

Make sure that you're following the Division of Responsibility (sDOR): In the sDOR, parents are responsible for *what, where,* and *when* food is served and kids are in charge of *if* and *how much* they eat (read page 41). If toddlers are served balanced, healthy meals and snacks at appropriate intervals, they will eat intuitively and learn to self-regulate their intake. Babies and toddlers rarely, RARELY overeat.

Don't restrict, forbid, or micromanage food intake: If your toddler feels that a desired food is restricted, it will create a desire for more. When available, they may eat more in anticipation of it being restricted afterward. Make sure to offer a variety of nutritious foods (including ones they love) at mealtimes and let your toddler have as much or as little as they'd like. Serve meals family style so kids get to serve themselves in proportions that feel right to them (yes, even toddlers!). They're always able to go back for more.

Give your toddler enough time to eat: Toddlers need at least 10 minutes to finish a meal. If they feel rushed, they may eat too fast (and subsequently too much). They should feel relaxed at the table and know that they have enough time to eat comfortably.

Minimize distractions: Screens and toys can impact the speed and amount that your toddler eats at a given time. These distractions can divert your toddler's attention away from their food and their tummy (internal hunger cues), which discourages mindful or intuitive eating.

Make it a teachable moment: Older toddlers will start to understand an association between a tummy ache and overeating if you can explain it in terms that they'll understand. At about age 2½ or 3, you can introduce the concept of "eating until your tummy is full" or "listening to your tummy" at mealtimes. If your toddler overeats and has a tummy ache, you can—without judging or making them feel bad—say something like "when we eat too much, our tummy hurts." And then when you see this happening again in the future, you can remind your toddler of the time that they overate and got a tummy ache.

CRISPY BAKED CHICKEN FINGERS

These are a staple food for many kids—but you don't have to rely on the boxed version. These are simple to make and actually take less time than baking frozen chicken fingers—they bake in just 15 minutes!

Makes 4 servings

1 egg

3 tbsp whole grain flour

½ cup whole grain panko (crunchy) breadcrumbs

3 tbsp grated Parmesan cheese

¼ tsp garlic powder

Pinch salt and pepper

2 chicken breasts (about 12 oz total), cut into strips

1. Preheat the oven to 400°F. Line a baking sheet with parchment paper.
2. In a small bowl, beat the egg.
3. In another small bowl, place the flour.
4. On a large plate, combine the breadcrumbs, Parmesan, garlic powder, salt, and pepper (and herbs, if using; see note).
5. One at a time, dip the chicken strips into the flour, then into the egg, then into the breadcrumb mixture to coat. Place on the prepared baking sheet.
6. Bake for 12 to 15 minutes, turning once, until the chicken reaches an internal temperature of 165°F.
7. Serve with your favorite dipping sauce.

Optional: If your child doesn't mind "green bits" in their food, add 1 teaspoon each dried parsley and dried oregano to the breadcrumb mixture.

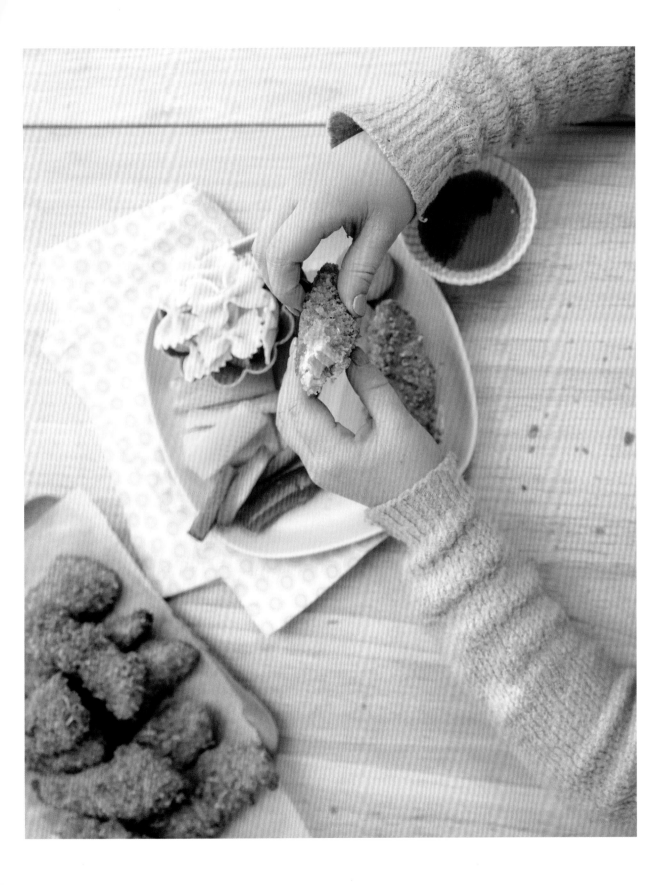

Is it okay to give my toddler dessert? How often and how much?

We agree, it's fun to watch the expression on a toddler's face when they taste something sweet! Perhaps it's birthday cake or Grandma's delicious homemade cookies. Joy and delight are words that come to mind—and there's good reason! But while your little one isn't going to suddenly turn into a cookie monster the second sugar hits their lips, it's important to be aware of how many treats they are eating.

Before 24 months: As mentioned on page 16, we don't recommend offering daily treats or desserts with added sugar until at least 24 months (birthday cake is the exception—c'mon, we're realists too).

After 24 months: It's okay to introduce the odd treat or dessert after your toddler's second birthday. Treats will likely be a part of your child's life no matter what—whether it's at birthday parties, holiday get-togethers, or at friends' or family members' houses. The key is to introduce treats at the right time, manage them in a healthy way, and teach your toddler to eat them mindfully.

> **WE GOT YOU!**
> When you stay calm and matter-of-fact about treats and desserts, it puts them on a level playing field with other foods and takes the excitement down a notch.

CARA SAYS: *Treats and desserts don't have to be sweet. While I prefer chocolate, my husband loves salty things, and my son and daughter inherited this quality. They may just pass up chocolate for pretzels, chips, tortillas, or any other salty, crunchy treats. (I totally don't get it.)*

SARAH SAYS: *I offer 3 to 4 "fun foods" (treats) a week, randomly and without strings attached. Sometimes it's after dinner, sometimes it's part of afternoon snack, and occasionally I even serve a small portion with a meal. We don't make a big deal of them! I've done this on purpose—I didn't want to make an association with mealtimes and dessert so that my kids expected it every night. Instead, it's a surprise and treat when it happens, and it doesn't affect their intake of food otherwise.*

Top Tips for Toddlers & Treats

OFFER RANDOMLY: Offer sweet foods when it makes sense to you and for your family, but do this randomly. Perhaps once or twice a week after a family meal, or maybe alongside a healthy snack for no particular reason. Don't make a big deal out of it. You don't want your child to associate treats with a particular day, time, or meal, or they will start to crave them at that time.

DON'T RESTRICT TOO MUCH: If toddlers feel treats are being withheld from them, it could trigger the "get it in while you can" mentality. You don't want your toddler "saving up" for or expecting treats.

AVOID USING AS A REWARD: For example, "If you're good in the grocery store, you can have a cookie," or "You were such a good boy at the doctor; would you like a cookie?" Trust us, we know how tempting it is to use this strategy to bribe or reward kids, but doing so only increases treats' desirability and puts them on a pedestal.

SEPARATE DINNER AND DESSERT: Rewarding your toddler with dessert foods because they ate their vegetables at dinner is communicating that vegetables are to be avoided and desserts to be desired, and may cause them to rush through the meal to get to the treat more quickly. This can work VERY well in the short term, but in the long term, you're not doing your toddler any favors.

DECIDE ON THE AMOUNT: There's no hard-and-fast rule about how often or how much when it comes to offering treats. It's important that nutrient-dense, whole foods fill precious tummy space first and foremost, and treats are the fun add-on. As the parent, without saying too much, you can orchestrate when treats are offered based on how you feel your toddler has eaten otherwise.

Jennifer, a mom of 3 boys, was having a dinnertime dilemma. Her 2 older kids would race through dinner to get to dessert. Something sweet after dinner became an expectation rather than an occasional treat, and she was fed up with her boys constantly asking "What's for dessert?" before dinner even started. She found that her boys never asked for seconds because the brownie after dinner could never compete with more broccoli. She also found that they ate very quickly, and dinner was over in about 5 minutes (even when it took her 30 minutes to prepare!).

We talked about different solutions to this problem. Jennifer liked giving the boys a sweet treat, so eliminating dessert wasn't a comfortable option for her—and that's okay! Remember, in the feeding relationship, the adult decides what to serve and when to serve it. She wasn't changing the "what," so we had to change the "when."

Jennifer tried something radically different. Instead of saving dessert (2 small cookies) for after the meal, Jennifer served them on the table alongside the other dinner foods. The boys were blown away! What was Mommy doing?! Of course, they ate the cookies first, but then an amazing thing happened. They sat through dinner without racing to the finish line, since they had already eaten dessert. They stayed at the table for 10 minutes instead of 5 minutes and enjoyed a family meal.

After a few weeks, the boys were calmer at dinner and even asked for seconds of broccoli when they were still hungry. Now Jennifer mixes it up. She likes to give the boys one small treat each day, but she's flexible with the timing. Sometimes it's at lunch. At other times, it's during or after dinner. And sometimes it's before dinner because . . . why not? She never gives enough dessert to fill their tummy or displace healthier foods, but just a small amount to make it fun.

Top 10 Tips

for toddlers (2 to 3 years)

Have a routine.
Offer meals and snacks at the same time each day to establish a pattern and avoid all-day grazing.

Eat as a family.
Be a role model for healthy eating while enjoying family time.

Make vegetables yummy.
Offer dips, try different textures, or serve as a soup.

Don't sneak the veggies.
Cook with your kids to show them the ingredients.

Wiggly kid? Bring back the high chair!
Kids can't sit for more than 10 to 20 minutes at a meal, and they need a properly positioned chair.

Offer vegetables often.
Kids will learn to eat vegetables with repeated exposure. You can be the role model.

Follow their appetite.
Remember the Division of Responsibility (sDOR). You serve healthy foods and let kids decide how much to eat.

Accept that messy eating is normal.
It's fine for kids to explore food, but it's also fine to set boundaries so it doesn't get out of hand.

Don't use treats as rewards.
A treat once in a while is fine, but not as a bribe or prize for good behavior.

Cook and shop together.
Get your kids involved in mealtimes.

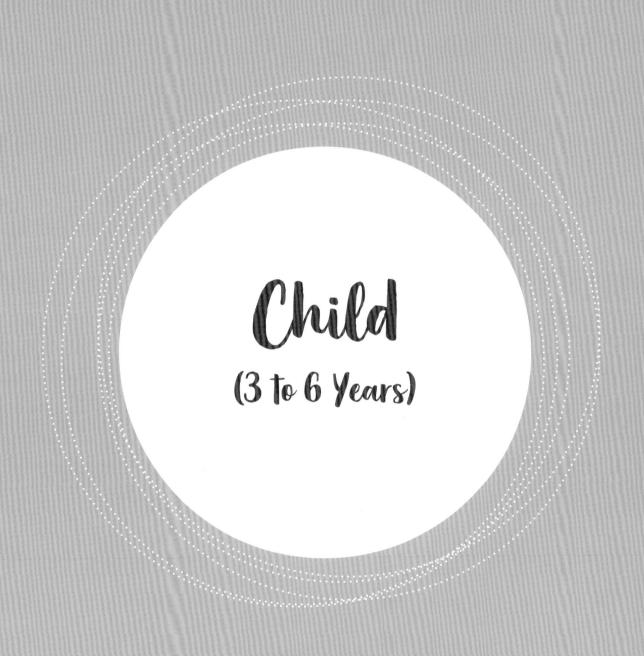

Child
(3 to 6 Years)

Introduction

For many parents, the biggest milestone in this age range is getting their child ready for their first day of school. Whether it's preschool or kindergarten, the day comes when you will hold their little hand, walk up to the classroom door, and say goodbye—you may shed some tears or you may totally celebrate! Or you may have a mix of emotions (which is true for most of us!). One thing it does mean (if this hasn't been the case for you already) is that your little one isn't going to be eating all of their meals at home anymore. Yikes—does this give you anxiety? If it does, you're not alone.

As always, your child will continue to look to you as their main role model for healthy eating. But at this stage, the foods that they see their friends eating will also have some influence on them. If your child's best friend has cookies and gummy bears at recess while your kid is eating carrot sticks and hummus, you are SO going to hear about it! Kids at this age also know what they like and tend to be vocal about it. It's time to involve your child in grocery shopping, food prep, and cooking so that they have some control over their food choices—they crave that at this age!

> As always, your child will continue to look to you as their main role model for healthy eating. But at this stage, the foods that they see their friends eating will also have some influence on them.

School-age kids are all over the place in terms of their interest in food. Some are totally distracted and can't seem to sit at the table for more than 2 minutes; some are intrigued by how ingredients blend together to form meals; some are experimental and are game to try anything; and others have 6 foods they enjoy (and only those 6!). There's no right or wrong—these kids are still learning!

The act of eating—chewing, swallowing, and knowing when they are full (when to stop eating)—is innate and doesn't really need to be taught or micromanaged. If we take the pressure off and just let them eat, they will usually do a great job! But not everything is intuitive. It's our job to guide and teach them about mealtime manners, eating at a table, choosing a variety of foods, and to provide a happy and positive eating environment so they can do all of that. And if they don't get it right away (maybe they're going through a picky phase or just not interested, or maybe they over-eat and feel sick after dinner!), it's all a learning process and you need to let them make mistakes, suffer natural consequences and above all, have patience.

In this chapter, we'll answer your questions about packing school lunches, cooking with your child, what to do when your child sneaks food, what to do if you're worried about your child's weight, and much more.

Nutrients

IRON
Iron continues to be important at this age. 3-year-olds require 7 milligrams of iron per day, while those aged 4 to 6 require closer to 10 milligrams per day. Offer iron-rich foods such as meat, fish, eggs, beans, or lentils.

VITAMIN D
Children aged 3 to 6 still require 600 IU (15 micrograms) per day. Since vitamin D is not found in many foods besides milk, egg yolks, and some fish, we recommend continuing to give your child a vitamin D supplement of 400 IU per day.

OMEGA-3 FAT
Studies have shown that omega-3 fat (specifically DHA and EPA), which is naturally occurring in oily fish such as salmon and trout, has beneficial effects on brain, nerve, and eye development in children. Offer oily fish at least twice a week. If your child doesn't eat fish, they may benefit from a daily omega-3 fish oil supplement.

How much DHA and EPA does my child need?

- **3 to 4 years old:** 100 to 150 milligrams per day
- **4 to 6 years old:** 150 to 200 milligrams per day

REALITY CHECK

If your child eats oily fish (such a salmon) that contains 500 milligrams of EPA and DHA combined, that can count for a few days' worth of intake. The per day rule can be spaced out over the week, where 2 servings of fatty fish can suffice.

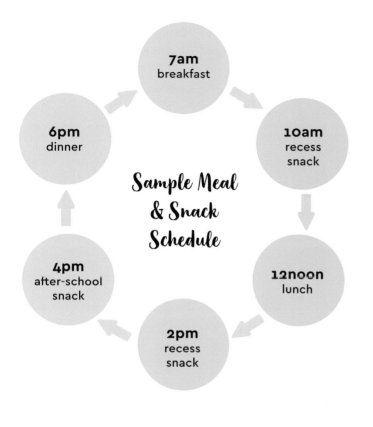

Sample Meal & Snack Schedule

7am breakfast

10am recess snack

12noon lunch

2pm recess snack

4pm after-school snack

6pm dinner

Your child's day

You should continue to have a consistent schedule for snacks and mealtimes, but may have to alter it slightly so it meshes with eating times at daycare or school. There will likely be 3 meals and 2 to 3 snacks. Some kids like to have a snack when they get home from school, or have one after dinner (maybe at 7:30 p.m.) because they go to bed a bit later compared to when they were toddlers (and they get hungry again). This will depend on when dinner is served or if there are any after-school activities. Only you can determine the right schedule for your household.

Food choices

At this stage, your child can eat mostly everything (we still watch out for choking hazards—see page 205), but that doesn't mean they will! There is a broad spectrum, from kids who enjoy a small handful of foods to kids who will try anything once. What's most important is that your child stays nourished by choosing foods that contain the nutrients their bodies require for normal growth and development.

CARA SAYS: *My children were raised in the same household with the same parents, same food choices and same guidance. Yet my daughter will try anything and loves to experiment with food, while my son is more cautious and wary, and prefers fewer foods than my daughter does. All kids are different and that's okay!*

CUT BACK ON ULTRA-PROCESSED FOODS

Here's the bad news: kids at this age tend to eat a lot of ultra-processed foods. And when we say a lot, we mean A LOT. The average American (over age one) gets a

Sample Meals And Snacks for 3-to-6-Year-Olds

Sample day 1	Sample day 2
Breakfast	
Oatmeal made with milk Banana Almond butter	Whole grain cereal with milk Strawberries
Morning snack	
Homemade muffin A few nuts	Cheddar cheese Whole grain crackers
Lunch	
Turkey sandwich Red peppers Apple slices Milk	Scrambled eggs Whole grain toast Tomatoes Grapes Milk
Afternoon snack	
Carrot sticks Hummus	Ants on a log (celery with peanut butter and raisins)
Dinner	
Chicken breast Whole grain pasta with sauce Broccoli Milk	Meatballs Brown rice Carrots Milk
Evening snack	
Blueberries Greek yogurt	Apple slices with a little almond butter

whopping 57.9% of calories from ultra-processed foods.[49] That means that more than half of their diet is filled with cookies, hotdogs, soft drinks, chicken nuggets, cake, and chips. Oh, man. We told you it was a lot.

After the US, Canadians are the second-largest buyers of ultra-processed foods in the world. Studies show that kids between the ages of 2 and 9 get 51.9% of their daily calories from ultra-processed foods. For context, Canadian adults get about 48% of calories from ultra-processed foods, so kids are eating even more junk than their parents![50]

Why is this a problem? A high intake of ultra-processed foods is linked to an increased risk of chronic diseases like type 2 diabetes, high blood pressure, and heart problems. On the flip side, diets that contain less ultra-processed food and more whole food can reduce the risk of obesity, type 2 diabetes, and heart disease. What your child learns to eat really does matter!

DEEP DIVE

On average, 3-to-6-year-olds require 1,000 to 2,000 calories per day. That's a huge range, right? As the chart below shows, it really depends on how active they are. These are called "estimated energy requirements" because they are just that—estimates. Do not count your child's calories—it isn't necessary, nor is it healthy! As long as you're following the Division of Responsibility (sDOR) (page 41) and setting appropriate mealtime boundaries, your child will eat as much as they need for proper growth and development.

ESTIMATED ENERGY (CALORIE) REQUIREMENTS FOR CHILDREN[51]

GENDER	AGE (YEARS)	SEDENTARY	MODERATELY ACTIVE	ACTIVE
Female	2 to 3	1,000	1,000 to 1,200	1,000 to 1,400
Male	2 to 3	1,000	1,000 to 1,400	1,000 to 1,400
Female	4 to 6	1,200	1,200 to 1,400	1,400 to 1,600
Male	4 to 6	1,200 to 1,400	1,200 to 1,600	1,600 to 1,800

- **Sedentary:** Only the light physical activity associated with typical day-to-day life. No sports or exercise.
- **Moderately active:** Physical activity equivalent to walking about 1½ to 3 miles per day, plus the light physical activity associated with typical day-to-day life.
- **Active:** Physical activity equivalent to walking more than 3 miles per day, plus the light physical activity associated with typical day-to-day life.

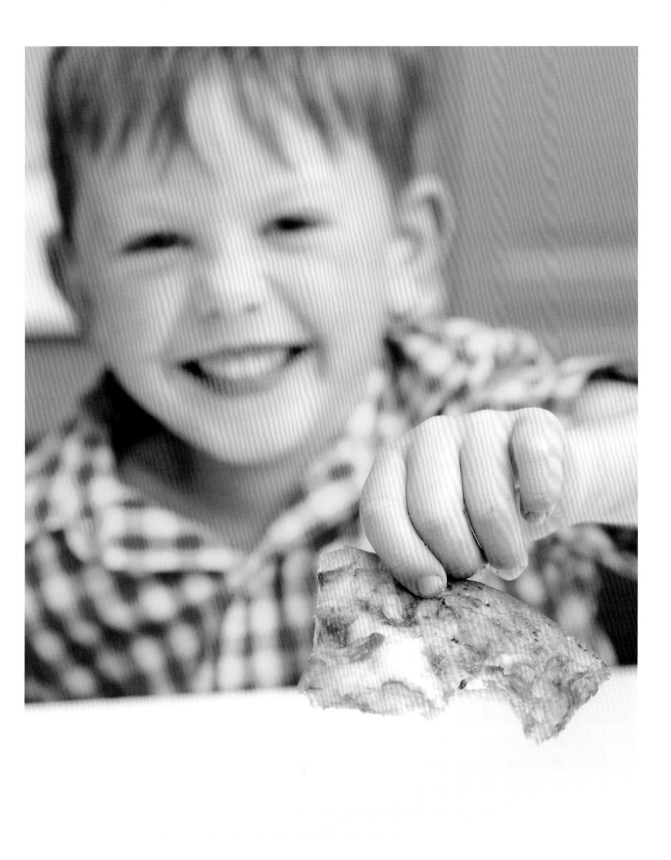

Imagine if someone told you there was a way to help your child get better grades, avoid teenage pitfalls of alcohol, smoking, and low self-esteem, stay healthy, and be a happier person all-round. Would you do it? Of course you would!

Well then, we have some important news to share! Family meals have all of those benefits—and more! Many studies have been conducted on the benefits of sharing meals, and the results are amazing.

Top 6 benefits of eating as a family

1. **Children make better food choices.** They tend to eat more vegetables and fruits, drink more milk rather than soft drinks, and eat less fried food.
2. **Children have more nutritious diets.** They also get more vitamins, minerals, and fiber, and less trans fat.
3. **Childhood obesity chances decrease.**
4. **Communication improves.** Mealtime conversations build better vocabulary skills in children and help them learn about current events. Time given to chatting about the day builds social connections and strong relationships.
5. **Children fare better in school and get better grades.**
6. **Family traditions are formed.** And role-modeling opportunities teach healthy eating and good manners.

And as your child grows into their teens, the benefits continue:

- Increased self-esteem
- Better success in school
- Lower incidence of eating disorders
- Less chance of drinking alcohol, smoking cigarettes, or using drugs
- Less school truancy
- Fewer episodes of violent behavior (fights)
- Fewer feelings of depression or thoughts of suicide

WE GOT YOU!

There truly are so many, varied benefits to eating together as a family. Aim to eat *at least* 4 meals together as a family, per week—but the more meals, the better! They don't just need to be dinner—breakfast, lunch, and brunch count too.

On page 304, we talk about how much ultra-processed food many kids are eating, and it makes sense that the numbers are staggeringly high because many of us are convinced that "kid food" is a thing. If you believe what restaurant menus tell us, a normal diet for a child is based on chicken fingers, hotdogs, pizza, soft drinks, and ice cream. Those are what are advertised to kids and offered in so many school lunches, so they must be right. Right? No, not so much.

WHAT FOODS SHOULD MY CHILD EAT MOST OFTEN?

You'll know by now that we always recommend whole foods first, and that nutritious processed foods are great too (but not to be confused with ultra-processed foods, see page 10). The foods listed below are nutrient-rich, and because kids have high nutrient needs but small stomachs, these foods should fill most meals and snacks:

- Vegetables
- Fruits
- Meat and poultry
- Fish and seafood
- Eggs
- Legumes and pulses: chickpeas, kidney beans, black beans, lentils, tofu, edamame, peanuts, etc.
- Dairy: milk, kefir, yogurt, cheese, cottage cheese, etc.
- Nuts: almonds, cashews, pecans, walnuts, nut butters, etc.
- Seeds: hemp, pumpkin, sesame, sunflower, chia, seed butters, etc.
- Whole grains: oats, quinoa, barley, rice, whole grain wheat (either as whole grains or made into bread or pasta), etc.
- Healthy oils: olive, avocado, sesame, etc.

SARAH SAYS: *We don't go out for dinner a lot with our kids, but when we do, we almost never peek at the kids' menu—we all order off of the adult menu instead, and we usually share 1 or 2 dinners between the 3 kids. They've never really known any different, and they're pretty open to new tastes and flavors because of this.*

CAULI-TOTS

These taste as good as tater tots but pack a nutritional punch. Your kids will gobble them up! Serve with dip, or on their own, as a side dish or snack.

Makes 24 tots

2½ cups finely chopped cauliflower (use a blender or food processor, or buy cauliflower rice)
2 large eggs, whisked
⅓ cup whole grain panko (crunchy) breadcrumbs
⅔ cup finely chopped onions
1 clove garlic, minced
2 cups grated Cheddar cheese
¼ tsp salt
Pinch pepper

1. Preheat the oven to 400°F. Line 2 baking sheets with parchment paper (or grease a mini muffin tin thoroughly as the tots may stick!).
2. Bring a pot of water to a boil and blanch the cauliflower for 5 minutes, then drain.
3. Place the cauliflower, eggs, breadcrumbs, onions, garlic, cheese, salt, and pepper in a medium-size bowl, and stir to combine.
4. Working 1 tablespoon at a time, scoop the mixture into small mounds and place on the baking sheets (or add to mini muffin cups).
5. Bake for 18 to 20 minutes, until golden brown on top. Rotate the sheets after 10 minutes for even cooking.

Tasks for Kids in the Kitchen

PRESCHOOL: Pour ingredients into a bowl; pick herbs off stems; tear salad greens into pieces; stir batter in a bowl.

KINDERGARTEN: Crack eggs; measure and level dry ingredients; spread butter; whisk a vinaigrette; peel hard-boiled eggs.

GRADE SCHOOL: Make pizza; peel fruits and vegetables; drain and slice tofu; form patties; thread food onto skewers.

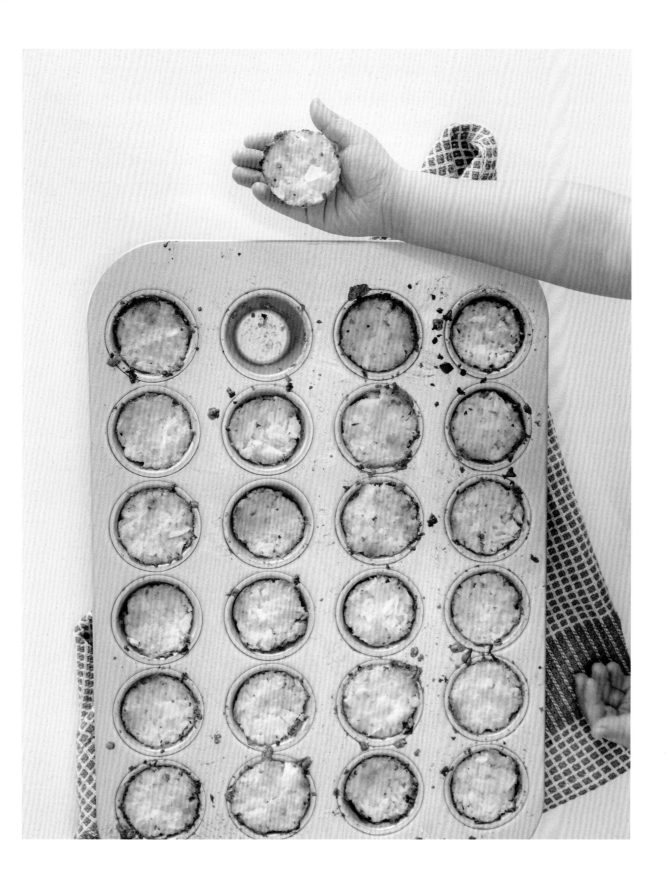

Are bedtime snacks okay for kids?

According to the Division of Responsibility (sDOR) (page 41), you are responsible for WHEN kids eat, so that's your decision. Some parents do offer a snack, and others don't—and either option is fine. It really depends on what time you have dinner and whether your child gets hungry again before bed. Our rule of thumb is that bedtime snacks can be offered if dinnertime and bedtime are at least 2 hours apart. Otherwise, dinner should be sufficient.

If a snack is always offered after dinner (let's say an hour after), and it's always a fan favorite (let's say yogurt), you better believe that your child will hold out for that yogurt and perhaps not eat as well at dinner. See how this can create picky eating issues?! For this reason, set boundaries around timing ("the kitchen is closed after dinner") and make sure to offer lots of variety if you do offer a snack. Also, switch it up and don't *always* offer a snack or your child will form an association between bedtime and snacks that could become very hard to break down the line.

And, remember to distinguish between snacks and treats (see page 16)—a bedtime snack isn't a reason to eat a chocolate bar or a bag of chips every night. Apple slices with some peanut butter or a small serving of Greek yogurt would be a better choice.

What should my child drink every day?

The first answer is water. It's neutral in flavor, readily available, sugar-free, and the best bet for everyday hydration. If your child enjoys milk, they can drink that every day too, in moderation. It's not mandatory, of course, but milk is a good source of calcium, vitamin D, and other nutrients. But do not exceed 2 cups daily, because milk is filling and can diminish your child's mealtime appetite (and displace other important nutrients in their diets). We recommend serving milk with meals rather than between meals for this reason.

What about juice? Oh, the ongoing saga of juice . . . It's good. Oh wait, it's terrible. What gives?! Juice is made from fruit, so it seems like it would be very healthy. But that's not really the case. When kids eat

> **WE GOT YOU!**
> You haven't ruined your kid if juice has been a regular part of their diet thus far. Just cut back and set some boundaries around it. Our rule of thumb is to not have it available at home, but allowing kids to enjoy it at parties, friends' houses, and for special occasions without strict limitations.

Make Water Fun

AWESOME WATER BOTTLE: Up your water bottle game with a color and/or design you know your child will like. Make sure your child knows how to open and close it on their own.

TRY A REUSABLE STRAW: Sometimes a playful straw (metal, bamboo, or silicone) gets a kid excited about what's in their cup.

ADD FLAVOR: Slices of fruit or a mint leaf can add a big splash of much-needed flavor (see page 139 for more ideas)

USE COOL CUBES: Get silly ice-cube tray shapes to make funky-shaped ice cubes. Or freeze pieces of frozen fruit to use instead of ice cubes.

MAKE "JUICE WATER": If you're trying to wean your child off juice, make them "juice water," which is basically 90% water and 10% unsweetened fruit juice. You may have to start at a higher percentage of juice, and gradually work your way down to a very small amount of juice, or try adding real fruit instead.

ADD FIZZ: Some kids enjoy mildly carbonated water (especially if you are trying to get them to drink fewer soft drinks). Add some fizzy water to plain water (half and half) to see if they like the bubbles.

BE A ROLE MODEL: If kids watch you sipping water, they are more likely to follow suit.

whole fruit, they get vitamins, minerals, and fiber all in one. They also begin to feel full, so it makes great sense as a satiating snack. But when kids drink juice, most of the fiber is lost in the processing phase, and some of the vitamins are lost too (vitamin C or ascorbic acid is often added back in). What's left is all sugar—about 6 teaspoons per cup of juice, the same as regular fizzy soda (see page 16)! And kids can keep sipping away and they never quite feel full from juice, right? That's not such a good idea. The high sugar content in juice contributes to increased calorie consumption and the risk of dental cavities.

Your best bet is to serve water instead of juice all of the time, and keep juice as a special-occasion drink (like at birthday parties or Sunday brunch). You could also try a fruit smoothie instead, where whole fruit (fresh or frozen)—fiber and all—is blended in!

REALITY CHECK

We're often led to believe that juice is healthy because it's made from fruit. But cup for cup, juice has the same amount of sugar as soft drinks like cola, root beer, or cream soda. Because juice may have some vitamins, it's marginally better than soft drinks, which are pure sugar. But both drinks have about 6 teaspoons of sugar per cup, so there's really no clear winner. Water is best.

DEEP DIVE: DRINKS & SUGAR

We are not fans of juice, but if you do want to offer it, here are the guidelines from the American Academy of Pediatrics.[52] The maximum daily intake of 100% juice products should be:

- 4 ounces (½ cup) for children aged 1 to 3 years (even this makes us cringe)
- 4 to 6 ounces (½ to ¾ cup) for children aged 4 to 6 years

Juice is not the only beverage that contains lots of sugar. Hmm . . . let's see, there's cola, iced tea, lemonade, fruit punch, sports drinks, milkshakes, soft drinks, hot chocolate, chocolate milk, etc. A cupful of any of these beverages is the nutritional equivalent to eating gummy bears. They should be seen as treats, not as everyday drinks. See page 37 for more about sugar.

CARA SAYS: *My son loves drinking "fancy water"—that's what he calls it when I add a few slices of cucumber and a sprig of mint, or some sliced strawberries. Making water more "fun" is a great way to ensure that kids stay hydrated.*

Should my child take vitamins, minerals, or other supplements?

We get this question a lot, and we wondered the same thing, especially when our own kids had their picky phases! Could we be sure they were meeting all of their nutritional needs from food alone? Well, there's no perfect answer that satisfies the needs of every child. Most of the time, kids who eat a good variety of foods will easily meet their nutrient needs with food alone. But if you find that your child is a finicky eater and has many restrictions, their diet may possibly be deficient in a particular vitamin or mineral. Here are some supplements to consider:

> **WE GOT YOU!**
> If you are unsure if your child is getting enough of the different groups (vegetables, fruit, protein, grains, etc.), keep a 2- or 3-day food diary of what your child is eating and then compare it with their requirements in the introduction to this chapter (page 307).

Multivitamins: If your child is growing well and you are feeding them a balanced and varied diet, and according to the sDOR (page 41), they're likely getting what they need from food alone and multivitamins are not needed. If your child is going through an extended picky eating phase though, a multivitamin might not be a bad idea. It's best to pick a multivitamin plus mineral (to include things like calcium and iron too) Seek guidance from your doctor or registered dietitian as needed, and read more more about picky eating on page 49.

> **WE GOT YOU!**
> Remember to buy supplements that are specifically formulated for kids, and keep them out of a child's reach— they often look and taste like candy, so kids may want to eat more than one.

Vitamin D: If we could suggest one vitamin to supplement your child's diet, it's vitamin D. Kids aged 3 to 6 require 600 IU. One cup of milk contains only about 100 IU of vitamin D, so if they drink 2 cups of milk and have a supplement of 400 IU, they will meet their vitamin D needs. Fortified milk alternatives (such as almond or soy milk) also contain vitamin D. Bottom line? Keep giving your child a 400 IU's vitamin D drop every day to be safe.

Calcium: If your child does not consume dairy-based foods or calcium-fortified equivalents (like soy or almond beverages), a calcium supplement may be warranted. Talk with your doctor or registered dietitian if you think this is the case, and read more about raising a vegan child on page 349.

Omega-3 fat: Experts suggest that children aged 3 to 4 get 100 to 150 milligrams of EPA and DHA, combined, per day, and kids aged 4 to 6 get 150 to 200 milligrams per day.

If your child doesn't eat any fish, a supplement is a practical idea. You can find omega-3 supplements for kids in liquid and chewable formats (and no, they don't taste like fish!).

Probiotics: Probiotics are "healthy" bacteria. There has been some promising research showing that probiotics may help shorten the duration and lessen the symptoms of colds, specifically with the *Lactobacillus* and *Bifidobacterium* strains.[53] And when your child starts preschool or kindergarten, you'll want anything that can help shorten a cold (read more on 263)! Look for supplements or yogurts that specifically carry both of those strains.

My child often eats a lot at mealtime. Should I worry?

Remember that your child is the best regulator of their own appetite. There will be days when they eat very little, and days when they ask for seconds and thirds (we call these "hungry days"). It's all normal.

CARA SAYS: *I find that growth spurts often align with my children's appetites, especially for my son. I remember when he was a baby, the weeks when he'd eat the most were the same weeks he'd outgrow his pajamas and onesies!*

So don't worry. Sometimes kids are growing and have a large appetite at meals, but that may be balanced out by eating less a few days later. You don't need to stop kids who want to have seconds (or thirds), but there is something you can teach kids about portions and mindfulness: Let's say you overeat and feel overfull after a meal, you could say something like "Ah, I think I ate too much tonight and now my tummy hurts. Next time I'll slow down and listen to my tummy more closely." This way your kids will understand that it is normal to overdo it sometimes, but you can learn from it.

SARAH SAYS: *I often put out a veggie plate with dip prior to dinner. My eldest son can have a huge dinnertime appetite, and I find that if he eats a couple of servings of veggies before we sit down together he can eat dinner slower and be more mindful of his portions. Bonus: He's eaten his veggies before dinner even starts!*

We find serving food "family-style" allows kids to have control over what they pick, while still reminding them (through the foods you serve) that a balanced meal includes vegetables, protein and grain. Offer enough variety so your child can build themselves a healthy plate (like the one on page 11). Help them by building *yourself* a balanced plate, so they can learn from your role modeling. Sometimes they will choose to eat all the things you serve, and sometimes they won't. That's okay! The Division of Responsibility (sDOR) (see page 41) reminds us of a parent's feeding jobs. Your job is to offer a balanced meal with a variety of nutritious foods, and it is your *child's* job to decide which of those foods to eat and how much of them to eat. Most kids are able to control their appetite and eat as much as they need to feel just full. If you start to meddle in their decisions, they will begin to doubt their own abilities to self-regulate, and stop trusting their own bodies. This is the last thing we want to do!

PROBLEM SOLVED: OVEREATING CONCERNS

Tina and Jack went to a dietitian for nutrition counseling when their son, Elliott, was 4. They were concerned that he was eating too much and that it might create poor eating habits down the road, and potentially lead to unhealthy weight gain. They were so concerned that they had started to restrict the amount of food he was eating as well as limit certain types of food. This had actually made matters worse—he was now sneaking food when his parents weren't watching and eating extremely fast at mealtime. Elliott had always been on the 75th percentile for height and weight, and still was.

The dietitian explained the Division of Responsibility (sDOR) and said that Elliott was likely eating intuitively, and perhaps just had a larger appetite than what his parents thought was normal. Tina and Jack breathed a sigh of relief. Elliott was actually quite similar to his parents—both were quite tall and had good appetites!

Tina and Jack were encouraged to stop micromanaging their son's intake, because this was likely making Elliott feel deprived of foods and driving him to feel as though he had to "get it in while he could" and sneak foods. They started following the sDOR, took the pressure off, let Elliott eat until his "tummy was full," and set appropriate mealtime boundaries (see page 41). Elliott stopped sneaking food, it became less of an issue or topic of discussion, and Tina and Jack could stop worrying, go back to enjoying family meals, and do their job of feeding, while Elliott could go back to doing his job of eating.

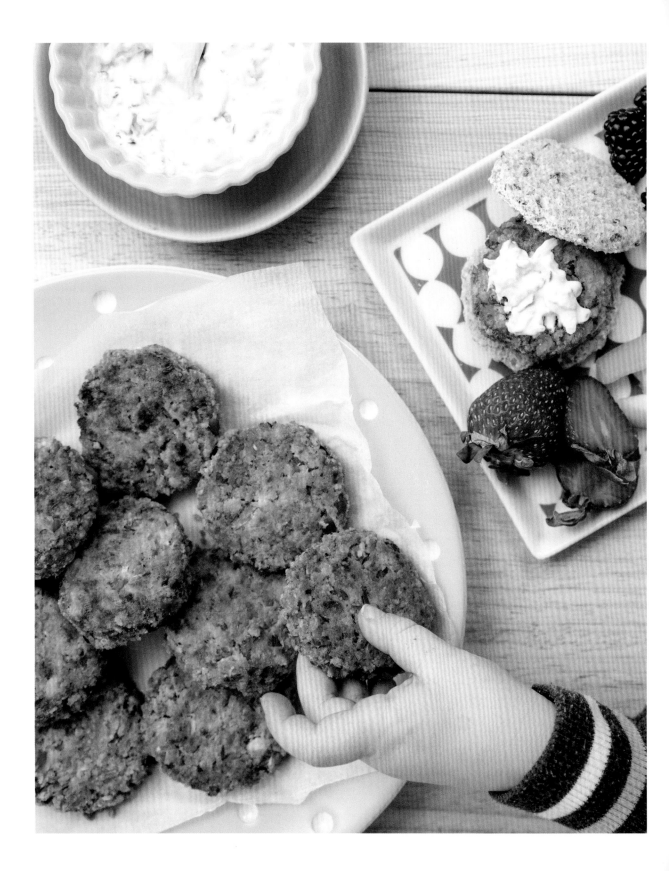

YUMMY SALMON BITES

These kid-size salmon bites are a powerhouse of protein and omega-3 fat. As your child gets bigger, so can the size of the bites—soon they will be eating salmon burgers! Serve with a dipping sauce like tzatziki (see page 285).

Makes 12 bites or 4 burgers

2 (5 to 6 oz.) cans salmon

2 tbsp mayonnaise

2 tbsp plain Greek yogurt

½ cup chopped onions, green onions, or chives

½ cup seeded and finely chopped red or yellow bell pepper

½ cup whole grain panko (crunchy) breadcrumbs

1 to 2 tbsp olive oil

1. In a large bowl, mash the salmon with mayonnaise and yogurt. Add the onions, peppers, and breadcrumbs. Stir to combine.

2. Use a tablespoon to scoop up 1 to 2 spoonfuls of the salmon mixture, and shape it into a flat bite-size pieces with your hands. Repeat to make all 12 bites (if you want to make burgers, use 3 to 4 tablespoons for each).

3. Place a nonstick skillet over medium heat and heat 1 tablespoon of the oil.

4. Fry the bites until browned, about 3 minutes per side, adding more oil to the skillet as needed (if making burgers, cook for an extra minute per side).

5. Serve with dipping sauce or on mini slider buns. Store salmon bites in the fridge for up to 3 days.

CARA SAYS: *It's vital to use a nonstick pan or cast-iron skillet for this recipe as the patties will be difficult to flip and will fall apart in a regular pan.*

How Can I Make Better Choices at the Grocery Store?

Grocery shopping can be tricky. Store shelves are filled with so many choices that it's easy to get overwhelmed when choosing what to buy. Add in the slick marketing that makes junk food sound healthy, and it's really hard to know what to add to your cart and what to skip. Here are some of the most common questions we hear when parents head into the grocery store.

Dairy

Is string cheese a good choice? The fun shape and pull-apart nature may make you think string cheese is a novelty item, but it is indeed real cheese. String cheese is the same as offering your child a few cubes of mozzarella or Cheddar. It's a wholesome snack filled with protein and calcium. Add it to your cart.

What about cheese slices? Individually wrapped cheese slices are ultra-processed and have more than double the amount of sodium compared to regular Cheddar cheese. Real (unprocessed) cheese is a better choice, even if you have to slice it yourself!

The yogurt section is overwhelming! How can I choose the best one? If you buy plain unsweetened yogurts, they are all good. For more protein, opt for plain Greek or Icelandic (skyr) yogurt. The harder part is buying flavored yogurts, because they contain added sugar (sometimes 3 to 4 teaspoons of added sugar per 4-ounce serving). Flavored yogurt is considered an ultra-processed food because of the added sugar, thickeners, stabilizers, and preservatives—but it also contains protein and calcium, so it's arguably better than gummy bears or chocolate bars. Flavored Greek yogurts tend to be the best choice as they are lower in sugar and higher in protein compared to regular flavored yogurts. Plus, they are so creamy and delicious! When shopping for flavored yogurt, buy brands with at least 2 of these attributes (but preferably all 5!): source of calcium, source of

> **WE GOT YOU!**
> The best choice is to buy plain yogurt and add your own fresh or pureed fruit (those unsweetened fruit and veggie pouches are perfect for this), or even a little drizzle of honey or maple syrup (just not 3 to 4 teaspoons of it!).

probiotics, source of protein—aim for at least 8 grams per 4-ounce serving, source of vitamin D, minimum sugar—no more than 12 grams per 4-ounce serving.

The good news is that companies are catching on and many now sell "low sugar" varieties. Look at the label to check these are truly low sugar, and not packed with artificial sweetener instead.

How about yogurt drinks and tubes? We'd place these on the "sometimes" list. They have a lot of sugar, but also may contain calcium and vitamin D, which kids require. So they are marginally better than candy, but not as good as, say, plain Greek yogurt with berries.

Bread

What kind of bread should I look for?
Sometimes it's difficult to get kids (and spouses!) on board with whole wheat or whole grain bread. Some don't like the brown color, while others are bothered by the seedy bits. But start early, and try, try again. It does contain more nutrition—fiber, vitamins, and minerals—than white bread.

Regardless of whether you opt for white or whole grain, it's better to buy fresh bakery bread, pita, buns, rolls, and bagels than ultra-processed bagged bread with preservatives. Check the ingredients and choose bread made with flour, water, yeast, salt, and sugar (some added grains and seeds are great too). That's how you would make bread in your own oven, right? The other ingredients in bagged bread—preservatives like calcium propionate and sodium stearoyl-2-lactylate—aren't needed to make tasty bread (they are just needed to make it last longer or ensure a consistent appearance loaf after loaf). Buy a fresh loaf and freeze it for a natural way to extend the shelf life.

> REALITY CHECK
>
> If you are buying whole grain bread in Canada, read labels carefully and look for the words "whole grain" on ingredients lists, rather than the words "whole wheat." In Canada, whole wheat flour is not 100% whole grain. It's milled slightly to extend shelf life, and the milling process removes some of the nutrient-dense parts of the grain, including vitamins and fiber. Whole grain is a better option. In the US, the terms "whole wheat" and "whole grain" are used interchangeably. This is strictly a Canadian thing!

SARAH SAYS: *My kids have never known anything but whole grain bread—we started at 6 months and haven't really deviated. In fact, when given the choice now, my kids always choose whole grain versus white because it's what is familiar!*

Meat

My kids love deli meat, but I've heard it's bad for them. Should you buy it? Deli meats have a bad reputation because they are high in sodium and often contain nitrates as preservatives. Nitrates are important because they ward off bacteria (trust us: it's better to have a hint of nitrates than any level of listeria, which is a nasty bacterium that causes serious illness). But the combination of sodium and nitrates in beef or pork deli meat (ham, roast beef, bologna, salami, etc.) is also linked to a slightly increased risk of colon cancer. So deli meats are fine once in a while, but should not be everyday staples.

Roast turkey or chicken deli meats are slightly better than beef- and pork-based ones because the link to colon cancer is in red (not white) meats. When buying deli meats, try to find lower-sodium options. Deli meats are too salty for infants and toddlers altogether, and fresh meats are a better option.

Pregnant women are advised to avoid deli meats (unless cooked to steaming hot) for the risk (however small) of listeria contamination. See more on page 82.

Mac and cheese

Is organic boxed mac and cheese healthier than conventional? Well, the organic companies certainly make it sound better! But is the organic version really healthier than the old blue box of mac and cheese that you grew up on?

Bottom line: it's a tie. Either of these boxed mac and cheese options is fine to enjoy once in a while as a meal or side dish. They are convenient and most kids love them! However, both are considered to be ultra-processed foods, which are not the most nutritious choice for everyday meals.

	Conventional boxed mac and cheese	Organic boxed mac and cheese	Winner?
Calories (per 2.5 oz)	250	270	Tie—it's so close!
Protein	9 grams	9 grams	Tie
Sodium	570 milligrams	540 milligrams	Tie—it's so close
Artificial color	None	None	Tie
Preservatives used	Yes	Yes	Tie
Organically farmed	No	Just the wheat	Organic
Ultra-processed food	Yes	Yes	Tie
Cost	$1	$1.25 to $2	Conventional

Snacks and treats

Are granola bars healthy or not? Well, it depends. A granola bar made from whole grain oats, nuts, seeds, and dried fruits with just a hint of added sugar can be a great between-meal snack that contains protein and fiber. But a chocolate-covered granola bar filled with marshmallows and chocolate chips should be considered a treat. It really depends on the ingredients in the bar. Ideally, the best options will have 6 grams of sugar or less per 30-gram serving. And if the bar is coated in chocolate, it's a chocolate bar!

Are organic cookies healthier than other cookies? Remember that organic is not a health logo; it just indicates how the ingredients were grown. Just like regular cookies, organic cookies are made with flour, sugar, and butter or shortening. A cookie is a cookie, whether it's organic or not. See more about organic food on page 18.

Are "vegetable chips" better than potato chips? You've probably noticed assorted bags of ruffled chips, sticks, and straws in subtle orange and green hues. The color usually comes from vegetable powders—like carrot, beet, or spinach—but the base of the chips is likely potato or corn, and they may contain a lot of salt or fat. These crunchy treats are totally fine to munch once in a while, but they should not be mistaken for vegetables (sorry, that pinch of spinach powder doesn't really count). They are the same as any other corn, potato, or tortilla chips.

Shopping on a budget

Many obstacles can get in the way of preparing healthy meals—and a tight budget or lack of easy access to fresh food can make feeding a family especially difficult. But, we've got you, and have some suggestions that may help.

Plan in advance: Figure out how much money you can afford to spend on food each month. Plan some meal ideas for the week, then make your shopping list and *stick to it* when you get to the store. Grocery shopping is a science, and yep, there are researchers who devote their lives to getting you to buy more when you're in the store. Shopping with a list will help you avoid the pitfalls of impulse shopping, stop you from wasting food, and make sure your dollars are spent wisely.

Plan for high nutrition, low cost options: The items in the table below offer the most nutritional value for the lowest cost.

Low Cost, High Nutrition Options		
Vegetables and fruit	**Grains**	**Protein**
Apples	Barley	Canned fish
Bananas	Bread	Canned or dry beans and lentils
Beets	Brown rice	Chicken thighs
Broccoli	Bulgur (cracked wheat)	Eggs
Cabbage	Corn flour	Evaporated skim milk
Carrots	Oats	Flank steak or chuck roast
Corn	Pasta	Ground beef
Onions	Popcorn kernels	Peanut butter and peanuts
Potatoes	White flour	Stewing meat
Squash	White rice	Tofu and edamame
Sweet potatoes	Whole wheat flour	White fish

Buy items on sale: Get fresh fruit and vegetables when they're in season or on sale. Cut them up and store them in the freezer. This works well for leafy greens, berries, squash, peas and corn. Likewise, buy whole grain bread on sale and freeze. Check flyers, apps and websites for coupons and sale items. But watch out for the word "special" on product displays. It may not mean that an item is on sale—it may just be a large display, and the price is the same as usual.

Buy larger sizes and prep at home: Instead of buying shredded or individually cut slices of cheese, choose blocks of cheese and shred or slice it yourself. Yogurt too; buy a large tub, which cost less per serving than buying mini-cups.

Look for substitutions: Sometimes you'll read a recipe that includes expensive, premium ingredients. Here's the thing: you can eat well without relying on expensive ingredients. The foods listed in the chart below cost less, and are just as nutritious (and delicious!).

♥ (WE GOT YOU!)

When you're buying vegetables and fruit, it doesn't matter if they are fresh, frozen or canned as they are all healthy options! If buying canned, go for low sodium varieties canned in water whenever possible (items canned in broth, oil or juice tend to contain lots of added salt or sugar). Bonus: Frozen and canned options last much longer than fresh vegetables and fruit, and there's less waste.

Affordable Alternatives

Instead of expensive . . .	Choose more affordable . . .
Ready-made granola	Rolled oats
Quinoa	Brown rice or millet
Acai or Goji berries	Raisins
Walnuts, almonds or pecans	Sunflower seeds or pumpkin seeds
Almond butter	Peanut butter
Canned albacore tuna	Canned skipjack tuna
Canned sockeye salmon	Canned pink salmon
Halibut	Haddock or tilapia
Ground beef	Tofu or brown lentils
Chicken breasts	Chicken thighs

Know your grocery store: Look at the top and bottom shelves in the grocery store: The most expensive brands are kept at eye-level, and great deals can be found if you shop the upper and lower shelves. Try no name or store brands of packaged foods; they are made by the same large food companies, but are packaged with different labels—meaning they are great quality and cost less. Also, many grocery stores have "points" cards, which earn you free groceries. Make sure to opt in to those programs.

IF YOU NEED HELP

Community Gardens: Many cities have local gardens where you can access low-cost or free fresh produce. Check your local community center or public health unit to learn about community gardens in your area.

Food Banks Canada: Some people think of food banks as the place to just get canned food or boxed mac and cheese, but more than 40% of food at food banks in Canada is actually fresh. You can get milk, eggs, bread, vegetables, and fruit too. There are 650 affiliated food banks across Canada. Find one near you at www.foodbankscanada.ca.

Salvation Army: Across North America, the Salvation Army has food banks that are open to assist you. Similar to shopping in a grocery store, you can browse and select the food you want, but there's no cost. They also offer nutritious free meals. For more information, go to www.salvationarmy.ca/what-we-do/food-services for the Canadian site or www.salvationarmyusa.org/usn/cure-hunger/ for the American site.

Feeding America: This nationwide network of food banks in the US gets nourishing food—from farmers, manufacturers, and retailers—to people in need. Find a food bank near you at www.feedingamerica.org/find-your-local-foodbank.

Special Supplemental Nutrition Program for Women, Infants, and Children (WIC): This US program provides federal grants to states for nutritious food and nutrition education for low-income pregnant and postpartum women. It also funds programs for infants and children up to age 5 who are found to be at nutritional risk. Learn more at www.fns.usda.gov/wic.

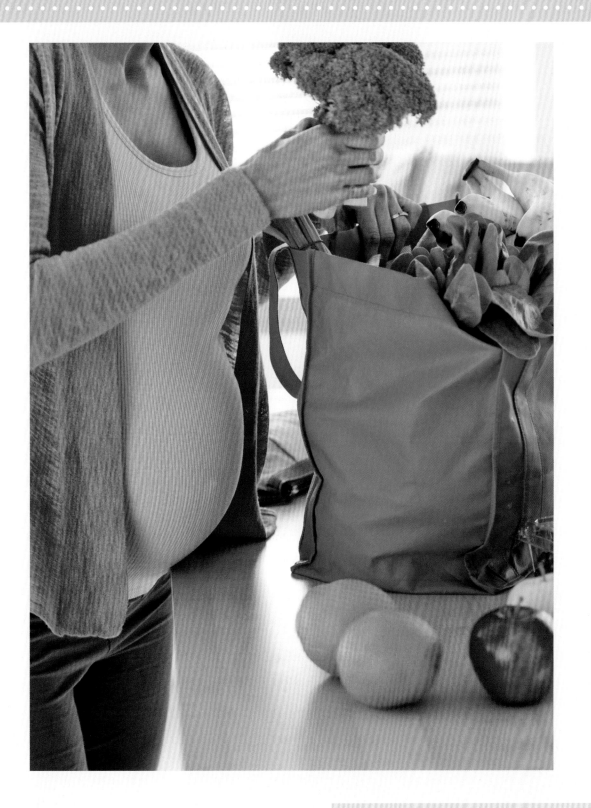

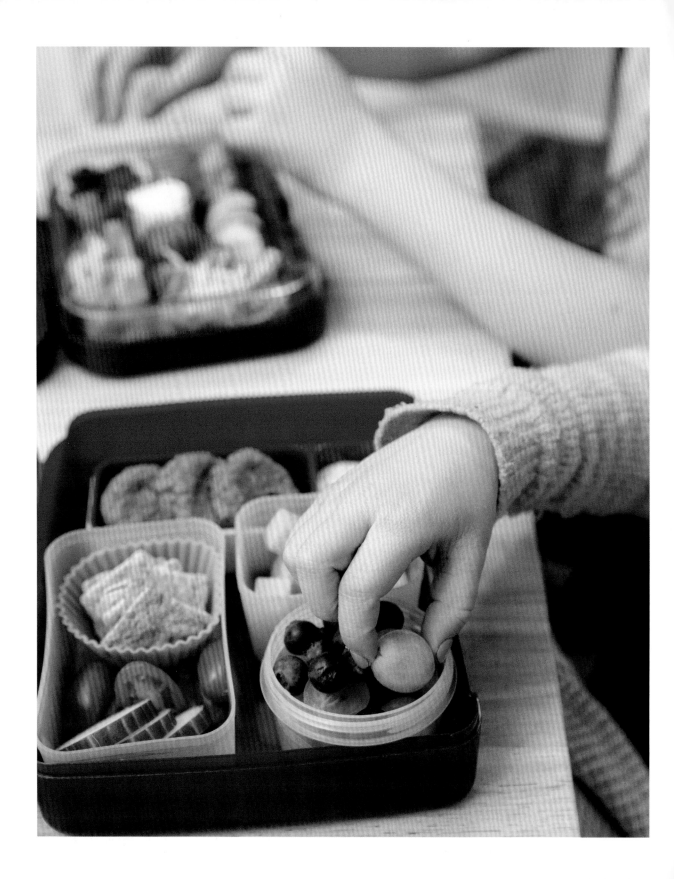

How Can I Make School Lunches that My Child Will Actually Eat?

One of the biggest milestones when kids start school is school lunches (um, that's a milestone for the parents AND the kids). Yup, 5 days a week, you may have to pour your time, effort, creativity, and nutritional knowledge into tiny containers and then cross your fingers. Can they open the lid? Will they eat it? Will your containers make it back home? It's a whole new world! After packing a combined 3,000 lunches between us (and growing!), we have some tips to make it easier for you. The key is to keep it simple (no overcomplicated Pinterest-like lunches here!) and to make yourself a solid lunch-packing strategy with a list of go-to options to choose from (see some suggestions on page 330). And turn to page 333 for our take on snacks for recess.

What you'll need

1. **Washable insulated lunch box or bag:** This helps keep containers cold (and altogether in one place!)
2. **Leak-proof containers or compartments:** These are ideal for storing different foods (we use bento-style lunchboxes for our kids)
3. **Thermos and ice packs:** Perfect for keeping hot foods hot, and cold foods extra cold
4. **Reusable cutlery:** We recommend you use a set that you don't mind losing (don't send your silverware as it may not come home!)

Be prepared

If you have time, pack lunch the night before and store it in the fridge overnight so that it's already cold when you pack it. Always add an ice pack to keep foods cold until ready to be eaten. For hot foods, you can't pack them the night before! That's a morning activity. Pour boiling water into the thermos first and let it sit for a couple of minutes to prewarm it. Pour the boiling water out of the thermos, place the hot food in the thermos, and seal. That way you know the food will stay warm for you kids some lunchtime.

And get your child to help pack their lunch—the more kids are involved in making it, the more likely they are to actually eat it! See our tips for getting kids into the kitchen on pages 357.

What to serve

You can make deciding what to pack for lunch easy, by thinking about the lunchbox being divided into 4 quadrants and filling each with one of these essential food groups:

1. **Protein-rich foods:** Options include meat, poultry, fish, eggs, milk, yogurt, cheese, beans, tofu, lentils, seeds, or seed butter.
2. **Whole grain:** Think whole grain bread, oatmeal, whole grain pancakes or waffles, leftover pasta, quinoa or barley, or corn tortillas.
3. **Vegetables:** Try/alternate any cooked or raw vegetable. A vegetable soup or tossed salad works well too!
4. **Fruit:** And always include fresh fruit or fruit salad.

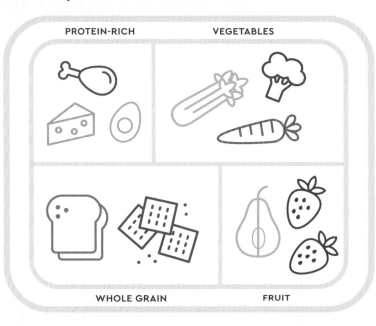

SARAH SAYS: *I make sure to include variety in every lunchbox I pack. My kids tend to eat much more when there's more to choose from, and it means that there's a nice balance of nutrients too! The more color and variety, the better!*

Ideas to Keep Lunchboxes Fun!

 BREAKFAST FOR LUNCH: Try homemade French toast, waffles, or pancakes, or a thermos of scrambled eggs and a multi grain bagel. Or try yogurt, fruit, and granola parfait—have your child add the granola (seeds, dried fruit, coconut, etc.) at school so it doesn't get soggy. And a fruit/vegetable/yogurt smoothie can also be fun, with some whole grain toast and seed butter.

THINGS ON SKEWERS: Cheese cubes, tomatoes, cucumbers, peppers, and turkey are so much more fun when they are on a stick.

FINGER FOODS: Make a lunch out of hors d'oeuvres! Add some of the following: whole grain crackers, cheese, hummus or other dips, vegetable strips, sliced grapes and other cut-up fruit, seed butter and protein/energy balls (see the recipe on page 336). Done.

 UNIQUE SANDWICHES: Roll sandwich fillings in a tortilla or stuff them between 2 pancakes or pieces of leftover French toast! Try a variety of fillings: grilled cheese, skipjack tuna melts, turkey, seed butter and banana, or egg salad.

 LOVE YOUR LEFTOVERS: Try a thermos of last night's homemade pizza, whole grain spaghetti bolognaise or mac and cheese, or think of ways to use up your cooked meat, fish or tofu for lunch—tucked in mini tacos or in sushi rolls can be fun!

Food safety

Lunch can get a little gritty, so you need to keep it clean. Here are some food safety tips:

- Empty and wash out the lunchbox as soon as the kids come home from school to avoid bacterial growth. Older kids can do this chore themselves!
- Wash those canvas lunch bags! They get used every day, and bits of food can get stuck in the corners. Put them in the washing machine weekly.

CARA SAYS: *I tossed my daughter's lunch bag into the dryer with the rest of the laundry. Did I mention that the cover was coated with plastic? Right. It was a picture of those Disney princesses, and let's just say they didn't like the dryer heat. Contorted melting faces of Cinderella and Snow White made my daughter cry (but then laugh). So please do wash your lunch bag, but let it air-dry!*

WHAT'S YOUR CHILD'S FAVORITE LUNCH TO BRING TO SCHOOL?

My kids love my macaroni and cheese. I do a homemade version with milk, Cheddar, and whole grain noodles, and they bring it to school in a thermos. —Edith

My daughter likes when I make wraps with sunflower butter and banana, then cut them into rounds to look a bit like sushi. —Billie-Jo

Usually leftovers. Chicken, rice, or pasta, and whatever vegetables we have. —Simone

Greek salad! Cucumber, tomato, feta cheese, and olives. Then I add some pita and hummus. —Diana

My kids both like to have little bite-sized nibbles. I use a bento-style lunchbox and add vegetables, dip, cheese cubes, crackers, fruit, etc. —Mallory

My son doesn't like sandwiches, so I have to be creative. Sometimes I do crackers, cheese, and cubes of chicken, or he likes warm leftovers in a thermos. That could be rice and chicken, chili with cornbread, or macaroni and cheese. —Lavonne

I make all sorts of fun things, but their favorite is a simple turkey sandwich. —Amanda

Often they get leftovers from dinner. Chicken korma or chana masala are popular. Sometimes it's a sandwich with meat or cheese. —Aliya

My little guy prefers a warm lunch. I send a thermos with chicken noodle soup, spaghetti and meatballs, or mac and cheese. —Kent

My daughter is learning to like salads. Usually I make quinoa or pasta as a base, and add beans, turkey, vegetables, and cheese. —Annie

They love leftovers! Pork or beef stir-fry with some rice. Vegetables and fruits in separate containers. —Li

A special lunch I make is breakfast-for-lunch. It's either pancakes or granola, yogurt, and fruit. —Sadie

What if lunch comes home uneaten?

Has this happened to you? After packing a delicious lunch, you go to clean the lunchbox at the end of the day and the food is STILL IN IT? It's sure happened to us! So why do some school-age kids skip lunch? There are 4 common reasons. And we're willing to bet that some detective work will get to the root of your problem. Ask your child the following questions:

Q: Did you enjoy the food in your lunchbox?

As a parent, you have the important job of selecting healthful foods for your child's lunchbox. But if children think some items are mushy, discolored, soggy, or just plain yucky, they're not going to eat very much.

Solution: Get your child's feedback: What do they want for lunch? Why didn't they like certain items? Give kids input in choosing foods and they will be more likely to munch their lunch. Bring your child to the grocery store and let them choose some nutritious favorites or get them involved in preparing and packing their lunch.

Q: Do you get enough time to eat, without being distracted?

Many schools offer a 20-minute lunch period, which seems like ample time to finish a mid-day meal. But classmates, loud voices, and putting on outdoor shoes can leave your child with just a few minutes to eat. Plus, few foods can compete with the lure of getting outside for cartwheels, freeze tag, and monkey bars.

Solution: Pack bite-size foods that are quick to eat. A sandwich is easier to eat than a thermos of steaming soup; cucumber rounds are quicker than stringy celery sticks. This is where bento-style lunchboxes come in handy—lots of colorful finger foods for the win!

Q: Are you able to open your lunchbox and containers?

For younger children, some lunchbox containers, lids, and zippers are too difficult for their small hands to open. When there's only one lunch monitor for a roomful of kids, it can be hard for little voices to ask for help. Some children may not be eating because they physically can't get to their food.

Solution: Before sending any new containers to school, test them out at home to ensure your child can open them. If they struggle, switch to more kid-friendly containers, or speak to the lunch monitor about helping your child with difficult lids.

Q: Are you hungry at lunchtime?

It may look like the lunchbox is coming home full, but perhaps your child is simply eating small portions. This may be because the portions you send are too large, or a morning snack was filling.

Solution: Kids have small stomachs and don't need large portions. Watch how much your child eats for lunch on weekends to gauge the correct portion to send during the week. If they fill up on their recess snack, ensure that it's nutritious. Send an apple and cheese rather than chips or candy. That way, even if lunch appetites are small, at least you know your child has eaten something nourishing while at school.

What snacks should I pack for recess?

More than a third of a child's daily calories comes from foods eaten between meals. That's a big chunk of the food that they eat each day! Nutritious snacks should be your go-to over sweet treats to ensure your child gets some vitamins, minerals, protein, and fiber at snack time, and has enough energy to fuel their day. A well-balanced snack will keep your child from developing that between-meal "hangry" (hungry + angry) mood, and will provide added insurance that they're getting the nutrients they need for optimal growth and development.

REALITY CHECK

Packing prepackaged snacks is easy and convenient (Bear Paws and Goldfish, anyone?), but there's a problem: lots of prepackaged snacks—like cookies, chips, and gummy candy—are ultra-processed foods and don't have the nutrients your child needs to fuel their busy school day. With smaller tummies, children get hungry between meals and require food as fuel. Sweet treats don't provide the nutrients that kids need for optimal energy levels and concentration skills.

HOW TO CHOOSE HEALTHY PACKAGED SNACKS

Sometimes you don't have time for homemade snacks, and that's okay. Not all packaged snacks are ultra-processed foods! We use packaged snacks as our plan B, and choose ones that are minimally processed, like milk made into yogurt (not ultra-processed, like white flour and jam made into Pop-Tarts). Pick packaged snacks that:

- **Do** contain mostly natural sugar (from fruit or milk), and not a lot of added sugar
- **Do** have at least 3 grams of fiber or protein, or ideally both!
- **Don't** have an ingredients list a mile long, with ingredients you don't recognize
- **Don't** have refined flour, sugar, or hydrogenated oil as the main ingredient
- **Don't** contain more than 180 milligrams of sodium per serving

Here are some great packaged options if you're short on time:

- Hummus
- Whole grain crackers
- Bean or lentil crackers
- String cheese
- Kale chips
- Roasted chickpeas

- Pumpkin or sunflower seeds (no shells)
- Greek yogurt cups
- Lower-sugar trail mix
- Lower-sugar granola bars
- Unsweetened fruit and/or vegetable sauces or pouches

Ultra-Processed Snack Swaps!

Swap these . . .	For these!
Chocolate- or yogurt-coated granola bars	Uncoated, lower-sugar, higher-protein, higher fiber granola bars
Fruit chews, gummies, or roll-ups	Unsweetened raisins, figs, or dried fruit
Fruit drinks or juice	Fresh fruit
Chips or pretzels	Air-popped popcorn (for 4 years and up)
Bear paws, cookies, or cereal bars	Homemade whole grain muffins or energy balls/bites
Chips with ranch dip	Vegetables with Greek yogurt dip

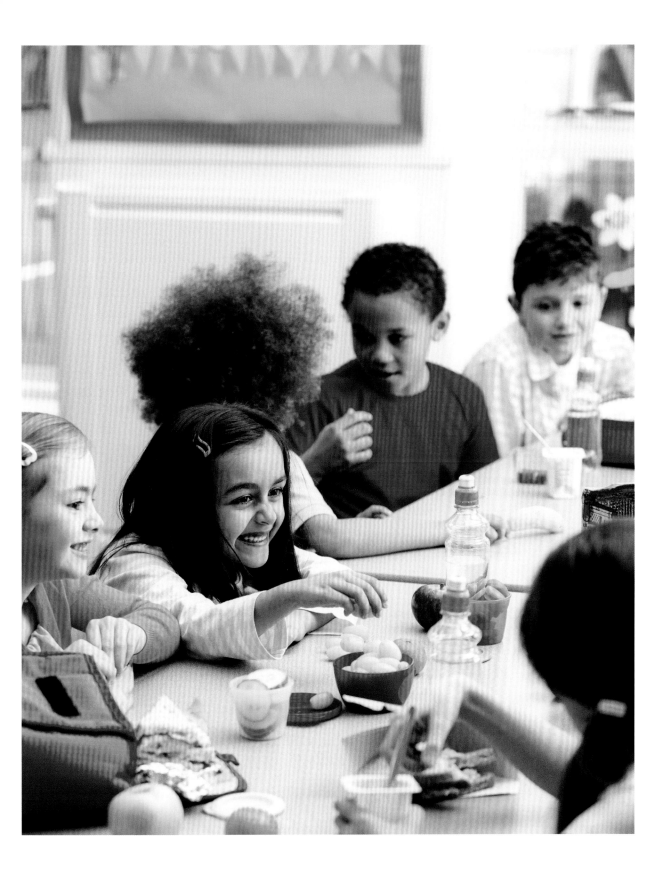

NO-BAKE GRANOLA ENERGY BITES

Your child can help you stir together these ingredients and roll them into bite-size balls. These are great for recess, lunchboxes, or after-school snacks. If your child's school has a no nuts policy, use soy or seed butter.

Makes 12 bites

1 cup rolled oats
½ cup any nut or seed butter (almond, peanut, soy nut, sunflower, pumpkin seed, etc.)
2 tbsp hempseeds or ground flaxseeds
2 tbsp honey
Your favorite add-ins (see variations below)

1. Line a baking sheet with parchment paper.
2. In a large bowl, combine the oats, nut or seed butter, seeds, honey, and your choice of add-ins. Stir to combine.
3. Using a rounded teaspoon, scoop out the oat mixture and roll it tightly into bite-size balls. Place on the prepared baking sheet. Repeat until the oat mixture is used up. It should make 12 bites.
4. Place the baking sheet in the freezer for 1 to 2 hours, then transfer the bites to a freezer-safe container for up to 4 months. You can eat them frozen or at room temperature!

ADD-IN VARIATIONS

Oatmeal raisin
½ tsp cinnamon
¼ cup raisins

Chocolate chip
¼ cup chocolate chips

Chocolate cherry
3 tbsp chocolate chips
2 tbsp chopped dried cherries

Tropical
¼ cup toasted coconut
½ tsp vanilla extract

Coconut almond
2 tbsp chocolate chips
2 tbsp coconut
2 tbsp chopped almonds

CARA SAYS: *You can double or triple this recipe to make dozens of energy bites, and freeze them. I pack 2 frozen bites per child in their lunchbox, and they are the perfect temperature when the recess bell rings (although my kids also like them frozen!)*

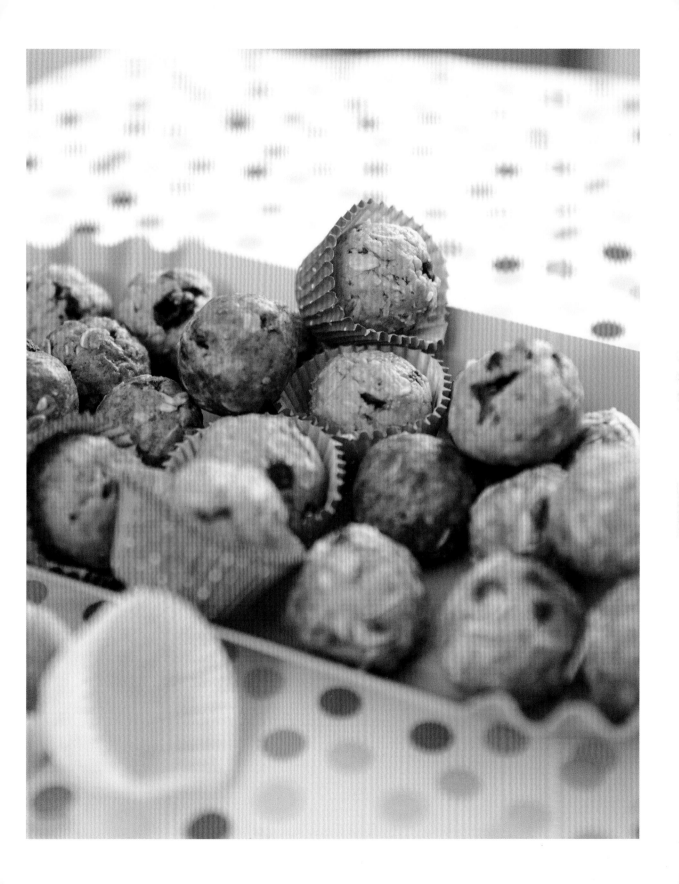

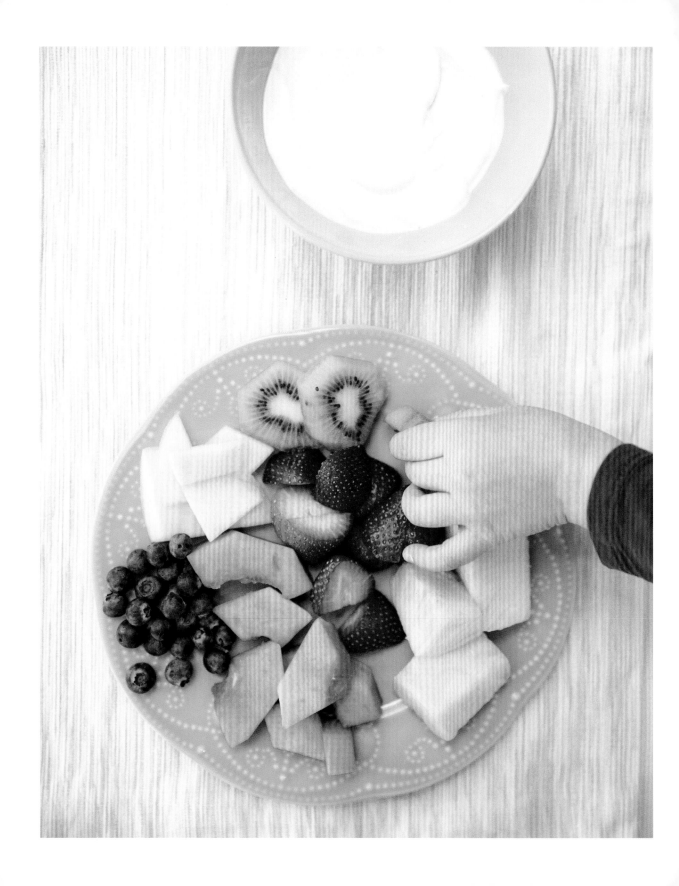

How can I control the foods my child eats at a playdate?

Here's a better question: why do you *want* to control the foods your child eats at a playdate?

Food allergy, intolerance, or special diet: If your child has a food allergy or intolerance, or follows a special diet (kosher, halal, vegan, etc.), then you need to talk to the playdate's parents about what they plan to serve your child to eat. Your child's health and safety are paramount, and it's your right as a parent to decide what you want another adult to offer them. Some parents make up business cards that their child brings with them to the playdate, so the other parent knows what not to serve and what to do in case of emergency (see below). If business cards are not your thing, simple communication with the playdate parent is always appropriate.

> **WE GOT YOU!**
>
> When you welcome other children into your home for a playdate, always ask their parents if there is anything you should know about food their child can or cannot eat. They'll thank you for it.

JOHNNY SMITH

TEL: 444-555-1212

FOOD ALLERGY: PEANUTS

I HAVE AN ANAPHYLACTIC ALLERGY TO PEANUTS.

IN CASE OF EMERGENCY:

1. GET THE EPIPEN FROM MY BAG AND INJECT IT INTO MY THIGH. HOLD FOR 10 SECONDS.
2. CALL 911.
3. CALL MY PARENTS AT 444-555-1212.

Questioning food choices: If you want to keep your child away from "bad" foods other parents or caregivers may serve (raise your hand if your parents or parents-in-law feel that it's their duty to fill your child's tummy with as much junk food as possible!), the answer is trickier. Often, well-meaning parents choose to completely restrict junk food, and their kids have no idea what Oreos, Kraft Dinner, or Coke taste like. Some parents want to keep it that way for as long as possible. But here's the thing: these foods are part of our culture—even though they're not the most nutritious options—and there will come a point when your child discovers them.

Try as you might, you can't be the food police as your child grows and develops (trust us, we both tried with our first children). Their future will be filled with drop-off birthday parties, playdates, class holiday parties, afternoons at Grandma's house, summer camps, school outings, and other occasions when they will have to make their own food choices. Junk food will be there. You can't ignore it, but you can educate them about it.

WE GOT YOU!

In the dessert question (see page 295), we talked about randomly having treats. Occasions like playdates, holidays, parties, and family visits are the perfect "random" times to have treats! Kids will learn to enjoy treats when offered at these occasions, because treats are not always available to them. NEVER equate guilt with eating treat foods. Try to hold off on negative comments about these fun foods—your child will pick up on your bad energy and question why a treat is a bad thing. It isn't, as long as treats are occasional and not all-the-time foods.

REALITY CHECK

Your job as the parent is to provide the majority of your child's meals and set them up to make wise choices when you're not around. If kids eat well the majority of the time, there is room for treats in the diet. They will miss out if you don't let them attend playdates because you are afraid of the food that's being served. That's your fear— don't make it theirs!

CARA SAYS: *When my daughter was 8, she wanted to try overnight camp. I looked at the website and was excited that she'd learn how to canoe, waterski, and play tennis. Cool! Then I got to the menu. Oh. My. Goodness. Not surprisingly, it was filled with traditional camp foods: hotdogs, hamburgers, chicken fingers, etc. And pop. And chips. And chocolate bars. And cookies. Let's just say, there was no kale or quinoa to be found. I was worried. Left to her own devices, how would my child fare with this kind of menu?*

But you know what happened? She was just fine. She ate the traditional camp food, and also found her way to the daily "salad bar," where she could get lettuce, sliced vegetables, chickpeas, pumpkin seeds, and fruit. She was used to eating vegetables at home, so her plate didn't seem right without them (those were her actual words!). The moral of the story is that if you set your child up with good eating habits at home, it will empower them to make nutritious choices even when you're not there. Trust your child.

SARAH SAYS: *I will fully admit it, I was a food micromanager when my firstborn started solids and entered his toddlerhood. As a dietitian and new mom, I was fairly diligent with what I served and how I served it. And when he was offered treats or sweets at his grandparents' or a friend's house, I cringed and sometimes even said something. But then I realized that this wasn't helping anyone—it was taking the fun out of Grandma's house and playdates, and it was sending the wrong message to my son. Sometimes you just have to let go and realize that it's not always going to be perfect, and that what happens at home most of the time is what really matters, nutrition-wise. Treats on special occasions are fun and okay (and normal), and you want your child to learn the same.*

My child eats about 6 foods. How can I expand their palate?

Kids are creatures of habit and tend to like what they like. (Does that sound familiar? Many adults are the same way!) But that doesn't mean that your child with a small repertoire of favorite foods won't ever try anything new. Turn to page 49 to read in full about tackling picky eating.

My child won't sit still at the dinner table. What can I do?

At some point in this 3-to-6-year-old range, your child will transition from their booster seat to an adult-size chair at the kitchen table. Most of the time, if a child won't sit still, it has to do with the chair they are in. It may be too low, so it is difficult for them to see their plate and reach their food if they don't stand up every few minutes.

If you are struggling with kids who resemble jumping beans, try this test: Have them sit at their chair in the same position that they would at dinner, and check their posture. They should be sitting with their hips, knees, and ankles all bent at 90-degree angles, like the corners of a square. If the chair is too low, the solution is to bring back that booster! If it's not the chair, there are many other reasons why your child may not sit still—turn to page 289.

I'm concerned my child is overweight. Should I put them on a diet?

You're certainly not alone if you're worried that your child is overweight—many parents share your concern and become anxious when they watch their "overweight" child devour their meal and then ask for seconds. What if they continue to gain weight (the unhealthy kind)? What if they get bullied at school because of it? What about chronic disease down the road? These are all valid concerns. But the short answer to dieting is: no. Here's the thing . . .

Children should not be on weight-loss diets: Period. End of story. A weight-loss diet means they will be restricting calories (energy), and a child cannot properly grow and develop if they are not eating enough food to meet their body's needs.

Children should not be on low-carb diets: Carbs are the body's main source of energy (see page 32). Don't take bread and pasta away from your child—that's not the answer to weight loss!

Children should not be on low-fat diets: Fat is essential for the normal development of the brain, eyes, and nerves. Kids can eat nuts, seeds, oils, etc.

(REALITY CHECK)

Going "on a diet" sets the stage for eventually going "off the diet," which leads to a vicious cycle of weight gain and weight loss and periods of restricted versus free-for-all eating. That is the last thing we want for our children! Much like adults, when kids feel restricted or deprived, they want MORE. They start sneaking or they "get it in while they can" (like at a friend's house), and this perpetuates the problem and creates lifelong eating issues.

There is no "perfect" size that all children need to be: Kids come in all shapes and sizes! If your mindset is that thin is the best and only option, flip to page 344 for some helpful advice.

Instead, trust the Division of Responsibility (sDOR): Set your child and yourself up with the sDOR (see page 41), and trust that it will allow them to eat the right amount of food to meet the needs of their growing body—at any age. That may mean that they are at the low end of the growth curve, or the high end. Bodies are all different, and that is not within a parent's control. And remember that their appetite fluctuates based on age, activity level, season, and gender.

If you are not practicing the sDOR yet, it might mean you have already formed the habit of controlling your child's food intake, but there is still time to reverse this behavior! You can start the sDOR at any age, though it will take older kids a bit of time to get used to it (and lots of patience on your part). Suddenly their parents aren't watching over them and instructing them on how much to eat. It may take a while until they discover their own ability to eat as much as they need and self-regulate, but it will happen in time! At first, they may overdo it on the foods that you were most restrictive on (um, pasta? bread? sweets?), but with guidance, they will learn to eat what their body needs. After a few weeks or months, they will begin to regulate their own food intake. A child should feel:

> **REALITY CHECK**
>
> Along with the sDOR, we want to encourage our children to be intuitive eaters (read more on page 44). This will set them up for a long-term healthy relationship with food.

- Like a competent eater
- Good about eating a variety of foods
- Able to independently make nutritious meal and snack choices
- Confident to eat at regular meal and snack times, and not ask for food between meals
- Hungry at the beginning of mealtime
- Able to stop eating when satisfied
- No stress at the meal table

Aim for a healthy lifestyle: If your child is significantly overweight, instead of jumping on the dieting rollercoaster (which it always is), you want your child to develop an overall "healthy lifestyle." This includes:

- Eating a variety of nutritious foods every day
- Including occasional treats and not putting any foods "off limits"
- Listening to their bodies and trusting their physical hunger and fullness cues so as to eat the right amount of the food that you offer
- Enjoying fun physical activity—at least 60 minutes per day
- Getting enough sleep each night
- Learning how to cope with stress in healthy, non-food-related ways—open to talking about their feelings and communicating with you when something is wrong

If you practice these tenets, your child can grow up with a healthy body image and the right skills to live a balanced and healthy lifestyle. They may be at an "ideal weight" according to scientific charts. Or they may be a few pounds underweight or overweight compared to the norm. But don't compare your child to others—instead, take the focus off the numbers and look at their overall health and lifestyle:

- Do they get 60 minutes of activity daily?
- Do they eat a variety of fruits and vegetables?
- Do they know that treats are "sometimes" foods?

These things matter more than the number on a scale. Your beautiful child is more than a number!

I'd love to help my child build body confidence, but how?

Most adults have struggled with body, weight, or self-esteem issues at some point in their life. Maybe it was a rude comment from a sports coach about losing some weight or bulking up that started the negative self-talk. Maybe it was comparing yourself to the beauty standards of models or actors (those pictures are often photoshopped, you know). If you have a weight bias that skinny is better, or have unrealistic desires for the "ideal body," you can easily pass those onto your innocent child. Don't let that happen!

Lucky for us, the negative diet approach that many of us grew up with is slowly being replaced with a new way of thinking. It's called mindfulness, mindful eating, intuitive eating (read more on page 44), or something similar, and it focuses on learning to LOVE and ACCEPT your body for what it is and for all of the wonderful things it can do—and to nourish that body with food and feel no guilt about it.

POSITIVE BODY IMAGE STRATEGIES
Do
- **Do** help your child focus on their abilities and personality rather than their physical appearance.
- **Do** focus on a healthy lifestyle, not a number on a scale. Shift your focus to healthy behaviors and away from the diet mentality—it's a much more positive approach.
- **Do** encourage your child to think critically about messages and images they see in the media.

- **Do** focus on ability and strength. Teach your child to love and accept their body for all of the wonderful things it provides them. Eyes that can see the world! Legs that can run and carry them to great adventures! Arms that can hug the people they love or lift heavy things!

- **Do** use the media to your advantage! When you feel your child will grasp the concept (maybe by age 6?), show them before-and-after pictures of famous people whose photos have been altered (search online for "photoshopped celebrities").

- **Do** speak kindly about yourself and your body. Do it out loud for your child to hear! Lead by example and they will follow suit.

REALITY CHECK

Children with a positive body image are more comfortable and confident in their ability to succeed. They don't obsess about calories, food, or weight. Imagine the freedom of that! If you read through this question and can't possibly see a way to be so positive about body image, consider working on this so you can be a body-positive coach to your kids. An intuitive eating (see page 44) therapist can help.

Don't

- **Don't** weigh your child (other than at doctor appointments) or make weight-related goals.

- **Don't** talk negatively about your own body in front of your child. Your child sees you as the most beautiful person in the world. If you constantly rag on your "big thighs" or your "fat butt," your child will not understand why the most beautiful person in the world doesn't see themselves correctly, and will begin to see you (and themselves) in a warped way too.

- **Don't** focus on the "perfect body," because there is no such thing. If your child always hears you talking about the size you want to be, they won't understand it. They think you're pretty perfect already, so take steps to be comfortable with the body you have.

Building self-esteem: Do's and don'ts

- **DO** focus on ability rather than physical appearance.
- **DON'T** weigh children or make weight-related goals.
- **DO** speak kindly about your body.
- **DON'T** talk negatively about anybody's body (yours or theirs).
- **DO** focus on a healthy lifestyle, not a number on a scale.
- **DON'T** overpraise. No one is perfect!
- **DO** let kids list what they love about themselves.

CARA SAYS: *There's a great self-esteem-building activity that I do with my kids, and maybe you'll want to try it too. I stand with each child (individually) in front of the mirror, and I ask them to tell me 5 things that they love about themselves. The kind of answers I hear include:*

- *I love that my arms are strong enough to do the monkey bars in the park.*
- *I love that my hands let me play guitar.*
- *I love that my ears let me hear the notes.*
- *I love that my legs let me run fast when I play soccer.*
- *I love that my calves are strong from drumming.*
- *I love that my arms can hug the people I love.*
- *I love that my hand can hold your hand when we walk to school.*
- *I love that my mouth can taste yummy food like pizza.*
- *I love that people laugh at my silly jokes.*
- *I love that I look a little bit like you, Mommy.*

I think my child is underweight. What should I be feeding them?

Despite high rates of childhood obesity, there's also the other end of the spectrum: About 4% of children are underweight. For children who are truly underweight, it may be a sign of a health problem and should be assessed by your child's doctor. They may offer a diagnosis or may simply encourage you to add extra calories to your child's diet in a healthy way.

(REALITY CHECK)

Being medically underweight is not the same thing as being slender or slim because of natural genetics. If your child is naturally small (maybe because you or your spouse are also slim or small), there's nothing wrong with that! And there is also nothing you can do to help them magically grow taller or become heavier. If they are eating well, are moving their body, and are generally happy, and the doctor has no issues with their weight, help them learn to love and accept their size (see page 344). If they are medically underweight it means the doctor has identified a problem and spoken to you about it.

If your child is medically underweight, add calories in a healthy way: Giving your child more calories from ultra-processed foods that are high in fat, sugar, and salt is not the right way to help gain a few pounds. Those foods do not provide the nutrients that your child needs for optimal growth and development.

If your child has a small appetite and is underweight, you need to make every bite count. What does that mean? Instead of them filling their small tummies with low-calorie foods like lettuce and cucumbers first, start their meals and snacks with the foods that are highest in calories: nuts, seeds, nut or seed butters, avocado, cheese, whole milk, or full-fat yogurt.

Put it into action: Let's say you are making your child toast. You could spread it with 25 calories from a tablespoon of hummus, 50 calories from a tablespoon of cream cheese, or 100 calories from a tablespoon of peanut butter. In this case, peanut butter is the best choice, because it provides the most calories for the same amount of food (and is really nutritious!).

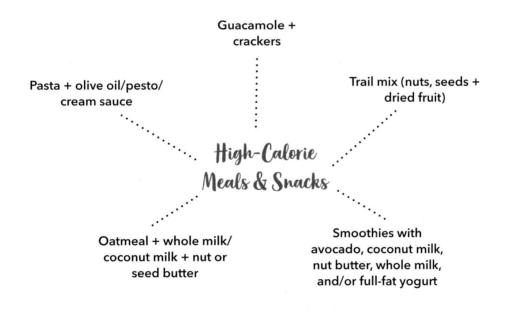

Guacamole + crackers

Pasta + olive oil/pesto/ cream sauce

Trail mix (nuts, seeds + dried fruit)

High-Calorie Meals & Snacks

Oatmeal + whole milk/ coconut milk + nut or seed butter

Smoothies with avocado, coconut milk, nut butter, whole milk, and/or full-fat yogurt

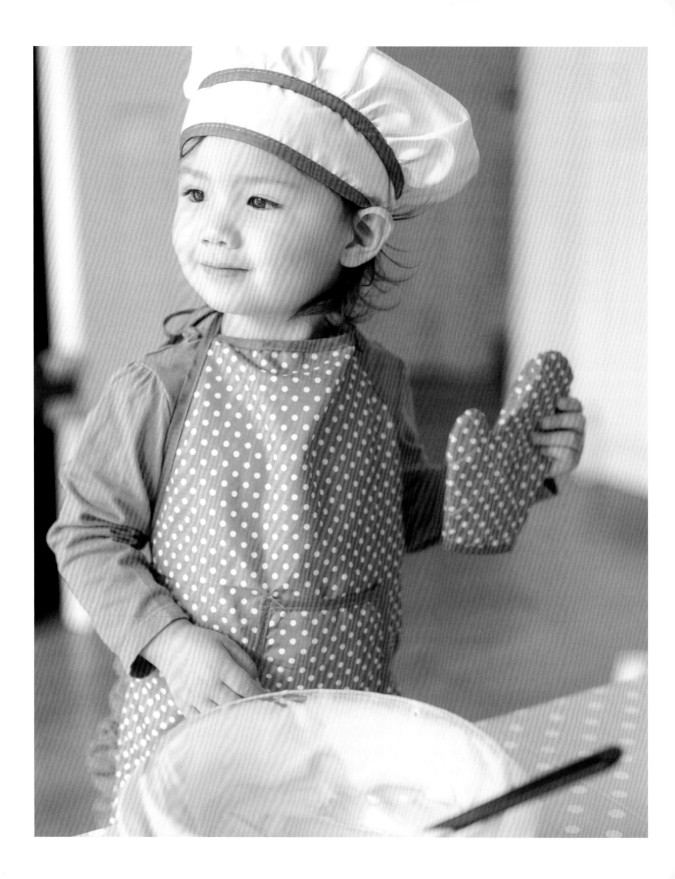

A vegetarian or vegan diet can definitely meet your child's nutritional needs as long as you properly plan. Turn to page 207 to learn the basics, and then read the information specific to older kids below.

CARA SAYS: *Your child may learn something at daycare or school that triggers a reaction that leads toward vegetarianism. For some kids, making the association that those cute pink piggies at the farm are where bacon comes from (and that the pigs have to die for it) is a huge eye-opening moment that totally freaks them out. Many kids go through a quick phase, then change their minds again. Support them through the learning process.*

Planning for nutrients

Iron: Recommendations for vegetarians are a bit higher than the standard because vegetarians require 1.8 times as much iron as non-vegetarians to compensate for the poor absorption of non-heme iron (see page 26):

- **Age 1 to 3 years:** 12.6 milligrams per day
- **Age 4 to 6 years:** 18 milligrams per day

Omega-3 fat (DHA and EPA): Skipping fish can mean a shortage of DHA, the nutrient that's important for brain health. Try omega-3-enriched eggs, which have 80 to 100 milligrams of DHA per egg. If you choose a vegan diet, talk to your doctor about a DHA supplement made from algal oil.

There's also a type of omega-3 fat called ALA, which is found in flax, hemp, chia, and walnuts. This type of fat does not have the same health benefits for brain, eye, and nerve development as DHA and EPA do, but some ALA is converted to DHA and EPA in the body (researchers suggest that less than 1% of ALA is converted to physiologically effective levels of EPA and DHA, but this number may be higher in vegetarians and vegans). Read more about omega-3 fat on pages 24, 301 and 367.

Calcium: If your vegetarian diet includes dairy products like milk, kefir, cheese, and yogurt, your child's calcium needs will be easily met. Vegan diets don't include dairy and need alternative calcium sources. See the list of calcium-rich foods on page 369–it includes beans, soy, leafy greens, broccoli, almonds, calcium-fortified plant-based beverages, and calcium-set tofu.

Vitamin B$_{12}$: If your child's diet includes eggs and dairy, vitamin B$_{12}$ needs will likely be met. Vegan diets require alternative sources of vitamin B$_{12}$, such as fortified soy or other plant-based beverages, fortified breakfast cereals, nutritional yeast, or a vitamin B$_{12}$ supplement. New to nutritional yeast? It's a yellow flaky condiment that is a great substitute for cheese, and is very high in vitamin B$_{12}$. It's now available in many grocery stores.

Vitamin D: Low serum vitamin D concentrations have been found with vegan and vegetarian children, so it's an important nutrient to watch, especially in the winter months in cold climates (vitamin D is the sunshine vitamin, see page 30). Depending on where you live and how much sunshine you get year-round, your children may need a vitamin D supplement. Few foods contain vitamin D—the short list is fish (which vegetarians don't eat), dairy (which vegans don't eat), and some mushrooms (which people don't tend to eat daily). We recommend vitamin D supplements for ALL kids (vegetarian or not), so this is easy advice: go for 400 to 600 IU vitamin D daily from supplements.

CARA SAYS: *My son is a self-proclaimed "flexitarian"—that means he chooses vegetarian meals most of the time, but is flexible enough to enjoy a burger or meatballs sometime. He is a huge fan of the savory and unique flavor of nutritional yeast, which tastes a bit like Parmesan cheese. He likes to sprinkle it on rice bowls, pasta, vegetables, and popcorn.*

I caught my child sneaking and hiding food. What should I do?

You start noticing food wrappers under your child's bed, or cookie crumbs in their bed sheets. You realize that your child is being dishonest and sneaking food. You might feel angry, confused, and concerned and your first instinct might be to address it promptly by disciplining your child, and setting even tighter boundaries around snacks and treats. Is this the right thing to do? How do you fix it?!

Although concerning, it's also an amazing opportunity to address any dysfunctional feeding dynamics going on (restricting or forbidding treats = sneaking and hoarding them *almost always*), create more trust, and foster open honest communication around food. This is a perfect time to help your child develop a healthy long-term relationship with food *without* feeling as though they need to sneak food, ever. Your first step is to figure out why they are sneaking food. Ask yourself:

- Is my child hungry, and not getting enough at mealtimes? Maybe they're going through a growth spurt?
- Are they emotional eaters and eating in the absence of hunger?
- Am I restricting certain foods or amounts of food?
- Am I limiting access to sweets?

The tricky part is when children confuse boredom or emotions with hunger. If you gently question your older child's (let's say 5- or 6-year-old's) hunger (maybe because they just finished eating a full dinner and it seems unlikely that they are actually still hungry), you can help them to tune in to their appetites and encourage them to identify true physical hunger, versus eating in the absence of hunger and/or emotional eating. This concept aligns well with encouraging your child to eat "intuitively" (read more on page 44).

WE GOT YOU!

It's really important to take a deep breath and know that there are ways to help your child from feeling they have to sneak food. If you approach it promptly, lovingly, and mindfully, you can turn things around.

We want to encourage our kids to be intuitive eaters, occasional emotional eating is a reality, and we shouldn't be too hard on our kids, or ourselves, for it. For example, when you're feeling down, you might crave and eat more "comfort foods," or when you're happy you may feel like celebrating with your favorite dessert. The goal is for them to be able to tune into their bodies, and honor their physical hunger and fullness cues *most* of the time. Eating for other reasons (sadness, boredom, happiness, excitement, etc.) will happen, and it's important to observe it, talk about it, and then do your best to re-focus them on their true *physical* hunger cues.

REALITY CHECK

Take a look at *what* foods your child is sneaking. Is it sweet treats you otherwise restrict or forbid? Research shows that restricting intake and limiting access to sweet foods increases children's preferences for those same foods. This is called scarcity, and it's when children feel food is restricted, so they want it more. Read more about managing treats on pages 295 and 353.

HOW CAN I FIX THIS?

Find a time to bring it up: Approach your child about it gently and lovingly, when both of you are calm and happy, and not during meal or snack time. Don't make it a huge deal, and try not to attack or get mad at them. Say something like "I noticed when I was cleaning your room that there were a few wrappers under your bed. I want you to know that you're not in trouble, but it's something we should talk about and figure out together." You don't want your child to feel threatened or like they're "bad" for sneaking food. You want them to feel safe to open up to you about it.

Ask them why, and show empathy: There are many reasons why kids sneak food, so it's important to find out why they're doing it first, so that you can solve the problem together. Leave it open-ended for them at first, but if they can't articulate their reasoning, offer thoughts like "Is your tummy still hungry after dinnertime?" or "Are there not enough foods that you like at meals?" or "Are you eating food when you feel sad, or bored, or mad?" or "Do you feel like I don't let you have these types of foods, so you need to sneak them instead?" Once you've gotten to the root of why it's happening, show empathy and compassion and acknowledge how they feel and why they're doing it.

Figure out a solution that works for both of you: Let your child know that they shouldn't ever have to feel as though they need to sneak or hide food. All foods can fit, and no foods are "forbidden." Try the following suggestions:

1. **If your child is still hungry after meals:** Make sure that you're involving your child in meal planning and preparation, and that they have a say in what is served. Ensure that there's at least one or two foods at the table that your child will eat, and that you're not restricting the amount that they can eat.

2. **If your child feels that certain foods are forbidden or highly restricted:** Let your child know that all foods are allowed, and that nothing is forbidden. Acknowledge that maybe some foods have been too-tightly limited (oops!) and come up with an amount that feels fair to both of you. Let your child know that *you as the parent* are still ultimately in charge of what food is served, and the timing of eating (meals and snacks), but that maybe, for example, you could offer a sweet treat more often than you have been. Or maybe you could add a little treat into school lunches (if you haven't been doing

♥ (WE GOT YOU!)
Try randomly offering dessert WITH dinner. Trust us! This might help. Read more about this, and its benefits, on pages 295 and 355.

that). Your child should always feel as though they can ask for a food, but they need to know that their request won't always be granted right then and there. The answer might be "yes," but not at that exact time. Parents are in charge of timing. Read again about the Division of Responsibility (sDOR) on page 41.

Read again about the Division of Responsibility (sDOR) on page 41.

I have a treat-obsessed child. How do I handle this?

When your child is about 3, treat may start to become a bigger deal—you know, when cookie tantrums become more frequent and they realize how delicious chocolate is? (And yes, it SO is.) It is normal for kids to want sweet, delicious desserts—after all, children have a biologically driven affinity to sweeter foods. But there has to be a limit. Not only will handfuls of sweets fill their tummies and displace their hunger for healthier foods, but sugary foods are also linked to increased disease risk as they get older.

What happens when a kid eats treats instead of snacks or meals? They don't get the sustainable energy they need to concentrate and thrive. Treats don't provide the nutrients that kids need, and if little tummies are filled with junk, there's less room for nourishing food. Read more about snacks versus treats on page 16, and more about sugar on page 34.

Read more about snacks versus treats on page 16, and more about sugar on page 34.

Top 5 tips for handling treat requests

1. **Say "yes" instead of "no".** Rather than no, a better response to a request for a treat is "Sure! You can have a treat today—let's decide when. If you have it now, that's it for today." When kids feel as though they CAN'T have something, they become frantic about having it NOW and ultimately a breakdown ensues. Simply saying yes instead of no can defuse the tantrum and urgency.

2. **Don't make treats a big deal.** Try to stay neutral when it comes to treats. If they get a loot bag from a birthday party or receive a lollipop after a haircut (why, right?! But it happens.), just go with it. Make it no big deal, and let them enjoy the treat with a regular meal or snack. This puts the treat on a level playing field with other foods.

3. **Eat the way you want your kids to eat.** Kids who are treat-obsessed may be observing their parents who eat the same treats (or, conversely, who strictly forbid them!)! It's important to address your own relationship with food, because you want to be a role model.

4. **Separate treats from parenting.** Don't use treats as rewards or bribes. Flip back to page 295 for more on this concept.

5. **Eat Dessert First.** Here's a radical idea that often works wonders with treat-obsessed kids. Serve dessert *with* dinner instead of afterward. Crazy, right?! But hear us out: providing a small treat (we're talking 2 little cookies, not a huge slab of double-fudge chocolate cake) alongside the main meal will put all of the dinner foods on an even playing field. Why does this work? It gives kids the choice of eating dessert before, during, or after the meal, which puts them in control. It makes them feel responsible and trusted, and eases suppertime tension. It can also help prevent your kids from racing through dinner to get to dessert and constantly ask "What's for dessert?"

   If you try this technique, the first couple of times you serve pudding or cookies WITH dinner, your kids will probably eat dessert first, and that's okay! After a few weeks when the novelty wears off, the sweet treat will just be another component of dinner. Some days the kids will choose dessert first, some days last, and some days they won't even finish it. That's when they've learned to normalize dessert as just another food they like, rather than an event.

Does my child need special foods when playing sports?

Physical activity is so important for children—they should be active for at least 60 minutes each day. That can be a full hour of play, or can be broken down into smaller increments. At this activity level, a normal, healthy diet is all that is required. Kids who "play" do not require any special supplements, protein powders, or sports drinks. They just need water and regularly timed meals and snacks (see page 302).

If your child belongs to the elite-athlete category and they are active for 2 or more hours most days, their nutritional needs are different than kids who play at the park or

---

REALITY CHECK

Water should always be on hand when kids are playing sports. Fluids help regulate body temperature, so it's vital to have around! Kids who are not elite athletes don't require sports drinks (such as Gatorade or Powerade), which are meant to provide electrolytes lost from sweat. So unless your kid is one in a million and is already an elite athlete (and really sweaty!), please skip the sports drinks. They provide extra calories, sodium, potassium, and sugar, which are not required for young children.

take lessons for fun skill-building. We're talking about AAA hockey players, elite soccer players, or competitive skaters, dancers, gymnasts, and the like—who aren't usually 3-to-6-year-olds! But if this is the case with your child, proper nutrition is vital, both so they will continue to grow and thrive and so they will perform to their highest potential in their sport. Seek advice from a dietitian if your child falls into this category.

What postgame snack should I bring to my child's sports/games ?

Little league sports teams are very convivial and sociable, and as a team parent, you will get sucked into the weekly juice-and-snack rotation. We're guessing you'll fall into 1 of 2 camps, found on any team . . .

One kind of parent: Yay! I get the chance to thread fruit onto kabob skewers and bake kale chips for all of the kids. They will love it!

Other kind of parent: Oh crap! I totally forgot! What do we have left over from Halloween? I'll just bring chocolate bars and fruit roll-ups!

Some parents are very conscious of what their kids eat and try to cut back on sugar, salt, or ultra-processed foods. They may not want other parents offering their kids juice and cookies after sport. Others are more lax and don't mind the postgame treat. Sometimes the competition between these parents is more heated than the action on the field. Of course, you have the right to say "no thanks" when your child is offered a snack that you do not want them to

WE GOT YOU!

What parent wouldn't like something taken off their to-do lists? If the postgame snacks are getting out of hand, you can always suggest to the coach that you cut the team snack altogether. That way, parents don't have to worry about getting snacks— and everyone can decide for themselves what kind of post-game snack is best for their child (or whether a snack is even needed).

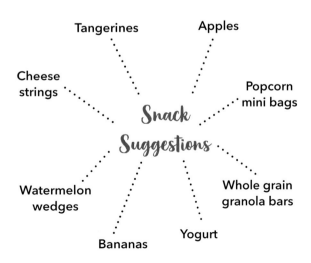

Snack Suggestions

Tangerines · Apples · Cheese strings · Popcorn mini bags · Watermelon wedges · Whole grain granola bars · Bananas · Yogurt

eat. But chances are they will feel left out, and you might have an awkward (and emotional) situation on your hands. And really, one snack on game day will not be detrimental to their overall healthy diet.

If your child enjoys sport, they should learn about the lifestyle that promotes athleticism too. Sport is fueled by nourishing food, not by ultra-processed food. Candy, chips, chocolate, and soda don't provide the right kind of energy to help working muscles power through activity, and they don't have the right nutrients for growth and development. If you are concerned about the snacks you see, talk to the coach about making changes and explain that physical activity and nutrition go hand in hand. Just as important as learning the rules of the game is learning how to fuel your body afterwards. When it's your turn to bring the team snack, try fruit and cheese strings. In some areas, the candy and pop after the game is so ingrained that the reaction you get may be: "Wow, oranges and cheese strings? Good idea! I never would have thought of that!"

> **REALITY CHECK**
>
> The World Health Organization recommends that children get at least 60 minutes of moderate- to vigorous-intensity activity daily. It doesn't need to be 1 straight hour—it can be 20 minutes 3 times a day or any other variation that works for your family. Playing in the park, running around, enjoying sports, and going to activities (dance, gymnastics, karate, swimming, etc.) are all examples of activity.

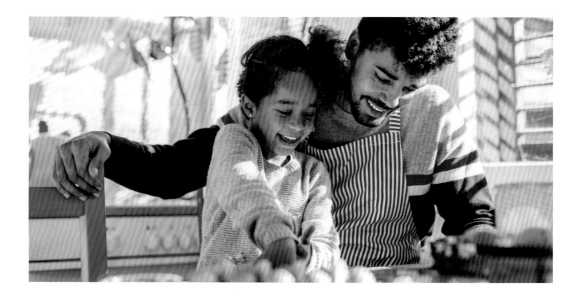

Imagine this: instead of cooking by yourself, you assign age-appropriate tasks to your child, and meal prep goes much faster. You might be thinking "Haha, yeah right . . . quicker?! C'mon . . ." But we promise it can happen! Our kids all help with age-appropriate tasks: the older ones peel carrots, slice vegetables, stir-fry, scramble eggs, and make salad dressing, while the younger ones rip lettuce and herbs, shuck corn, and pop peas out of the pod. See page 308 for some more age-appropriate ideas.

Yes, there's a learning curve that will last a few weeks, but after that you'll be so proud of your child's newfound skills. And kids are more excited to try a variety of foods when they've helped prepare them. Trust us, it truly can be fun and rewarding to involve kids in meal prep! (Oh, but it does get messy. That's why dishcloths and brooms exist.) Kids will shift in and out of interest with helping—some days they'll really want to help, and other days they'll have no interest. Make it fun, and have an open-ended invitation for them to help you, but don't pressure them.

Top 5 reasons for cooking with kids

1. **Improves math skills.** It's nearly impossible to cook without doing a little math. Cooking teaches fractions, addition, geometry, and more. Those skills don't just belong in textbooks; they have a practical, everyday application!

2. **Helps with reading.** Kids who are starting to read can practice on so many things in the kitchen. Recipes, food packages, nutrition labels, instructions—there are words everywhere!

3. **Builds self-esteem.** Being able to make a meal provides a sense of accomplishment, and hearing compliments on the outcome makes the experience even better.

> **WE GOT YOU!**
> Back to that whole "mess" thing. Seriously—you will have oil and flour in crevices that you didn't know existed. But remain calm and patient. Kids are learning, and a bit of mess is naturally going to be part of it. If you are planning an elegant dinner party, it's not the ideal time to involve your child in the kitchen!

4. **Shares new cultures.** Introduce meals and ingredients from different countries and use a globe or atlas to give context. Make foods from different cultural or religious holidays to widen your child's global breadth.

5. **Provides health protection.** Understanding how to cook from a young age exposes your child to vital information about nutritional content, food preparation,

food safety and whole versus processed foods. And giving them the ability to cook usually means that they will consume less fast food as adults. Parental win!

SAFETY FIRST

The stove is hot. The knives are sharp. Raw chicken may contain bacteria. The kitchen is not a playroom! Before you start cooking, teach your child some safety rules:

- Tie long hair into a ponytail.
- Wash your hands before you start cooking, and any time after you touch raw meat, fish, poultry, or eggs.
- Never cut raw vegetables on the same cutting board used for raw meat.
- Never taste anything raw that is meant to be baked, such as cookie dough or cake batter. Raw eggs may carry salmonella and raw flour may carry E. coli.
- Do not touch whirring electric beaters, hot pans, or stovetops.
- Wear oven mitts when touching something hot (and only with supervision).
- Don't wear scarves or loose sweaters near an open flame of a gas stove.
- Keep pot handles turned inward so you don't accidentally bump them.
- Learn the proper way to hold a knife, a vegetable peeler, a grater, or anything else that has a blade on it.
- Use a sturdy kitchen stool if you're not tall enough to see over the counter.
- Don't climb on the counters to reach for items.

> **REALITY CHECK**
>
> Here's the most important rule to save your sanity: plan for kitchen time when you're not rushed to get a meal prepared, so you can calmly supervise. Don't cook with your child when you are stressed or rushed—you'll just end up losing your patience, and no one will enjoy the experience. And leave time to clean up. (Did we mention it's messy? Don't say we didn't warn you!)

I'm a newly single parent. How do I survive dinnertime now?

As if meal planning and preparation wasn't hard enough, now you're doing it as a single parent (either part time or full time), and it just got that much harder. Here are our tips for mealtime success as a single parent. Because, if you're running the show solo, help—although not always necessary—is always appreciated.

I never thought I'd be a single parent, but then again, who does? Although my kids now have a happier mom and dad, I do miss the teamwork that comes along with having a live-in co-parent. Someone to help with making meals, brushing teeth, and reviewing homework. Parenting often feels like a juggling competition. Just when you've finally figured out a good balance, life can throw another ball your way. And if I thought mealtime was a struggle before, I had no idea what I was in for as a solo parent.

Prepare freezer meals to maximize time: This is a one-size-fits-all tip for all families, whether you're single parenting or not. Batch-cooking recipes to stock up your freezer is a wonderful way to ease the 5 p.m. "witching hour." If you cook and freeze in advance, when the time comes, all you have to do is defrost and reheat. This means less stress and more quality time with the kids. Win-win.

WE GOT YOU!
Freeze and label your soups and sauces into family-size portions AND single servings. Because when the kids are with their other parent, you still need to feed and nourish yourself.

Menu plan in advance: All family schedules will be different, so this tip is going to take some trial and error. Aim to prepare larger meals earlier in your week with the kids so that you can repurpose leftovers for your remaining meals. For example, the roasted chicken you cook on Wednesday can turn into chicken quesadillas, chicken soup, or chicken pizza!

Leverage leftovers like crazy: Food wastage has been the toughest part of meal planning as a single parent. It can take a lot of practice to prepare the right amount of food when you are used to cooking enough food to feed a family of 5 with leftovers for lunch the next day. Through trial and error, you will discover your new normal and rely heavily on your freezer in the meantime. You can freeze just about everything, from shredded cheese and bread to browning bananas and overripe avocados! Read more about reducing food waste on page 247.

Embrace the one-pot meal: All you need is one pot or sheet pan, some simple ingredients, and about half an hour, and voila, you've made a delicious dinner that your kids will love (well, most of the time anyway—you know kids!). This kind of meal cuts down on dishes, time, and stress. It simplifies mealtime and also (typically) creates some leftovers that are great for school lunches the next day. And it leaves more time for hanging out with your kids.

Keep mealtime boundaries: Whatever you do, don't forget to keep your regular mealtime boundaries. Parental guilt happens to all parents, because let's be real, parenting is hard. But when you've gone through a separation or loss, you may feel an extra sense of guilt about the family unit and overcompensate with leniency, treats, and catering to everyone's likes and dislikes. We all do it sometimes. Single parenting—especially in the beginning—can be hugely emotional and hard, and sometimes it's just easiest to give in. But the best thing you can do for your kids is to keep as much stability and "normality" as possible (and structure is part of this and will make them feel more in control).

> ♥ **WE GOT YOU!**
> Now . . . remember that you can't control what goes on at the other parent's house (as frustrating as that can be) and that you only have control over what happens at your house. Your kids are resilient and will learn how to adapt as long as you stay consistent.

SARAH SAYS: *I have learned so much about myself in the process of my separation. I have found that my inner strength is stronger than I could have imagined, that my friends and family love me unconditionally, and that my kids will be okay. So, if a meal isn't perfect, if you become overwhelmed, or if you are feeling like you need a break that's okay! Forgive yourself and move forward.*

Top 10 Tips

for children (3 to 6 years)

1   **Serve whole, unprocessed foods most often.**
Cut back on ultra-processed foods.

2   **Assemble a balanced lunchbox.**
Add vegetables, fruits, whole grains, and protein-rich foods.

3   **Serve water as the main beverage.**
Juice and soft drinks are treats–like candy!

4   **Teach the "balanced plate."**
Fill half with vegetables and fruits, a quarter with grains, and a quarter with protein.

5   **Stay active.**
Kids should have at least 60 minutes of physical activity every day.

6   **Cook with your child.**
Teach them some age-appropriate kitchen tasks and remain calm about the mess!

7   **Do not put kids on weight-loss diets.**
Live a healthy lifestyle instead.

8   **Foster good self-esteem.**
Inspire your child to list what they love about themselves.

9   **Know that vegetarian or vegan diets are safe.**
Assure adequate protein, iron, and vitamin B_{12}.

10   **Be flexible, not restrictive.**
Food is never the enemy.

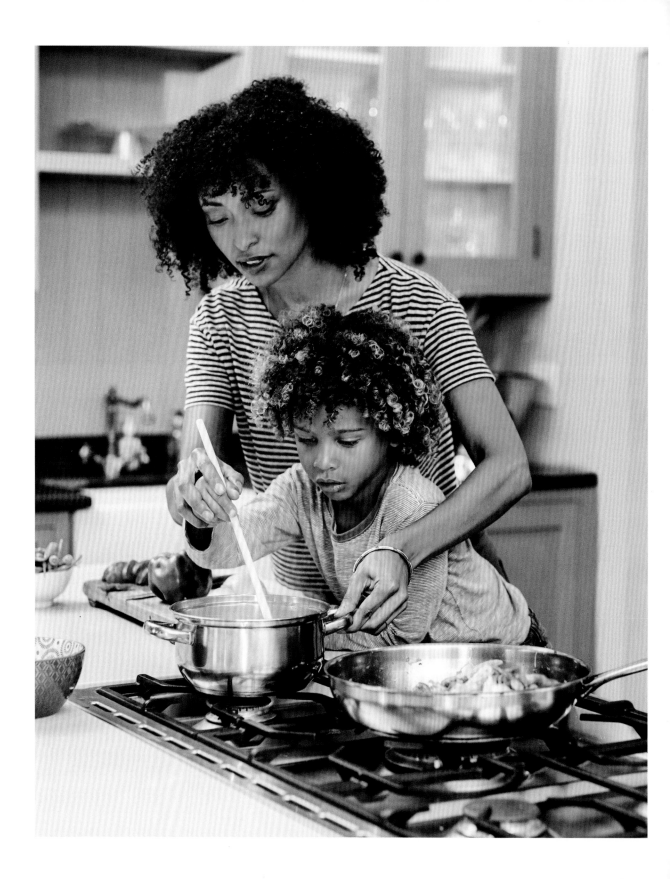

Conclusion

So there you have it. All the nutritional info you need from the time you find out a baby is one the way, up until your little 6-year-old is making you toast and scrambled eggs for Mother's Day (likely with bits of shell in those eggs)!

Hopefully this book has helped you take a closer look at what you eat and what you feed your child. You now know a bit more about what you should be eating and serving most often—and that's whole foods like vegetables, fruits, fish, poultry, meat, dairy, beans, nuts, seeds, and whole grains. Given this extensive list, maybe you've been inspired to rely a bit less on ultra-processed food and add more whole foods to your family's diet. Every small change adds up! Tomorrow it's a sweet potato instead of French fries—and maybe next month you'll add broccoli to your repertoire.

> **One of the best things you can do for your child is to help them develop a healthy relationship with food.**

Beyond *what* your family eats, we hope this book has also made you think about *how* you eat. How you teach your child to eat—encouraging them to nurture their intuitive appetites, and trust their own growing bodies—is an incredibly important job. No matter how old your child is, always keep the Division of Responsibility (sDOR) (page 41) in mind. Your job is to determine what food to serve, plus where and when to serve it. It's your child's job to determine how much to eat, or whether to eat at all.

You are a role model. How you think about, talk about, and serve food will influence how your child feels about food. If you eat vegetables, they will follow suit. And of course, if you gorge on chips and cookies, they will follow suit with those too. One of the best things you can do for your child is to help them develop a healthy relationship with food. With some navigation they can grow into young adults who are able to grocery shop for healthy food, prepare nutritious meals, and one day feed their own family. Imagine. Yup, it's a long way off. But the choices you make now are setting the stage for their lifelong relationship with food! As your child grows, just continue to shop, prep, cook, and eat together. You've got this!

Nutritional Breakdowns

We're definitely not advocates of counting every gram of protein or milligram of calcium that you consume. That would be stressful—and close to impossible to accomplish! But there may be times when you require some extra information about daily nutrients. Perhaps you think you need to get more iron in your family's diet, but aren't sure how much. Or maybe your doctor told you that your calcium intake is too low and you're not sure which foods to eat more of. That's what the charts on the following pages are for: to act as a guide for specific questions about nutrients. Measurements, unless otherwise noted, are per day.

Protein

DAILY INTAKE
Adults

19 years and over: 0.8 to 1.0g per 1kg (2.2lbs) of body weight. This means about 10% to 35% of your diet should be made up of protein. (Yup, this is a big range! And some people on high-protein diets get even more than this. There's no exact right number for everyone.)

Pregnant: About 1.1g per 1kg (2.2lbs) of body weight per day, minimum

Breastfeeding: About 1.3g per 1kg (2.2lbs) of body weight per day, minimum. (You need more protein at this stage because you are supporting the growth of a baby, producing breastmilk, and/or healing from delivery or C-section.)

Children

0 to 6 months: At least 9g (coming from breastmilk and/or formula)

7 to 12 months: At least 11g (a combo of breastmilk and/or formula + solids)

1 to 3 years: At least 13g

4 to 8 years: At least 19g

FOOD	SERVING SIZE	PROTEIN (G)
MEAT AND ALTERNATIVES		
Meat, poultry, or fish, cooked	2½ oz	18 to 23
Egg	2 large	13
Beans, peas, or lentils, cooked	¾ cup	12 to 15
Tofu, firm	½ cup	11
Nuts or seeds	¼ cup	4 to 8
Nut or seed spreads	2 tbsp	4 to 8
MILK, DAIRY AND ALTERNATIVES		
Greek yogurt	¾ cup	14 to 18
Cheese (Cheddar, Swiss, mozzarella, etc.)	½ cup shredded	12 to 14
Cottage cheese	½ cup	12
Soy beverage	1 cup	8
Cow's milk, any type (skim, 1%, whole)	1 cup	8
Plain yogurt	¾ cup	6 to 10
GRAIN PRODUCTS		
Bread	1 slice	2 to 5
Pasta, rice, quinoa or other grain, cooked	½ cup	2 to 5
Breakfast cereal	½ cup to 1 cup	3 to 4
Oatmeal	¾ cup	3 to 4
FRUITS AND VEGETABLES		
Fruits	1 fruit or ½ cup	1 to 2
Vegetables	½ cup or 1 cup lettuce	1 to 2

Dietary Fat

DAILY INTAKE
Adults
Total fat intake should be about 20% to 35% of our calorie intake. If you eat 2,000 calories per day, that would be 45 to 75g of fat.

Children
There is no official recommendation, but 20% to 35% of your child's overall diet can come from fat. If they eat 1,000 calories a day, that's 23 to 38g of fat.

FOOD	SERVING SIZE	FAT (G)
MEAT AND ALTERNATIVES		
Mixed nuts	¼ cup	18
Peanut butter, natural	2 tbsp	16
Regular ground beef, cooked	2½ oz	11
Salmon, cooked	2½ oz	10
Egg, cooked	2 large	10
Chicken breast with skin, cooked	2½ oz	6
MILK, DAIRY AND ALTERNATIVES		
Cheese, Cheddar	½ cup shredded	20
Butter	1 tbsp	12
Milk, whole	1 cup	9
Cream cheese	1 tbsp	5
Yogurt, plain, Greek style (2%)	¾	4
GRAIN PRODUCTS		
Bread	1 slice	2
FATS AND OILS		
Any oil	1 tbsp	14
SNACKS		
Plain tortilla chips	15 chips	9
Snack crackers	8 crackers	7
Granola or cereal bars	1 bar	2 to 5

Omega-3

DAILY INTAKE

There is no set government standard for how much DHA and EPA you should get each day, but some independent health organizations have suggested 250 to 500mg per day for adults including pregnant women, and 50 to 100mg per day for children, depending on their age.

FOOD	SERVING SIZE	ALA (MG)	EPA/DHA (MG)
FISH & SEAFOOD			
Salmon, farmed Atlantic or chinook	2½ oz	70 to 130	1300 to 1770
Herring, cooked	2½ oz	50 to 110	1600
Salmon, wild Atlantic	2½ oz	260 to 280	1300 to 1400
Sardines, canned	2½ oz	170 to 370	740 to 1000
Salmon, sockeye	2½ oz	50 to 90	870 to 930
Trout, cooked	2½ oz	60 to140	700
Tuna, albacore	2½ oz	50	650
Tuna, light, skipjack or cooked shrimp	2½ oz	0	210
EGGS			
Omega-3 enriched egg	2 large	500	160 to 200
Regular egg	2 large	0 to 60	70
NUTS & SEEDS			
Chia seeds	¼ cup	7500	0
Flaxseeds (ground)	¼ cup	6600	0
Hempseeds	¼ cup	3500	0
Walnuts	¼ cup	2300	0
FATS AND OILS			
Flaxseed oil	1 tsp	2460	0
Walnut oil	1 tsp	480	0
Canola oil	1 tsp	420	0
Omega-3 margarine made with canola oil	1 tsp	340	0
Soybean oil	1 tsp	310	0

Iron

DAILY INTAKE

Adults
Men 10 and older: 8mg
Women 19 to 50 years: 18mg
Post-menopause: 8mg
Pregnant: 27mg
Breastfeeding: 9mg

Children
0 to 6 months: 0.27mg
7 to 12 months: 11mg
1 to 3 years: 7mg
4 to 8 years: 10mg

FOOD	SERVING SIZE	IRON (MG)
MEAT AND ALTERNATIVES		
Beans, white, kidney, navy, pinto, black, etc., cooked	¾ cup	2.6 to 4.9
Lentils, cooked	¾ cup	4.5
Tofu, firm	1 cup	3 to 4
Peas, chickpea/garbanzo, black-eyed, or split, cooked	¾ cup	2 to 3.5
Beef, cooked	2½ oz	1.4 to 3.3
Edamame/baby soybeans, cooked	½ cup	1.9 to 2.4
Nuts - cashew, almond, hazelnut, etc.	¼ cup	1.3 to 2.2
Lamb, cooked	2½ oz	1.3 to 2.1
Chicken, cooked	2½ oz	0.4 to 2.0
Egg, cooked	2 large	1.8
Pork, cooked	2½ oz	0.5 to 1.5
Tuna, light, skipjack canned in water	2½ oz	1.2
Turkey, cooked	2½ oz	0.3 to 0.8
GRAIN PRODUCTS		
Oatmeal, instant, cooked	¾ cup	4.5 to 6.6
Cream of wheat, cooked	¾ cup	5.7 to 5.8
Ready-to-eat breakfast cereal, all types	½ to 1 cup	4.0 to 4.3
Pasta, enriched, cooked	½ cup	1.2
VEGETABLES AND FRUITS		
Spinach, cooked	½ cup	2.0 to 3.4
Potatoes, with skin, cooked	1 medium	1.3 to 1.9
Apricots, dried	¼ cup	1.6
Peas, green, cooked	½ cup	1.3

Calcium

DAILY INTAKE

Adults

Men 19 to 70 years: 1,000mg

Men 70 years +: 1,200mg

Women 19 to 50 years: 1,000mg

Women 51 years +: 1,200mg

Pregnant: 1,000mg (1,300mg if <19)

Breastfeeding: 1,000mg (1,300mg if <19)

Children

0 to 6 months: 200mg

7 to 12 months: 260mg

1 to 3 years: 700mg

4 to 8 years: 1,000mg

FOOD	SERVING SIZE	CALCIUM (MG)
MEAT AND ALTERNATIVES		
Tofu, prepared with calcium sulfate	¾ cup	302 to 525
Cow's milk, any type	1 cup	300 to 320
Sardines, canned, with bones	2½ oz	180 to 286
Salmon, canned with bones	2½ oz	179 to 212
Beans, white or navy, canned	¾ cup	93 to 141
Tahini/sesame seed butter	2 tbsp	130
Almonds, dry-roasted, unblanched	¼ cup	93
DAIRY AND ALTERNATIVES		
Cheese (Cheddar, Colby, Gouda, mozzarella, etc.)	1½ oz	250 to 500
Rice, almond, cashew, or coconut beverage, fortified with calcium	1 cup	315 to 325
Soy beverage, fortified with calcium	1 cup	320
Yogurt, plain	¾ cup	263 to 275
Cottage cheese	1 cup	146 to 265
Yogurt, plain, Greek style	¾ cup	180 to 212
Yogurt, soy	¾ cup	206
Kefir	¾ cup	198
VEGETABLE AND FRUIT		
Greens (collards, kale, turnip greens, etc.)	½ cup	100 to 180
Orange juice, fortified with calcium	½ cup	155
Broccoli	1 cup	36

Dietary Fiber

DAILY INTAKE

Adults
Men 19 to 50 years: 38g
Men 51 years +: 30g
Women 19 to 50 years: 25g
Women 51 years +: 21g
Pregnant: 28g
Breastfeeding: 29g

Children
1 to 3 years: 19g
4 to 8 years: 25g
Boys 9 to 13 years: 31g
Boys 14 to 18 years: 38g
Girls 9 to 13 years: 26g
Girls 14 to 18 years: 26g

FOOD	SERVING SIZE	FIBER (G)
LEGUMES		
Beans (kidney, pinto, cannellini, etc.), cooked	1 cup	15
Chickpeas, cooked	1 cup	11
Lentils, cooked	1 cup	9
Edamame, cooked	1 cup	8
VEGETABLES AND FRUITS		
Pears	1 medium	5
Potato with skin on	1 medium	4
Raspberries	½ cup	4
Apple, orange, or banana	1 medium	3
Brussels sprouts, broccoli, or cauliflower	½ cup	3
Prunes	¼ cup	3
Strawberries or blueberries	½ cup	2
Most other vegetables	½ cup	1 to 2
NUTS AND SEEDS		
Flax seeds	2 tbsp	8
Chia seeds	2 tbsp	7
Almonds, pecans, or peanuts	2 tbsp	2
Peanut butter	2 tbsp	3
GRAIN PRODUCTS		
High fibrer bran cereal	1/3 cup	12
Whole wheat pasta, cooked	1 cup	6
Shreddies or Raisin Bran	1 cup	6

Food	Serving Size	Amount
Quinoa, cooked	1 cup	5
Brown rice, cooked	1 cup	4
Popcorn, air popped	3 cups	4
Oatmeal	1 cup	4
Whole grain bread	1 slice	2

Vitamin D

DAILY INTAKE

Adults

600 IU (read more on page 30)

Children

0 to 12 months: 400 IU

1 to 8 years: 600 IU

FOOD	SERVING SIZE	VITAMIN D (IU)
MEAT AND ALTERNATIVES		
Salmon, sockeye/red, canned, raw, or cooked	2½ oz	394 to 636
Salmon, chinook, coho, or pink	2½ oz	340 to 450
Snapper, cooked	2½ oz	392
Mackerel, Pacific, cooked	2½ oz	343
Salmon, Atlantic, or chum, cooked	2½ oz	210 to 245
Halibut, herring, or trout	2½ oz	144 to 208
Tuna, albacore, raw, or cooked	2½ oz	99 to 106
Egg, yolk, cooked	2 large	57 to 88
Tuna, albacore, canned with water	2½ oz	60
MILK AND ALTERNATIVES		
Cow's milk, any type	1 cup	104
Milk, goat's, fortified with vitamin D	1 cup	100
Rice, oat, or almond beverage, fortified with vitamin D	1 cup	85 to 90
Soy beverage, fortified with vitamin D	1 cup	86
Yogurt, fortified with vitamin D	¾ cup	58 to 71
FATS AND OILS		
Margarine	1 tsp	25 to 36
VEGETABLES AND FRUITS (this food group contains very little of this nutrient)		
Orange juice, fortified with vitamin D	½ cup	50

Folate or Folic Acid

DAILY INTAKE

Folate is the name for the naturally derived form of this vitamin found in foods, and folic acid is the name for the form found in supplements.

Adults
400mg
Women of child-bearing age: 600mg

Children
Babies 7-12 months: 80mg
Children 1-3 years: 150mg
Children 4-8 years: 200mg

FOOD	SERVING SIZE	FOLATE (MG)
MEAT AND ALTERNATIVES		
Beans, pink, pinto, navy, black, white, kidney, or great northern, chickpeas, cooked	¾ cup	140 to 265
Edamame/baby soybeans, cooked	½ cup	106 to 265
Lentils, cooked	¾ cup	265
Sunflower seeds, without shell	¼ cup	77 to 81
GRAIN PRODUCTS		
Pasta, white, cooked	½ cup	88 to 113
Bread, white (made with fortified flour)	1 slice	64
Bread, whole wheat	1 slice	11
VEGETABLES AND FRUITS		
Spinach, cooked	½ cup	135
Asparagus, cooked	4 spears	130
Artichokes, cooked	½ cup	90
Broccoli or Brussels sprouts, cooked	1 cup	89
Avocados	½ fruit	81
Beets, cooked	½ cup	72
Lettuce, romaine or mesclun	1 cup	70
Orange juice	½ cup	33
Spinach, raw	1 cup	61
Potatoes, with skin, cooked	1 medium	55

Resources

INFORMATION ABOUT FEEDING CHILDREN
AboutKidsHealth (SickKids): www.aboutkidshealth.ca/nutrition
ChopChop Family (cooking with kids): www.chopchopmag.org
Dietitians of Canada: www.unlockfood.ca
Ellyn Satter Institute (Division of Responsibility (sDOR)): www.ellynsatterinstitute.org
Healthy Children (from the American Academy of Pediatrics): www.healthychildren.org
Jill Castle (childhood nutrition expert): www.jillcastle.com
KidsHealth: www.kidshealth.org
Sally Kuzemchak (Real Mom Nutrition): www.realmomnutrition.com

Helping Your Child with Extreme Picky Eating by Katja Rowell, MD and Jenny McGlothlin, MS, SLP. **Plus corresponding Facebook page:** www.facebook.com/extremepickyeating

GUIDELINES AND POLICIES FOR FEEDING CHILDREN
American Academy of Pediatrics: www.aap.org
Canadian Paediatric Society: www.cps.ca
World Health Organization: www.who.int/en

FOOD ALLERGIES
American College of Allergy, Asthma and Immunology: www.acaai.org
Food Allergy Canada: www.foodallergycanada.ca
Food Allergy Research and Education (FARE): www.foodallergy.org

INTUITIVE EATING
Intuitive Eating website: www.intuitiveeating.org
Intuitive Eating by Evelyn Tribole, RD and Elyse Resch, RD

INFORMATION FOR PREGNANCY AND BREASTFEEDING
La Leche League: www.lllc.ca (Canada) and www.lllusa.org (US)
MotherToBaby: www.mothertobaby.org
Office on Women's Health: www.womenshealth.gov
US Food and Drug Administration: www.fda.gov/consumers/free-publications-women/medicine-and-pregnancy

Acknowledgements

WE WOULD LIKE TO THANK THE FOLLOWING:

The amazing team at Appetite, Penguin Random House Canada: Lindsay Paterson, publishing manager, our friend and fellow mom! We could not have made it through this process without your sensibility, honesty, keen eye, patience and constant support! And to Robert McCullough, publisher; Leah Springate, designer; Erin Cooper, typesetter; Susan Burns, managing editor; Carla Kean, production director; Lana Okerlund, copyeditor; Eva van Emden, proofreader; Wendy Thomas, indexer; Charlotte Nip, publishing intern.

Our creative team behind the scenes: Sylvia Kong, our wonderful food stylist; Shannon Hutchison, our talented food photographer; Diana Matthews, patient recipe tester (and perfecter!); Sarah's kids—Ben, Lylah and James—for being our cute (and well-behaved!) models and taste testers; Carsen and Anna Perkins, for allowing us to use Carsen's photos in the book; and a special thanks to our dietitian friend, Melanie Ksienski, for coming up with the name "Food to Grow On!"

Our sponsors, for having faith in this idea, investing in the process, and kindly donating copies of the book to many families:

- Egg Farmers of Canada, www.eggs.ca
- California Almonds, www.almonds.com
- Peanut Bureau of Canada, www.peanutbureau.ca
- The Helderleigh Foundation, www.thehelderleighfoundation.org

And finally: To our dietitian colleagues, social media communities, friends, and family for their wisdom, kindness and support.

References

1. E. Martínez Steele et al., "Dietary Share of Ultra-Processed Foods and Metabolic Syndrome in the US Adult Population," www.ncbi.nlm.nih.gov /pubmed/31077725; Bernard Srour et al., "Ultra-Processed Food Intake and Risk of Cardiovascular Disease," www.ncbi.nlm.nih.gov/pmc /articles/PMC6538975/; Fiolet T et al.,"Consumption of Ultraprocessed Foods and Cancer Risk," www.ncbi.nlm. nih.gov/pubmed/29444771.

2. Jean-Claude Moubarac, "Ultra-Processed Foods in Canada: Consumption, Impact on Diet Quality and Policy Implications," www.heartandstroke.ca /-/media/pdf-files/canada /media-centre/hs-report-upp -moubarac-dec-5-2017.ashx.

3. Jorge Fernandez-Cornejo et al., "Genetically Engineered Crops in the United States," www.ers.usda.gov/webdocs /publications/45179/43668 _err162.pdf.

4. M.F. Bouchard et al., "Prenatal Exposure to Organophosphate Pesticides and IQ in 7-Year-Old Children," www.ncbi.nlm.nih.gov /pubmed/21507776;Eskenazi B. et al., "Organophosphate Pesticide Exposure, PON1, and Neurodevelopment in Schoolage Children from the CHAMACOS study,"

www.ncbi.nlm.nih.gov /pubmed/25171140; Polańska K, Jurewicz J, Hanke W, "Review of Current Evidence on the Impact of Pesticides, Polychlorinated Biphenyls and Selected Metals on Attention Deficit / Hyperactivity Disorder in Children," www.ncbi.nlm.nih .gov/pubmed/23526196.

5. Gary D. Foster et al., "A Randomized Trial of a Low-Carbohydrate Diet for Obesity," www.nejm.org/doi /full/10.1056/NEJMoa022207.

6. World Health Organization Guideline, "Sugars intake for adults and children," www.who.int/nutrition /publications/guidelines /sugars_intake/en/.

7. "World Health Organization Guideline: Sugars Intake for Adults and Children," apps. who.int/iris/bitstream/ handle /10665/149782/9789 241549028_eng.pdf.

8. "Most Americans Should Consume Less Sodium," Centers for Disease Control and Prevention, www.cdc.gov /salt/index.htm.

9. Centers for Disease Control and Prevention, "Top 10 Sources of Sodium," www.cdc .gov/salt/sources.htm.

10. "Intuitive Eating Studies," www.intuitiveeating.org/ resources/studies/

11. Betty Ruth Carruth et al., "Prevalence of Picky Eaters Among Infants and Toddlers and Their Caregivers' Decisions About Offering a New Food," jandonline.org /article/S0002- 8223(03)01492-5/fulltext.

12. *American Psychiatric Association, Diagnostic and Statistical Manual of Mental Disorders*, 5th ed. (Washington: American Psychiatric Association Publishing, 2013).

13. Katja Rowell and Jenny McGlothlin, *Helping Your Child With Extreme Picky Eating* (Oakland: New Harbinger Publications, 2015).

14. Katja Rowell and Jenny McGlothlin, *Helping Your Child With Extreme Picky Eating* (Oakland: New Harbinger Publications, 2015).

15. Nancy Zucker et al., "Psycho-logical and Psychosocial Impairment in Preschoolers with Selective Eating," pediatrics.aappublications.org /content/pediatrics/136/3 /e582.full.pdf.

16. Paul J. Turner et al., "Fatal Anaphylaxis: Mortality Rate and Risk Factors," www.ncbi .nlm.nih.gov/pmc/articles /PMC5589409/.

17. Elana Lavine and Moshe Ben-Shoshan, "Anaphylaxis to Hidden Pea Protein: A Canadian Pediatric Series," www.jaci-inpractice.org

/article/S2213-2198(19)
30175-8/abstract.

18 Government of Canada, "Safe
Cooking Temperatures,"
www.canada.ca/en/health
-canada/services/general-food
-safety-tips/safe-internal
-cooking-temperatures-chart
.html.

19 P. Middleton et al., "Omega-3
Fatty Acid Addition During
Pregnancy," www.cochrane.org
/CD003402/PREG_omega-3
-fatty-acid-addition-during
-pregnancy.

20 Government of Canada,
"Omega-3 Fatty Acids and
Fish During Pregnancy,"
www.canada.ca/en/public
-health/services/pregnancy
/omega-3-fatty-acids-fish
-during-pregnancy.html.

21 Maria Elisabetta Baldassarre,
"Rationale of Probiotic Supplementation during Pregnancy
and Neonatal Period,"
www.ncbi.nlm.nih.gov/pmc
/articles/PMC6267579/.

22 Vanessa Garcia-Larsen et al.,
"Diet During Pregnancy and
Infancy and Risk of Allergic or
Autoimmune Disease: A
Systematic Review and Meta-
analysis," www.journals.plos
.org/plosmedicine/article?id
=10.1371/journal.pmed
.1002507.

23 Carolyn Tam, Aida Erebara,
and Adrienne Einarson,
"Food-Borne Illnesses During
Pregnancy: Prevention and
Treatment," www.ncbi.nlm
.nih.gov/pmc/articles
/PMC2860824/.

24 T.A. Desrosiers et al., "Low
Carbohydrate Diets May
Increase Risk of Neural Tube
Defects," www.ncbi.nlm.nih
.gov/pubmed/29368448.

25 World Health Organization,
"Guideline: Sugars Intake for
Adults and Children"; World
Health Organization, "WHO
calls on countries to reduce
sugars intake among adults
and children," www.who.int
/mediacentre/news/releases
/2015/sugar-guideline/en/.

26 M.E. Lamar et al., "Jelly Beans
as an Alternative to a
Fiftygram Glucose Beverage
for Gestational Diabetes
Screening," www.ncbi.nlm
.nih.gov/pubmed/10561636.

27 Frazier A., et al., "Prospective
Study of Peripregnancy
Consumption of Peanuts or
Tree Nuts by Mothers and the
Risk of Peanut or Tree Nut
Allergy in their Offspring,"
www.pubmed.ncbi.nlm.nih
.gov/24366539

28 Adrienne J. Lindblad and
Sudha Koppula, "Ginger for
Nausea and Vomiting of
Pregnancy," www.ncbi.nlm
.nih.gov/pmc/articles
/PMC4755634/

29 T.M. Bayley, "Food Cravings
and Aversions During
Pregnancy: Relationships with
Nausea and Vomiting," www
.ncbi.nlm.nih.gov/pubmed
/11883917.

30 Jackie Trillet and Chastity Hill,
"Eating and Drinking in
Labor," www.journals.lww.com
/jpnnjournal/Citation/2016
/04000/Eating_and_Drinking
_in_Labor__Reexamining_the
.2.aspx.

31 A. Ciardulli et al., "Less-
Restrictive Food Intake
During Labor in Low-Risk
Singleton Pregnancies: A
Systematic Review and Meta-
analysis," www.ncbi.nlm.nih
.gov/pubmed/28178059.

32 Dushyant Maharaj, "Eating
and Drinking in Labor:
Should It Be Allowed?"
www.sciencedirect.com
/science/article/pii
/S0301211509002929.

33 50 Nancy C. Sharts-Hopko,
"Oral Intake During Labor: A
Review of the Evidence,"
www.journals.lww.com
/mcnjournal/Abstract/2010
/07000/Oral_Intake_During
_Labor__A_Review_of_the
_Evidence.5.aspx.

34 Eileen Behan, "Losing Weight
While Breast-feeding,"
www.eatright.org/health
/pregnancy/breast-feeding
/losing-weight-while-breast-
feeding.

35 C.L. Wagner et al., "The
Safety of Mother's Milk® Tea:
Results of a Randomized
Double-Blind, Controlled
Study in Fully Breastfeeding
Mothers and Their Infants,"
www.ncbi.nlm.nih.gov
/pubmed/30005170.

36 A. Bumrungpert et al.,
"Effects of Fenugreek, Ginger,
and Turmeric
Supplementation on Human
Milk Volume and Nutrient
Content in Breastfeeding
Mothers: A Randomized
Double-Blind Controlled
Trial," www.ncbi.nlm.nih.gov
/pubmed/30411974.

37 Kate Smolina et al., "The
Association Between
Domperidone and
Ventricular Arrhythmia in the
Postpartum Period,"
onlinelibrary.wiley.com/doi
/full/10.1002/pds.4035.

38 J.A. Mennella, G.K.
Beauchamp, "Maternal Diet
Alters the Sensory Qualities
of Human Milk and the

Nursling's Behavior," www.ncbi.nlm.nih.gov /pubmed/1896276.

39 Julie A. Mennella, Coren P. Jagnow and Gary K. Beauchamp, "Prenatal and Postnatal Flavor Learning by Human Infants," www.pubmed .ncbi.nlm.nih.gov/11389286/.

40 Kym Spring Thompson and Judith E Fox, "Post-Partum Depression: A Compre- hensive Approach to Evaluation and Treatment," www.ncbi.nlm.nih.gov/pmc /articles/PMC3083254/.

41 J. McDonald et al., "Alcohol Intake and Breast Cancer Risk," www.ncbi.nlm.nih.gov/pmc /articles/PMC3832299/

42 American Heart Association news story, "Breastfeeding Boost: Nursing May Help Mothers Improve Heart Health," https://www.heart .org/en/news/2019/01/10 /breastfeeding-boost-nursing -may-help-mothers-improve -heart-health#; Sanne A. E. Peters et al., "Breastfeeding and the Risk of Maternal Cardiovascular Disease: A Prospective Study of 300 000 Chinese Women," www.ahajournals.org/doi/10 .1161/JAHA.117.006081.

43 American Academy of Pediatrics, "Baby Led Weaning Does Not Increase

Choking Risk When Modified for Safety," www.aap.org/en-us /about-the-aap/aap-press -room/pages/Baby-Wed -Weaning-Does-Not-Increase -Choking-Risk-When-Modified -for-Safety.aspx.

44 National Institute of Allergy and Infectious Diseases Summary for Parents and Caregivers, "Addendum Guidelines for the Prevention of Peanut Allergy in the United States," www.niaid.nih.gov /sites/default/files/peanut -allergy-prevention-guidelines -parent-summary.pdf.

45 Food Allergy Research & Education, "Facts and Statistics," www.foodallergy .org/life-with-food-allergies /food-allergy-101/

46 American College of Allergy, Asthma & Immunology press release, "New Study Suggests 21 Percent Increase in Childhood Peanut Allergy Since 2010," www.acaai.org /news/new-study-suggests-21 -percent-increase-childhood -peanut-allergy-2010.

47 Adrian R. Martineau et al., "Vitamin D Supplementation to Prevent Acute Respiratory Tract Infections," www.bmj .com/content/356/bmj.i6583.

48 B.O. Rennard et al., "Chicken Soup Inhibits Neutrophil Chemotaxis In Vitro,"

www.ncbi.nlm.nih.gov /pubmed/11035691.

49 Eurídice Martínez Steele et al., "Ultra-Processed Foods and Added Sugars in the US diet: Evidence from a Nationally Representative Cross-Sectional Study," www.bmjopen.bmj.com /content/bmjopen/6/3 /e009892.full.pdf.

50 Jean-Claude Moubarac, "Ultra-Processed Foods in Canada: Consumption, Impact on Diet Quality and Policy Implications," www.heartandstroke.ca/- /media/pdf-files/canada /media-centre/hs-report-upp -moubarac-dec-5-2017.ashx.

51 Dietary Guidelines for Americans, "Appendix 2. Estimated Calorie Needs per Day, by Age, Sex, and Physical Activity Level," www.health.gov /dietaryguidelines/2015 /guidelines/appendix-2/.

52 Melvin B. Heyman, Steven A. Abrams, "Fruit Juice in Infants, Children, and Adolescents: Current Recommendations," www.pediatrics.aappublications .org/content/pediatrics/139/6 /e20170967.full.pdf.

53 Q. Hao, B. R. Dong, T. Wu, "Probiotics for Preventing Acute Upper Respiratory Tract Infections," www.ncbi.nlm.nih .gov/pubmed/25927096.

Index